ENCYCLOPAEDIA OF
TISSUE CULTURE

Encyclopaedia of
Tissue Culture

Volume 2

M.S. Ahmad

ANMOL PUBLICATIONS PVT. LTD.
NEW DELHI - 110 002 (INDIA)

ANMOL PUBLICATIONS PVT. LTD.
H.O.: 4374/4B, Ansari Road, Darya Ganj,
New Delhi-110 002 (India)
Ph.: 23278000, 23261597

B.O.: No. 1015, Ist Main Road, BSK IIIrd Stage
IIIrd Phase, IIIrd Block
Bangalore - 560 085 (India)
Visit us at: www.anmolpublications.com

Encyclopaedia of Tissue Culture

First Published, 2006

ISBN 81-261-3084-9 (Set)

PRINTED IN INDIA

Printed at Mehra Offset Press, Delhi.

Contents

Preface

A cell is the smallest unit of the body of a living or non-living object. And a combination of cells is called 'tissue'. Tissues are of different kinds and of different shapes and sizes. Some are cylindrical; some are circular; some are long and some others are short in length. Besides, some are soft; some are medium and hard. In common parlance, they form the flesh, blood and bones.

With the advancement in Science and Technology, experiments were also made in this branch of Biology. Replacement of tissues is the major thrust area. Plastic surgery is an example in this connection. With the help of this technology, faces can be changed to any extent. This technology has proved to be a boon for the victims of fire or terrorist attacks.

Like animals, plant tissues also hold a great importance. New to newer experiments are being made at different botanical labs to increase the produce of hybrid plants of varied characteristics. It is a bright career-field and a lot has yet to be done in future.

Encyclopaedia of Tissue Culture attempts at bringing all the relevant and uptodate information on this subject. This multi-volume work includes various aspects of tissue culture at length. Students, scholars, academics, doctors and the general readers would find it equally useful and beneficial.

Comments and suggestions sent by sincere readers would be of great importance to us.

— Editor

1

Tissues and Cells

Several techniques are employed for cell study. Different techniques have different levels of resolving power and have been evolved in course of time according to needs of more detailed study. Depending upon these techniques and the structures, they reveal, different areas of study have been arbitrarily defined. These details are listed in Table. It should be realised that there is some overlapping in the classes made, so that same method can be used for two areas or the same area may utilise more than one method.

Analysing Power

The term 'resolving power' or resolution refers to the ability of a system to separate details and it has nothing to do with the magnification. In a particular system, the image formed may not be magnified at all but may be resolved into details. Similarly, in another system the image may be magnified with no further resolution. The resolving power of a lens is defined as the smallest distance between two objects, which can be identified as separate images by the aided eye. The resolving power of a microscope is given by the following relationship:

$$h' = \frac{0.61\lambda}{n'\sin\theta} \quad n'\sin\theta = \text{N.A. (numerical aperture)}$$

where, = smallest distance between two points resolved.

λ = wavelength of light used; (400-750) nm for visible light used in compound microscope (Fig.)

n' = refractive index of the medium between the object and objective

(usually air, with refractive index-1)

θ' = angle which the marginal rays form with the axis (Fig.)

When θ is 90°, $\sin\theta$ (sin 90°) will be equal to unity and if n'=1 (as in case of air), N.A. (numerical aperture) will be unity.

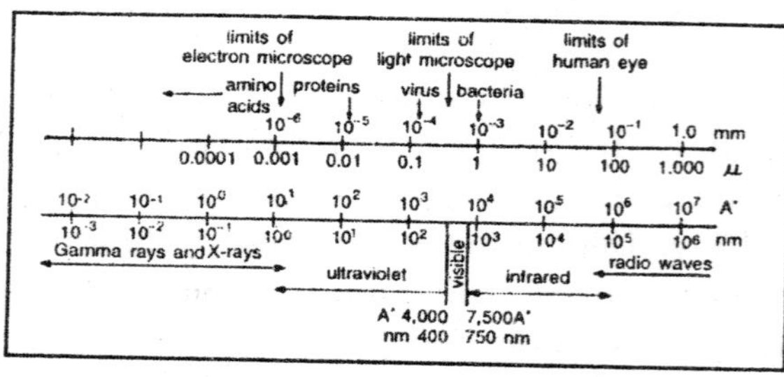

The electromagnetic spectrum on a linear log scale, shown in four units (mm, μ, nm, Å = angstrom): at the top are given the limits of light microscope, electron microscope and human eye; also shown are sizes of bacteria, virus and macromolecules (amino acids and proteins).

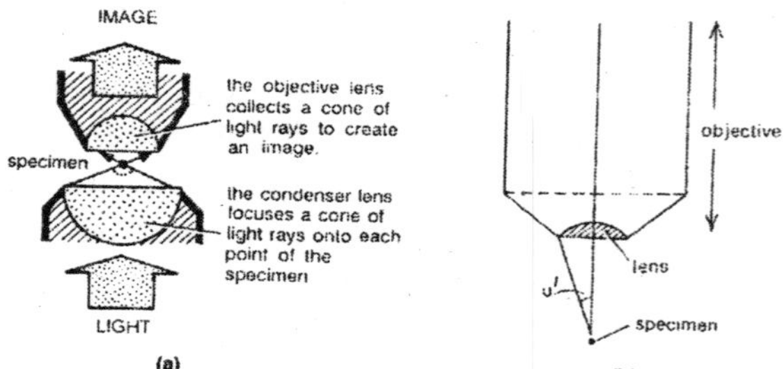

A part of objective showing the angle which the marginal rays entering the objective form with the axis.

Since maximum limit of θ is 90°, N.A. can not be more than one, if air is the medium. However if the space between object and objective is occupied by oil (immersion oil) having higher refractive index, the value of N.A. can increase. Therefore, the resolving power (R) of the microscope will depend upon the wavelength of light used and on the numerical aperture of the objective.

(i) $h' \alpha \lambda$ (ii) $h' \alpha \dfrac{1}{N.A.}$:

(h' is the smallest distance resolved)

Thus, the distance resolved will decrease, with an increase in N.A. and with a decrease in wavelength. Based on the above principle, it is known that an unaided eye can resolve 0.025 mm to 0.1 mm. Lines closer than this will not be resolved. A compound microscope normally resolves up to 275 nm or 0.275 microns (micron or

$$\mu = \frac{1}{1000} \text{ mm; } 1 \text{ nm} = 10^{-6} \text{ mm} = 10\text{Å})$$

Since the wavelength of light (electron beam) used in electron microscope is very low (.005 nm), the resolution reaches up to 1.0 nm. In other words, we may say that, while human eye resolves up to 100 μ., an electron microscope can resolve up to .001 μ (Fig.).

Fixation, Sectioning and Saining of Tissues for Light Microscopy: For a study of cell structure, tissues need to be treated with a fixative, in order to immobilise, kill and preserve cells. The fixation makes the cells permeable to stains and cross-links macromolecules within the cell, so as to stabilise and lock them in their natural position and state. The fixatives earlier used included organic solvents like alcohol, but more efficient fixatives used now, include aldehydes like formaldehyde and glutaraldehyde which form covalent bonds with free amino acids of proteins, thus cross-linking adjacent proteins.

After fixation, tissues are often sectioned into thin slices or sections (1-10) μ m thick) either manually with a razor blade or with a microtome (a machine with a sharp metal blade that works like a meat slicer). The tissue is often soft and fragile and therefore to facilitate sectioning by microtome, it is often embedded in a supporting medium like wax or resin. The supporting medium is used in liquid state, so that it will permeate and surround the embedded tissue.

The medium is then hardened to a solid block, which is conveniently sectioned with a microtome (Fig.). However, while sectioning manually using a razor blade, no embedding in a supporting medium is required. Sometimes, to avoid fixation and embedding, that may disrupt the cell structure in an undesirable manner, the tissues may be rapidly frozen and the frozen tissue may be sectioned with a cryostat (freeze microtome) maintained at a low temperature in a cold chamber. The disadvantage of freezing, however, is that ice crystals formed during freezing may disrupt the fine structure of the cell.

The sections obtained as above need to be stained with dyes, because most of the structures in these sections can not be easily distinguished from each other without such staining. A number of dyes having specific affinity for subcellular structures are available for staining the sections. For instance, hematoxylin has affinity for negatively charged molecules thus permitting the study of the distribution of DNA, RNA, and acidic proteins in a cell.

Other dyes are Malachite green, Sudan black, Coomassic blue, Safranin, etc. Dyes are also available, which have specific affinity for DNA, RNA or proteins. For instance, Basic fuchsin (feulgen stain) locates DNA, Azure B locates RNA and naphthol yellow S or mercuric bromophenol blue locates proteins. The technique is often described as histochemistry and cytochemistry.

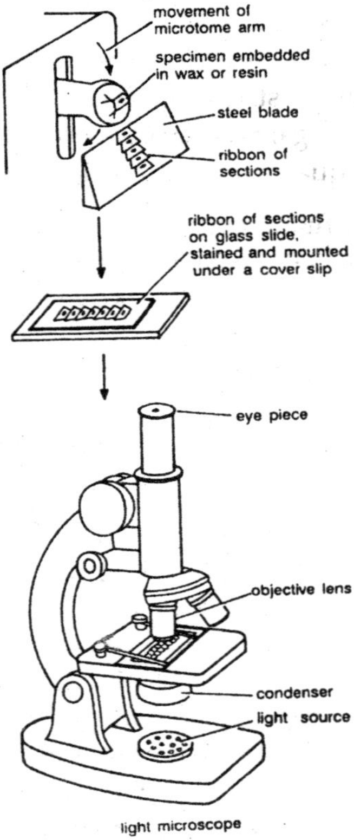

Preparation of sections for examination in the light microscope (redrawn from Alberts et al.: Molecular Biology of the Cell, 1994).

Fluorescent Microscopy, Phase Contrast Microscopy, Interference-contrast Microscopy and Dark Field Microscopy : For locating macromolecules like specific proteins within the cell, sometimes simple staining with ordinary dyes does not serve the purpose and sensitivity of the technique needs to be enhanced. Fluorescent dyes, which absorb light at one wave length and emit it at another wavelength, are used to increase the sensitivity. These fluorescent dyes help in the study of the distribution of a variety of molecules with the help of a fluorescent microscope (Fig.), which makes use of a filter, that permits light of only a specific wave length to reach the specimen being viewed, and uses another filter which blocks all the light except the wavelengths emitted by the fluorescing dye. The molecule or structure to which fluorescing dye binds, thus seem to glow against a dark background, so that molecules even in minute quantities can be detected.

Sometimes, a fluorescent dye may be linked to an antibody (specific to a protein) to make it highly specific staining reagent. Fluorescein (emitting green light when excited with blue light) and rhodamine (emitting deep red light when excited with green yellow light) are two such dyes. By using two or more different antibodies linked to two or more such dyes, distribution of two or more specific molecules (for which antibodies are used) within a cell can be studied.

Since fixing and staining or freezing the tissues may distort cell structure, sometimes it is desirable to examine the cells, while they are still alive. This is facilitated with the use of phase-contrast microscope and differential- interference-contrast microscope. Both these microscopes exploit the principle of the change in the phase of light wave, when the light passes through a relatively thick or dense part of the cell such as nucleus. The extent of the change in phase depends on the refractive index of the structure within the cell and thus may allow the determination of the density or thickness of the cell inclusion being studied.

A device simpler than the above, to examine living cells is dark-field microscopy, in which light rays are directed on the specimen from the side, so that only scattered light enters the microscope lens. Consequently, the cell appears as an illuminated object against a dark background. The above three approaches (phase-contrast, interference and dark-field microscopy) allow the study of movements of chromosomes during cell division, cell migration and movement of other cell structures within the cell. Microcinematography (time-lapse motion pictures) and video recordings are used to study these motions.

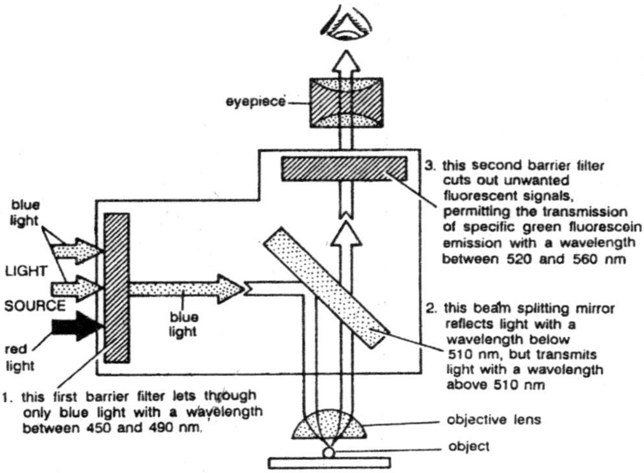

The optical system of a modern, fluorescence microscope: note the presence of two barrier filters, a dichroic (beam splitting) mirror and an objective with high numerical aperture (redrawn from Alberts et al.: Molecular Biology of the Cell, 1994).

Electronic Imaging Systems and Image Processors

In recent years, electronic imaging systems and associated image processors have been extensively used with light microscopy, which firstly allow observations on cells for long periods at very low light intensity (prolonged exposure to bright light damages the cells due to heat produced) and secondly allow detection of small differences in light intensity against a bright background.

In this device, a highly sensitive video camera is attached to the microscope and the image formed by the camera is digitised and fed to a computer device for processing the image to get a variety of information otherwise not available. This also improves the contrast and resolution. This device allows us to see objects like components of cytoskeleton (*e.g.*, microtubules), and also allow preparation of karyotypes automatically from preparations of chromosomes (using chromosome image analysing system or CHIAS).

Confocal Scanning Light Microscopy

When we study a tissue in section, the information on three dimensional structure of the tissue or the cell or the components of the cell is lost. This is sometimes overcome by examination of a series of serial sections followed by reconstructing the three dimensional structure. Computer based imaging can be another solution. However confocal scanning microscope allows direct examination of three dimensional structure of an object. In this microscope, a strong source of light (laser) focuses a spotlight onto a single point at a specific depth in the specimen. The fluorescence emitted is collected and electronic image is formed at the entry point of a detector. This allows examination of a series of sequential sections by scanning the object through focusing light at different depths of the object, without cutting sections; the images are stored in a computer, permitting reconstruction of a three dimensional image. This is comparable to CAT scanning generally done in hospitals by a radiologist to study human body.

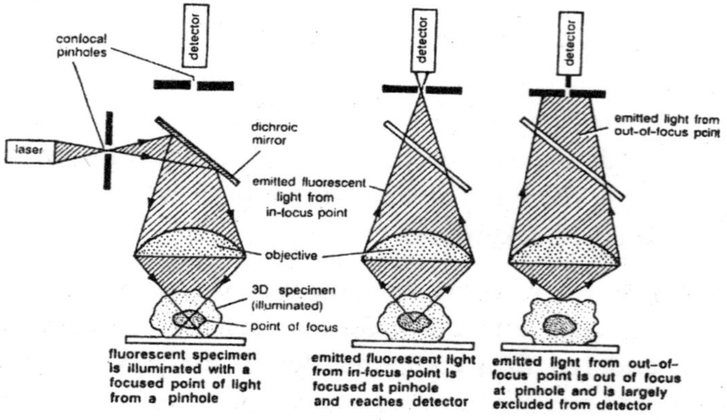

The optical system used in a confocal scanning fluorescence microscope: compare with system for fluorescence microscope shown in Fig. note that the emitted fluorescence from a specific point in the specimen is focussed at a pinhole, which is confocal with a pinhole used to illuminate this specific point in the object (redrawn from Alberts et al.: Molecular Biology of the Cell, 1994).

In confocal scanning microscope, the pinhole aperture at the detector is confocal with the illuminating pinhole (Fig.), so that light from the source focuses on a point in the object and emitted light from the object then focuses at the pinhole at the detector. The light from regions out of the plane of focus is largely excluded from the detector. This confocal scanning microscope has been successfully used for the study of the three dimensional structure of numerous complex objects including the network of cytoskeletal fibres in the cytoplasm and the arrangement of chromosomes inside the nucleus.

The Electron Microscopy

In electron microscope, electrons are propelled by a charge of 50,000 volts and the illumination is focused by electromagnetic lenses instead of conventional glass lenses (Fig.). The electromagnetic lenses mean that the electron beam is allowed to pass through an electromagnetic field created by electromagnets. It does the same job of converging the beam as the ordinary glass lens does in the light microscope. Because of such high resolving power of an electron microscopic and because the sub-cellular particles lie much below the level of resolution by a light microscope, the electron microscope has become an indispensable equipment for cytological studies.

The electron microscope was built for the first time in 1931 by Ernst Ruska of West Berlin, who shared the 1986 Nobel Prize in Physics with G. Binning, and H. Rohrer, 'who developed scanning tunneling microscope (in 1981), which will open new field for the study of the structure of matter. Preparation of specimens for electron microscopy (fixation, sectioning, staining, shadowing, negative staining, etc.) Since the specimen examined in an electron microscope is subjected to very high vacuum, it can not be examined in living state. Further, the techniques of fixing, sectioning and staining used for light microscopy are not suited to electron microscopy. The material

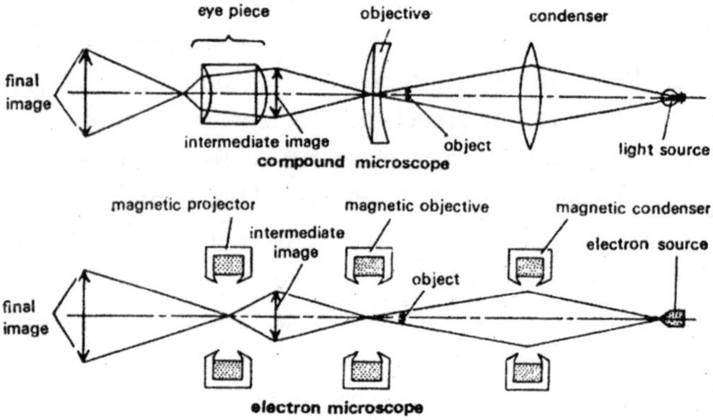

A comparison of optical systems involved in a compound microscope and an electron microscope.

is fixed first with glutaraldehyde and then with osmium tetroxide, the former cross-linking the proteins with their neighbours, and the latter binding and stabilising the lipid bilayers and proteins. The specimens are cut into very thin sections (50-100 nm as against 1000-10,000 nm for light microscopy), about 1/200 of the cells thickness, since the electrons have very limited penetrating power. This is made possible by dehydration followed by permeation of material with a monomeric resin, giving a solid block of plastic, which is cut with a glass or diamond knife on an ultramicrotome. The thin sections obtained are placed on a small circular metal grid for viewing in the microscope (Fig.).

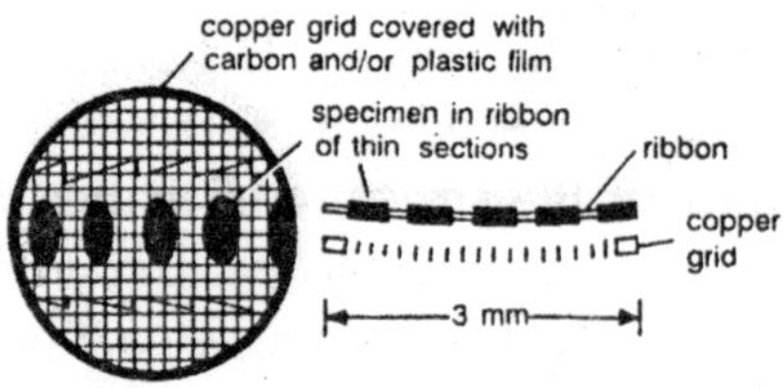

A copper grid used to support the thin section specimen to be examined in the transmission microscope.

In electron microscope, the contrast depends on atomic number of molecules in the specimen. Since most specimens have carbon, oxygen, nitrogen and hydrogen each having small atomic number, they are impregnated with salts of heavy metals like uranium and lead with high atomic numbers (this is described as staining). The degree of contrast depends on the degree of such an impregnation or staining, which can be done either before or after sectioning.

Sometimes, for electron microscopy, the specimen (whole mounts or sections) after fixation and drying is sprayed with a heavy metal, which makes a thin film. The metal is sprayed with an oblique angle, so that the coating is thicker in some regions than in others; the process is called shadowing.

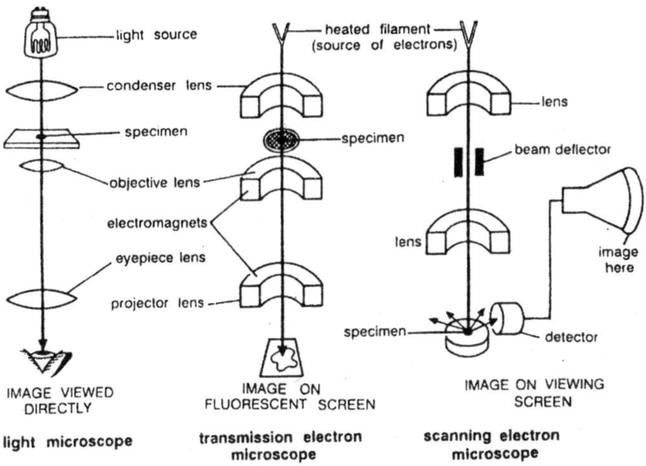

A comparison of principal features of a light microscope, a transmission electron microscope and a scanning electron microscope (redrawn from Alberts et at.: Molecular Biology of the Cell, 1994).

Transmission Electron Microscopy (TEM) vs Scanning Electron Microscopy (SEM)

The design of electron microscope, described briefly above, is similar to that of light microscope, except that it is much larger in size, is upside down and utilises electromagnetic lenses (Fig. above). The specimen is stained with an electron dense material, so that some of the electrons are scattered and the remainder are focused to form an image either on a photographic plate or on a phosphorescent screen. Since the scattered electrons are lost from the electron beam, the dense regions of the specimen show up in the image as areas of reduced electron flux and looks dark.

The TEM can also be used to study the surface of a specimen. For this purpose, a thin film of heavy metal (*e.g.*, platinum) is evaporated onto the dried specimen from an oblique angle so that a coating is deposited, which is thicker in some places than in others - a process called shadowing. Due to shadow effect, the image gives a three dimensional appearance. This can be satisfactorily done for thin or small specimens, in which electrons can penetrate directly. In thick specimens, organic material of the cell must be dissolved after shadowing, so that only a thin metal replica of surface of the specimen is left. This replica is reinforced with a carbon film and placed on a grid and examined in TEM.

In contrast to TEM, where electrons pass through the specimen to form an image, in scanning electron microscope (SEM) the electrons are scattered or emitted from the surface of the specimen. The specimen is fixed, dried and coated with a thin layer of heavy metal. This specimen is then scanned with a very narrow beam of electrons.

The quantity of electrons scattered or emitted from each successive point on the metallic surface is measured and used to control the intensity of a second beam, which moves in synchrony with the primary beam and forms a highly enlarged image on television screen. The SEM technique provides great depth of focus and because the quantity of electrons scattered depends on the angle of the surface to the beam, the image gives a three dimensional appearance. However, only surface features can be examined with SEM and the resolution is low (10nm), while in TEM as well as in confocal scanning microscope, the internal structure can also be studied. Therefore

SEM is used for study of surface rather than the subcellular structures.

Freeze-fracture and Freeze-etch Electron Microscopy: The type of thin metal replicas, which are used in TEM have also been profitably utilised in Freeze-Fracture and Freeze-Etch Electron Microscopy, which help to visualise the interior of cell membrane without fixing the cells. For freeze-fracture electron microscopy, living cells are first frozen in liquid nitrogen (-196°C) in the presence of a cryoprotectant (antifreeze), which prevents distortion due to formation of ice crystals. The frozen block is cracked with a knife blade. The fracture often passes through a plane passing through the hydrophobic middle of lipid bilayers, thus exposing the interior of cell membrane. The fracture faces are shadowed with platinum, the organic material is dissolved away and the replicas are floated off and viewed in the electron microscope. The presence of bumps on replicas indicate the presence of transmembrane proteins.

Another related technique for examining the exterior or interior of cells is freeze-etch electron microscopy, where living cells are frozen extremely rapidly (*e.g.*, by slamming the specimen against a copper block, cooled with liquid N_2). The frozen specimen will now be embedded in ice and can be fractured with a knife as above.

The fractured pieces will remain embedded in ice with fractured face exposed. The ice level around the cell, and to a lesser extent even within the cells, is lowered by sublimation in vacuum (freeze drying), so that margins both outside and inside the fractured face will appear etched (Fig.). The surfaces exposed by etching are then shadowed, as above, to make a platinum replica, which can be examined under an electron microscope to reveal internal as well as external structure of the cell, so that three dimensional organisation of the cell can be studied.

Cryoelectron Microscopy: Recently methods have been developed, where specimens can be examined, without fixation, staining or drying, to study the interior of a three dimensional structure (*e.g.*, viruses, etc.) with much higher resolution than what is possible with shadowing or negative staining. In this technique called cryoelectron microscopy, a very thin (~ 100 nm), rapidly frozen and hydrated sample is prepared on a grid. This frozen sample on a grid is kept at –160°C in the vacuum of the microscope, where it can be viewed directly without fixation, staining or drying.

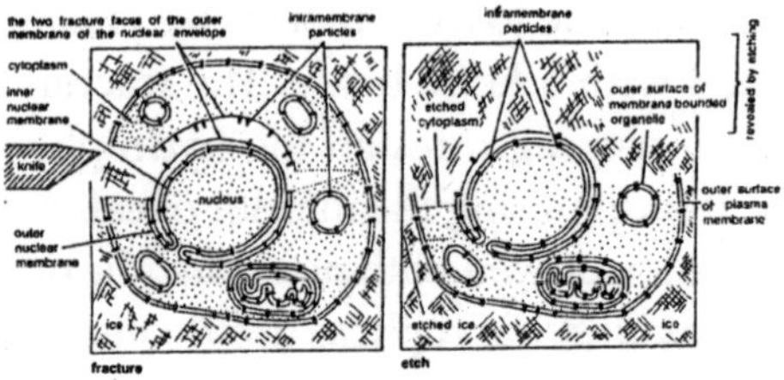

Two steps in the preparation of a specimen in freeze-etch electron microscopy; following these steps a replica of frozen surface is prepared and examined in a transmission electron microscope (redrawn from Alberts et al.: Molecular Biology of the Cell, 1994).

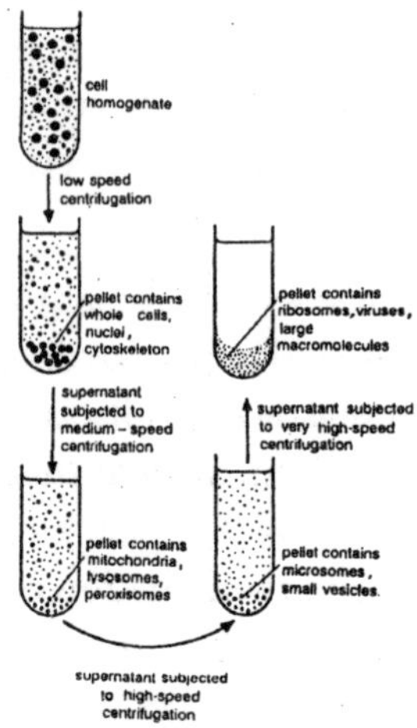

Different steps in cell fractionation by centrifugation (low speed = 1000 × g for 10 min; medium speed = 20,000 × g for 20 min; high speed = 80,000 × g for 1 hour; very high speed = 150,000 × g for 3 hours).

Methods of Cell Division

Various components of cell can be studied after their isolation by cell fractionation methods, which involve homogenisation (destruction of cell boundary) followed by separation, based on specific gravity, etc. The cells are often homogenised in aqueous media, which are usually sucrose solutions of various concentrations. A standard cell fractionation method is shown in Figure.

Preparative Ultracentrifugation

The tissue (*e.g.*, liver of an animal) is first homogenised in 0.25M sucrose solution and is then subjected to differential centrifugation. The method of differential centrifugation utilises different levels of centrifugal forces with the help of standard centrifuge or ultracentrifuge (Fig.). The centrifugal force is exercised with the help of speed at which the tubes containing the cell extract are made to rotate. For instance, at a lower speed, nuclei and intact cells will sediment, while at higher speed mitochondria and at still higher speed ribosomes, Golgi complex and other membranes will sediment (Fig.).

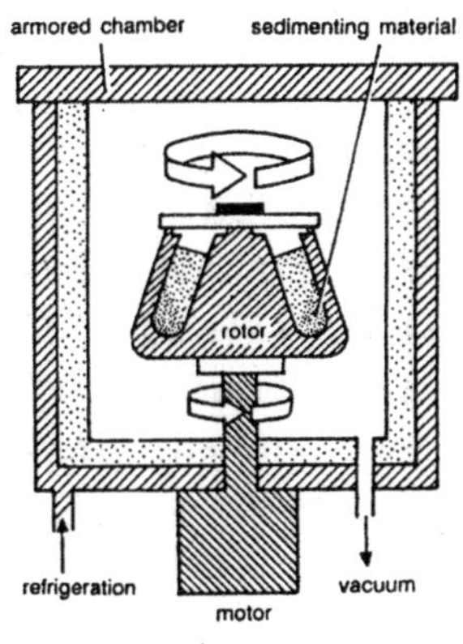

A preparative ultracentrifuge, showing details of structure; sample is contained in tubes carried by a rotor, which rotates generating centrifugal force causing particles to sediment; sample, is maintained at 4°C; vacuum prevents heating due to friction.

A classical cell fractionation will separate the cell components into four fractions, namely:

(i) nuclear fraction,

(ii) mitochondrial fraction,

(iii) microsomal fraction and

(iv) soluble fraction.

It should be noticed that cell fractions do not represent cell organelles, which form only a part of a particular fraction. For instance, mitochondrial fraction of liver, mainly represents mitochondria, while that of brain is fairly heterogeneous. Similarly a microsomal fraction does not consist of what are sometimes erroneously called "microsomes", but consists of broken endoplasmic reticulum, ribosomes, Golgi complex and other membranes.

For separation of different RNA's, DNA, etc., another improved technique of centrifugation is used, which is called gradient centrifugation.

Velocity Sedimentation vs Equilibrium Density Gradient Sedimentation

In the first step of cell fractionation, homogenate is a suspension and cell components are separated on the basis of their size by centrifugation. In the second step, for finer separation, homogenate is placed as a layer on top of a salt solution that fills centrifuge tube. When centrifuged, the components move with different speeds (depending on their size) and form a series of bands during a process called velocity sedimentation.

However, when the solution above has a higher density than the solution below, there is convective mixing, making, the process ineffective. To improve effectiveness, the centrifuge tube is filled with a gradient of sucrose prepared using a special device. In this density gradient, the denser solution is at the bottom and its density gradually decreases towards the top. In such a sucrose density gradient, cell components separate as distinct bands, which can be collected effectively.

The sedimentation rate depends on the size of components and is described as sedimentation coefficient or svedberg units (S value). The centrifuge tubes can rotate at speeds of up to 80,000 rpm (rpm=rotations per minute), producing a force equivalent to 500,000 times that of gravity, so that even small molecules like tRNA can sediment and separate from other components. On the basis of knowledge of sedimentation coefficients, size and composition of different components of the cell can be determined.

In another modification, during ultracentrifugation, molecules can also be separated on the basis of their buoyant density, independent of their size and shape. In this case a very high concentration of the solution of sucrose or caesium chloride is used in the form of very steep density gradient in the centrifuge tube.

The components of the homogenate, in this case do not move with different speeds (depending on size and shape) as in velocity sedimentation, but each component moves down and reaches a position, where the density of the solution is equal to its own buoyant density (irrespective of its size and shape). At this point, the component floats and moves no further, so that a series of distinct bands are formed, not according to S value, but according to buoyant density, which is highest at the bottom and lowest at the top (Fig.).

The process is called equilibrium sedimentation and allows separation of molecules having heavy isotopes (with ^{13}C or ^{15}N). The method was developed in 1957 by Meselson and Stahl to separate heavy DNA with ^{15}N from DNA with' ^{14}N to provide evidence for semi-conservative DNA replication.

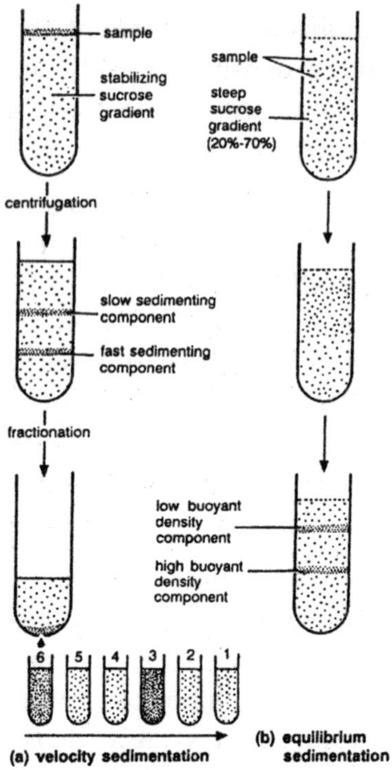

A comparison of velocity sedimentation and equilibrium sedimentation: note that in velocity sedimentation the sample is layered on surface and the components sediment at different velocities according to their size; in equilibrium sedimentation on the other hand, a solution is used and components can move up and down in a gradient to reach an equilibrium, (redrawn from Alberts et al.: Molecular Biology of the Cell, 1994).

Chromatography

Chromatography is the most common method of separation of cell constituents. Following four types of chromatography are available for this purpose: (i) adsorption or column chromatography, (ii) ion exchange chromatography; (iii) gel filtration chromatography and (iv) affinity chromatography.

Adsorption Chromatography: In adsorption chromatography, the cell extract is passed through a column of inert material packed in a glass or steel tube. Most commonly used column materials include finely divided solids such as charcoal, silica, alumina, calcium phosphate, hydroxyapatite, etc. The effluent solution is continuously collected in small fractions of 1.0 to 2.0 ml.

The protein in each fraction is estimated by measuring the absorption at 280 nm using a UV spectrophotometer. The enzyme is also assayed in each fraction. Various spleen enzymes such as basic RNase, acidic RNase, acidic DNase, phosphodiesterase, phosphomonoesterase, etc. are often separated from each other using adsorption chromatography. For large scale chromatographic separation of enzymes, the process is accelerated by using motors and other mechanical devices for packing the column, for loading the enzyme on the column and for eluting the enzyme.

Ion Exchange Chromatography: In ion exchange chromatography, generally a cellulosic ion exchange (consisting of small beads carrying either a negative or a positive charge) is taken in the column. The cell constituents are separated according to their charges. The resolution is quite high and the technique can facilitate large scale protein purification. This has been successfully employed for insulin purification, plasma fractionation and for purification of many other enzymes.

Gel Filtration Chromatography: In this chromatography, various proteins are separated on the basis of differences in their molecular sizes. This type of chromatography is also known as molecular exclusion chromatography or molecular sieve chromatography.

The basic arrangement for gel filtration chromatography is similar to that for adsorption chromatography. A column made up of glass or steel is taken and packed with a gel (Fig.). The most commonly used gel is 'sephadex' which is a cross-linked dextran produced by certain strains of bacteria. Several types of sephadex, namely G-10, G-30, G-50, G-100, G-150.

G-200, etc. are available, which differ according to their pore sizes.

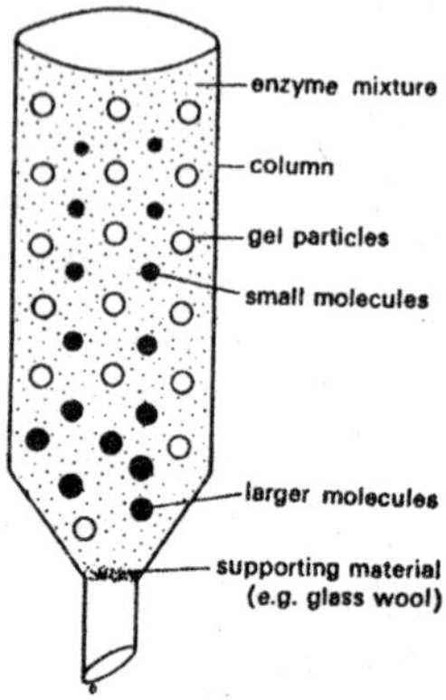

An arrangement for gel filtration chromatography to purify an enzyme.

When a mixture of cell constituents like enzymes or proteins is poured on top of the column, different proteins move downwards according to their molecular sizes and come out from the column in order of decreasing sizes; the larger molecules are eluted first. The elution volume is logarithmically proportional to the molecular size. Gel filtration chromatography can also be used for determining the molecular weight of a protein by calibrating the column with proteins of known molecular weights.

Affinity Chromatography: In this method, cell constituents like enzymes are purified according to their specificity for a particular substrate or cofactor. One component of the mixture containing enzyme binds covalently to the solid support of the column, and the other components percolate down through the column. The basic requirements for affinity chromatography are the same as in adsorption or gel filtration chromatography but the packing gel must have some component which can bind with one component of the mixture.

Many commercial gels available for affinity chromatography contain functional groups attached to the 'spacer arms' of the gel. The "spacer arm" is a chemical linkage between the functional group and the gel or matrix proper, so that the binding between functional group and the enzyme is kept away from the gel. Thus the steric hindrance will be unlikely to prevent binding of the specific enzyme to the column (Fig.).

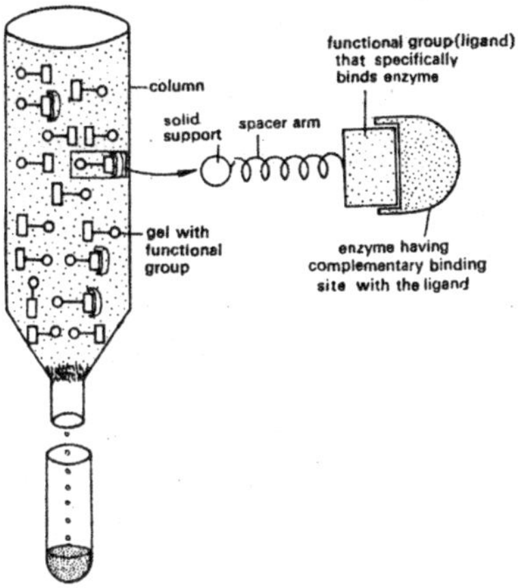

An arrangement for affinity chromatography, showing the role of functional group having affinity with the enzyme.

Electrophoresis Method

Electrophoresis is a technique in which molecules (enzymes, proteins, amino acids, nucleotides and nucleic acids) are separated by differences in their net charge in the presence of an externally applied electric field. This technique is routinely used in enzyme purification and isozyme separation in the laboratories although it has found only limited application at large scale, since the technique is time consuming and is a bit expensive.

Various types of instrumental approaches have been used to separate and purify charged molecules using electrophoresis. However, the most common method for purifying enzymes, is through electrophoresis on polyacrylamide gel.

Polyacrylamide is a polymer of acrylamide and methylene bisacrylamide and when prepared as a gel it is transparent, thermostable, non-ionic and extremely regular in structure. The gel may be taken either in the form of a column or a slab, although the latter is preferred over the former (Fig.).

The protein mixture is loaded in the gel and the components are separated under a direct current of constant voltage. The migration rate of the various components of the mixture is dependent upon their charge and molecular weight.

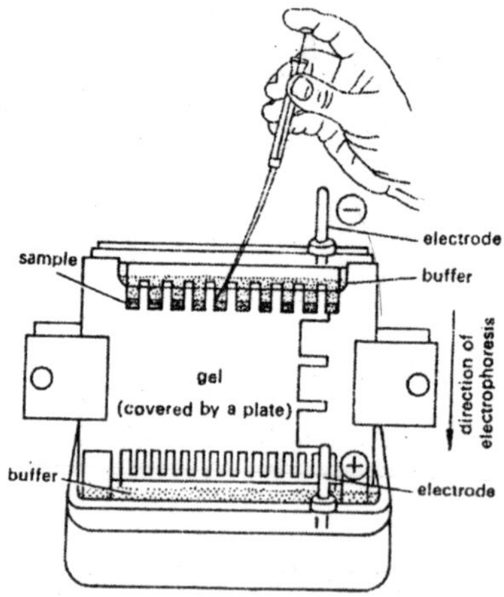

An arrangement for vertical polyacrylamide gel electrophoresis technique for separation of macro-molecules.

A variation of the above polyacrylamide gel electrophoresis, is the sodium dodecyl sulfate-polyacrylamide gel electrophoresis (SDS-PAGE), which is used to determine the molecular weight of proteins. In this method, the separation is caused by the serving action of the gel.

The proteins migrate through the gel depending on their shapes and mass to charge ratio. Gel electrophoresis is also used to separate various isozymes of a given enzyme. Isozymes perform the same catalytic function but differ in their regulatory and some kinetic aspects.

SDS Polyacrylamide-gel Electrophoresis (SDS-PAGE) (One Dimensional)

Electrophoresis was originally used to separate proteins in a mixture either in an aqueous solution or in a solid porous matrix such as starch. SDS -PAGE, is a modified version of the original electrophoresis technique, and was developed in mid-1960s, to facilitate better separation and analysis of proteins.

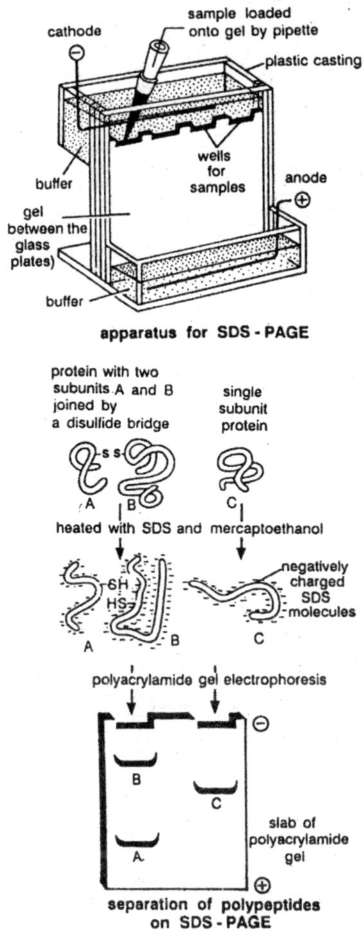

Apparatus for SDS-PAGE and separation of molecules through PAGE using SDS.

The proteins are not held in an aqueous solution, but are held in a solution, which includes a powerful negatively charged detergent called sodium dodecyl sulphate (SDS). SDS binds to hydrophobic regions of protein molecules and causes them to unfold into extended polypeptide chains.

It also releases these chains from their association with other proteins or lipid molecules. Another reducing agent, mercaptoethanol is added to break any S-S linkages, so that subunits of a multi-subunit protein can be separated and analyzed. The gel used in SDS-PAGE is a cross-linked gel of polyacrylamide in the form of an inert matrix through which proteins migrate. This gel is prepared by polymerisation from monomers, just before using. The pore size in this gel can be adjusted to retard the passage of the protein of interest. Through this gel, when a mixture of SDS-solubilised proteins is electrophoresed by applying a voltage, proteins migrate towards the positive electrode.

Since native structure of protein is unfolded by SDS and mercaptoethanol, the proteins of same size behave similarly and proteins of different sizes form a series of discrete bands. The gel can be stained with a dye such as Coomassic blue and major proteins can be visualised as stained bands. Minor bands can also be seen by treating the gels with a silver stain. Since polypeptides are separated due to size and since subunits are also separated, molecular weights and subunit composition of a protein complex can be determined by SDS-PAGE (Fig.). Membrane proteins, cytoskeleton proteins, seed storage proteins, etc. have been successfully analyzed using SDS-PAGE during 1970s and 1980s.

Two-dimensional PAGE: In one dimensional electrophoresis, bands sometimes overlap, so that only a limited number of proteins (up to 50) can be resolved, but if after completing electrophoresis in one direction by a method called isoelectric focusing, the proteins are separated further in another direction (at right angle to the first direction and in presence of SDS), as many as 1000 proteins can be separated as a two dimensional protein map.

In this method, the sample is dissolved in a small volume of a solution containing non-ionic (uncharged) detergent (no SDS is added) along with mercaptoethanol and urea (denaturing agent). Consequently, all polypeptide chains are denatured and dissociated, but the intrinsic charge remains unchanged (in SDS-PAGE the intrinsic negative charge is enhanced).

The polypeptide chains are now separated by a procedure called isoelectric focusing, which depends on the principle that the charge of the protein varies with pH of the solution (at high pH it is negatively charged and at low pH it is positively charged). Furthermore, at a specific pH (called isoelectric point), a particular protein has no net charge, so that at this point it will fail to migrate in an electric field.

Thus for isoelectric focusing, proteins are electrophoresed in a narrow tube with polyacrylamide gel having a pH gradient established by a mixture of buffers. Each protein migrates to its own isoelectric point and stays there giving first dimension of the two dimensional PAGE. If this narrow gel containing proteins already separated in one dimension is again subjected to electrophoresis in a direction at right angle to the direction of the first separation, up to 2000 polypeptide chains can be resolved. While subjecting to electrophoresis in the second dimension, the narrow gel with proteins already separated in one dimension is soaked in SDS and placed on one edge of an SDS-PAGE-gel slab, through which each polypeptide chain then migrates and forms a discrete spot.

Only those proteins can remain unresolved, which have identical size and identical isoelectric point, a situation, which is rather rare. Staining procedures or autoradiography can be used for detection of these resolved proteins, so that even proteins that differ by a single amino acid can be resolved.

Antibodies coupled with radioisotopes, specific enzymes or fluorescent dyes can also be used for detection of specific proteins, following a procedure called western blotting or immuno-blotting.

X-Ray Diffraction and NMR Spectroscopy

Amino acid sequences in proteins and nucleotide sequences in nucleic acids can sometimes be used to predict the secondary structures of these molecules. For instance helix structure of a transmembrane segment of a protein can be predicted from its amino acid sequence. Similarly, the clover leaf model of tRNA was predicted from the nucleotide sequences of a number of tRNA molecules. But these sequences did not allow us to predict the three dimensional structures of these macromolecules. X-ray diffraction and nuclear magnetic resonance (NMR) spectroscopy have been used extensively for the study of three dimensional structures of cellular macromolecules, particularly the proteins and nucleic acids.

In x-ray crystallography, the macromolecule should be available in a crystal form and x-rays (wave length=0.1 nm = diameter of hydrogen atom which is much smaller than other electromagnetic radiations) are allowed to pass through crystal sample. Most of the x-rays pass through, but small fraction is scattered by the atoms in the sample. If these atoms are well ordered, the diffracted x-rays may reinforce and make diffraction spots to be recorded by a detector. By looking at the spots in the x-ray diffraction patterns, information about the positions of atoms in the crystal can be deduced. From this information (available in the form of a complex three dimensional electron density map) and the information about the amino acid/nucleotide sequences of a macromolecule, three dimensional structure can be deduced using a computer device.

NMR spectroscopy (proposed by Jeener in early 1970s) has been used largely to analyze the structure of small molecules like small proteins or protein domains. It does not need the sample in crystalline form, but only in the form of a solution that is placed in a strong magnetic field. Certain atomic nuclei, particularly hydrogen nuclei, have a magnetic moment or a spin (which means intrinsic magnetisation, like a bar magnet), so that they align along the magnetic field in which they are placed.

However, if radio frequency (RF) pulses of electromagnetic radiation are applied from outside, the atomic nuclei which were aligned to the surrounding magnetic field are changed to a misaligned excited, state. These misaligned excited nuclei, when relaxed to their aligned state, they emit RF radiation, which can be measured and displayed as a spectrum. The nature of these emitted radiations depends on the environment of each hydrogen nucleus, so that if one hydrogen nucleus is excited, it will influence the absorption or emission of radiation by other nuclei in the neighbourhood. Therefore, the signals from hydrogen nuclei in different amino acid residues will differ.

The shift, in these signals can be measured and used to obtain information about distances between different parts of a small protein molecule. When this information is used with the information about amino acid sequences, three dimensional structures can be obtained for molecules of 15,000 - 20,000 daltons molecular weight. In future molecules with molecular weights of up to 30,000-40,000 daltons will hopefully be analyzed by NMR, but bigger molecules can not be examined by this method. Many functional domains of proteins and complex carbohydrate side chains of glycoproteins have been examined using NMR spectroscopy.

Radioisotope Tracer Technique and Autoradiography: Radioisotopes are often used to detect the presence of specific molecules and to determine their quantity within the cell. This is possible because radioisotopes emit radiations, which can be easily detected. One of the earliest uses of radioisotopes in cell biology involved tracing of the pathway of carbon during photosynthesis. For this purpose, Chlorella (a unicellular alga) cells were maintained in an atmosphere of labelled CO_2 ($^{14}CO_2$) and were exposed to sunlight for sometime. At different intervals the soluble contents of these cells were separated by chromatography and examined. This helped in the detection of small molecules containing ^{14}C derived from $^{14}CO_2$. This facilitated in tracing the path of carbon from CO_2 to sugar during photosynthesis.

The resolution of the above radioactive tracer technique could be further improved by using pulse-chase labeling protocol. In this technique, radioactive material (the pulse) is added for a very short period and then washed. This is followed by replacement of radioactive material by non-radioactive material (the chase). Thereafter, samples are taken at regular intervals and radioactivity is located in the cell or in the tissue organ by autoradiography (see below). This helped in studies like tracing the pathway, that is followed by secreted proteins from ER to the cell exterior.

The technique of autoradiography involving the use of radioactive elements has also been very useful for the studies like duplication of chromosomes. In this technique, cells are exposed to solutions having molecules with radioactive elements, (*eg.* ^{3}H- thymidine, ^{3}H-uridine). The cells are then incubated for variable periods or grown in a medium containing no radioactive molecules. These cells are then fixed and the preparation is overlaid with a thin film of photographic emulsion and left in the dark for a few days. The emulsion gets exposed to radiations emitted and is then developed to show the position of radioactivity in the form of developed silver grains. Autoradiography is also used to locate the position of specific bands in the gels/filters in molecular biology experiments.

Intracellular Electrodes, and Light-Emitting Indicators: The concentration of different ions (Ca^{2+}, K^+, Cl^- H^+) in different regions of the cell play an important role in regulating a variety of cell functions. This could be shown through a study of ion concentrations in different regions of the cells using microelectrodes. A microelectrode is a glass tube with a tip (having diameter of a fraction of a micrometer) filled with a conducting solution (*e.g.*, KC1).

This microelectrode may be inserted into the cytoplasm through the plasma membrane and used for measuring the concentrations of various inorganic ions. In order to measure the concentration of a specific ion, it is also necessary to use a material that is permeable only to that ion, whose concentration needs to be measured.

This material is placed between the test solution (the cell) and a solution containing known concentration of that ion. A reference microelectrode is also inserted into the interior of the cell (Fig.). Recently, microelectrode technique has also been used to study the movement of ions through ion channels. The technique is described as patch clamp technique.

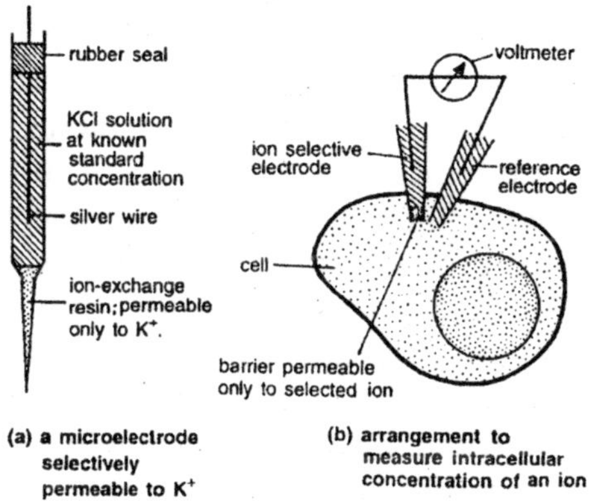

An ion-selective microelectrode and its use to measure the intracellular concentration of a specific ion like K^+ (redrawn from Alberts et al.: Molecular Biology of the Cell, 1994).

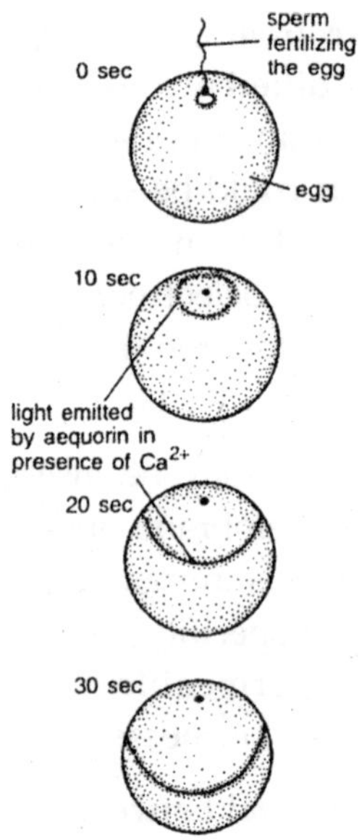

Egg of a fish, which was injected with aequorin before fertilization; a wave of release of Ca^{2+} is indicated by luminescence of aequorin, which spreads across the egg starting from the site of sperm entry (redrawn form Alberts et al. Molecular Biology of the Cell, 1994).

The above microelectrodes, however, are not suitable for measuring rapid and transient changes in the concentration of cytosolic Ca^{2+} as responses to extracellular signals. This can be studied through the use of ion-sensitive indicators, whose light emission reflects the local concentration of the ion. Some of these indicators are luminescent (emitting light spontaneously), while other are fluorescent (emitting light on exposure to light). A commonly used luminescent indicator is ae quorin, which is a protein isolated from certain marine jellyfish. Aequorin emits light in the presence of Ca^{2+} ions and responds to changes in Ca^{2+} concentration in the range of 0.5 mM to 10 mM. For instance, if aequorin is injected into an egg, this protein aequorin emits a flash of light, when a sperm enters and fertilizes the egg. This emission of light indicates sudden localised release of Ca^{2+} into the cytoplasm, on fertilization of the egg (Fig.).

There are also fluorescence indicators like quin-2 and fura-2 which are widely used for determining the concentration of Ca^{2+} ions. These indicators bind Ca^{2+} ions tightly and are excited at slightly longer wavelength when they are free of Ca^{2+}, than in their Ca^{2+} bound form. In view of this if ratio of fluorescent intensities at two excitation wavelengths is worked out using fluorescence microscope, this will indirectly give a ratio of Ca^{2+} free indicator and Ca^{2+} bound indicator. This allows determination of the concentration of free Ca^{2+} in a specific region of a cell. Fluorescent indicator for measuring concentrations of other ions like H^{+} are also available.

Introducing Molecules into Cells for Studies of Intracellular Dynamics: Studies in cell biology are also facilitated by introducing a variety of molecules into living cells. One of these techniques, described as fluorescent analogue cytochemistry, involves microinjection of molecules tagged with a fluorescent dye.

The fate of the injected molecule can be followed in a fluorescent microscope, when the cell grows and divides. For instance, if tubulin is thus tagged and injected into the cell, it will be incorporated into microtubules, and the microtubule dynamics can be followed in a living cell. Similarly, antibodies, if injected, can block the function of specific molecules. For instance, anti-myosin-II antibodies, have been shown to stop cell division even though the nuclear division occurs normally. This suggested that myosin is mainly involved in the division of cytoplasm, but not in the nuclear division.

Macromolecules can also be introduced into the cells when the cells are permeabilised with the help of an electric shock or a chemical treatment. Large pores are transiently created and are automatically sealed within a few minutes, thus permitting time for the entry of macromolecules. One such technique is electroporation, commonly used for introducing DNA into the cells for production of transgenic plants.

Macromolecules can also be enclosed into vesicles, which may be made to fuse with the plasma membrane of cell to allow introduction of these molecules within the cell.

The above techniques of introducing molecules into a cell do not allow a molecule of choice to be introduced at the desired place within the cell at a specified time. In order to facilitate this, caged molecules are used. These caged molecules are inactive photosensitive molecules, which can be activated by a strong pulse of light from a laser. A microscope can be used to focus the light pulse on any tiny region of the cell, to control where and when the active molecule is delivered.

For example, tubulin protein labeled with caged fluorescein has been incorporated into microtubules of the mitotic spindle. After such an incorporation, when a small region of the spindle was illuminated with laser, labeled tubulin became fluorescent, so that its movement along the spindle could be followed.

2

Variety of Tissues

Multicellular organisms have a wide variety of cells, all ultimately derived from the zygote in sexually reproducing forms. These cells differ in shape and function. Gland cells are specialised for secretion, muscle cells for contraction and nerve cells for conduction. The early stages of development have relatively similar cells. The cells of the blastula, for example, show relatively little variation. The process by which cells gradually specialise and undergo change in shape and function is called *cell differentiation.* Differentiation of cells begins during gastrulation and continues through tissue formation. After the cells become well differentiated, they cannot go back to the undifferentiated form.

It must be remembered that though the cells of an individual vary greatly, they are identical as far as their genes are concerned. The DNA molecules are identical in all the cells, since they have been derived from the DNA molecules of the zygote. The problem of cell differentiation therefore is: how can an identical genetic complement give rise to such a wide variety of structure and function? In other words, how can one cellular genotype result in so many different cellular phenotypes?

The nucleus and the cytoplasm have mutual control over each other and are, therefore, interdependent. The cytoplasm with its ribosomes is the site of protein synthesis and provides energy to the cell. Nuclear DNA provides the template for the synthesis of messenger RNA. A discussion on cell differentiation should therefore consider how the nucleus controls the cytoplasm, and conversely, how the cytoplasm controls the nucleus. Differentiation results from the interaction of the nucleus and the cytoplasm.

Cytoplasmic Factors: Mosaic and Regulative Eggs

The eggs of animals can be divided into two types with reference to the stage at which determination takes place (Fig.). In *mosaic* or *determined* eggs, determination takes place at the time of fertilization.

The cytoplasm can be divided into different areas which form definite regions of the embryo. Each part of the cytoplasm develops into a particular part of the embryo. If a part of the cytoplasm of the egg is removed from a molluscan egg, the embryo that develops is deficient in some part. Differentiation has taken place early in the egg. Mosaic eggs

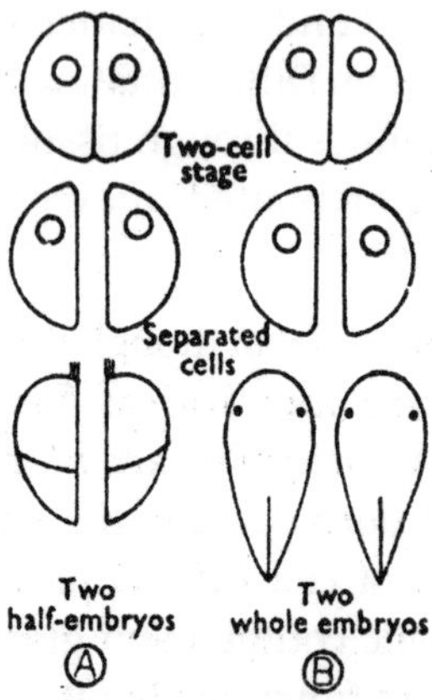

Diagrams showing the development of (A) mosaic egg and (B) regulative egg.

are found in annelids, insects and molluscs. If a two-cell stage is separated into two cells, each cell will give rise to a half embryo.

In *regulative* or *undetermined* eggs, found in echinoderms and vertebrates, determination takes place at a later stage. If the two-cell stage is separated into two cells, each forms a *complete embryo* of half the normal size. Separation of the cells in the four cell stage will give rise to four embryos. The cytoplasm of the egg has not yet been determined. In the 16-cell stage, however, if the blastomeres are separated, each forms only 1/16 of the embryo, showing that determination has taken place.

Nuclear Command of Cytoplasm

The early experiments of Boveri and Balbiani demonstrate nuclear control of the cytoplasm. *Boveri* removed nuclei from sea urchin eggs. These eggs were then fertilized by spermatozoa of another species. The resulting hybrid (*merogonic hybrid*) resembles, in certain characters, the species providing the nucleus. This suggests that development is directed by the nucleus. *Balbiani* showed that if amoebae are enucleated they survive only for a short time. They do not show growth and are incapable of reproduction. If a nucleus of the same species is implanted within three days, the *Amoeba* becomes normal and reproduces. If the transferred nucleus is from another species, the *Amoeba* is activated , but does not divide so readily.

Hammerling's experiments (1966) also demonstrate nuclear control of cytoplasm. He studied nucleocytoplasmic relationships in the marine alga *Acetabularia*. This alga consists of a single giant cell nearly six cm long. It is divided into the three parts, *rhizome stalk* and *cap*. There is single large *nucleus* in the *rhizome*. If the stalk is cut, the nucleated rhizome can regenerate the missing part.

Two species of *Acetabularia*, *A. crenulata* and *A. mediterranea* can be distinguished by the differences in their caps. Transplantation experiments have shown that the morphology of the cap is determined by the nucleus. The stalk of the *A. crenulata* was transplanted on the nucleated rhizome of *A. mediterranea.* In the first generation a new hybrid cap was formed, with characters intermediate between the caps of the two species. The hybrid stalk was then grafted on the *A. mediterranea* rhizome. The new cap formed had the phenotype of the *A. mediterrenea* cap. In this experiment, the *cytoplasm* was provided by the stem of *A. crenulata.* The shape of the cap was, however, of the *A. mediterranea* type because the *nucleus* was of *A. mediterranea.* Thus the genome of the nucleus controls morphogenesis. This is done through messenger RNA which is formed by the nucleus, and which probably induces differentiation of the cap.

Influence of the Cytoplasm on the Nucleus

In the gall midge *Mayetiola destructor*, the zygote contains 40 chromosomes (Fig.). The zygote nucleus divides thrice to give rise to eight nuclei which are evenly distributed in the egg cytoplasm.

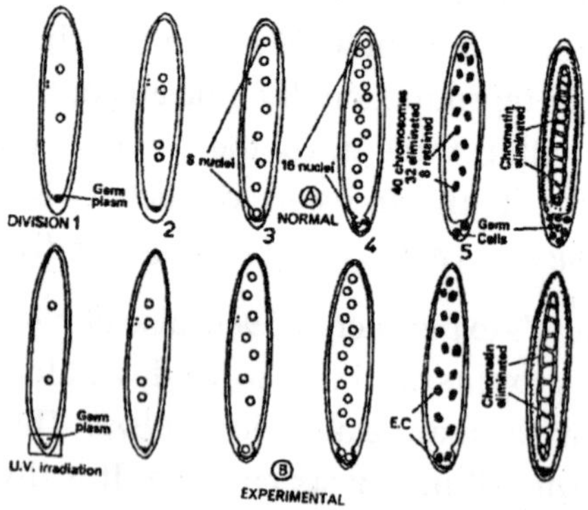

Influence of the cytoplasm on the nucleus in the gall midge Mayetiola destructor. (A) Normal nuclear divisions in the eggs. (B) Nuclear divisions after ultraviolet irradiation of the germ plasm at one end of the egg.

One of the eight nuclei moves towards the posterior pole and comes to lie in the *germ plasm* there. During the fourth division 16 nuclei are formed, of which two *(primary germ cells)* are separated by a constriction of the germ plasm at the posterior pole. During the peculiar fifth division 32 of the 40 chromosomes are eliminated from the nuclei, leaving 8 chromosomes in each nucleus. The 32 chromosomes of each somatic-cell dissolve and are eliminated. No chromosome elimination, however, takes place in the two germ cells which retain the full number of 40 chromosomes. Thus the behaviour of the nuclei is determined by a cytoplasmic factor.

Bantock irradiated the posterior germ plasm of the egg with ultraviolet rays, before the nuclei had migrated there. He found that the germ plasm nuclei also undergo chromosome elimination at the fifth division. They retain only eight chromosomes, as in somatic nuclei. Gall midges developing from eggs treated with ultraviolet rays are sterile, and have no reproductive cells in their gonads. It can be concluded that under normal conditions, the germ plasm affects the two posterior nuclei and prevents chromosome elimination in them. After ultraviolet irradiation, however, the germ plasm can no longer control the nuclei, and chromosome elimination takes place.

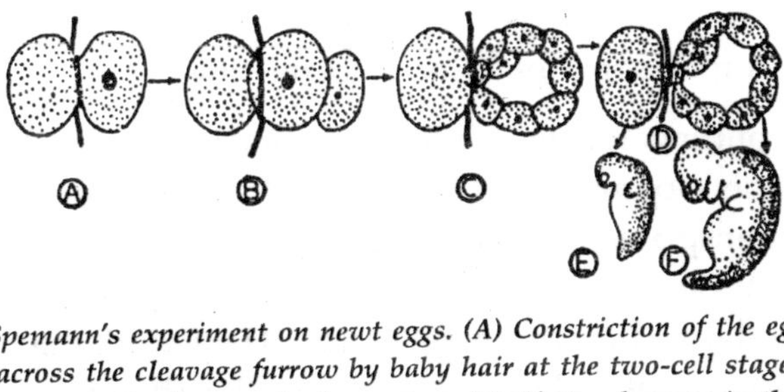

Spemann's experiment on newt eggs. (A) Constriction of the egg across the cleavage furrow by baby hair at the two-cell stage. (B) and (C) Cleavage in the nucleated half. No cleavage in the anucleate half. (D) Migration of the nucleus from the developing half into the anucleate half, (E) Delayed but normal development from the left half. (F) Normal embryo development from the right half.

An experiment by Spemann on the eggs of the newt demonstrates the influence of the cytoplasm on the nucleus (Fig.). In the two-cell stage, the egg is constricted by a hair along cleavage furrow in such a way that both nuclei are on one side. The part with the nucleus continues to divide, but there is no division in the part without the nucleus.

At some later stage of division, a nucleus slips through the protoplasmic bridge, from the dividing part to the enucleate part. This part then starts dividing and develops normally. The experiment demonstrates that a nucleus which has been derived after several divisions of the zygote is still capable of supporting normal development.

In Spemann's experiments both halves develop normally only if they receive a part of the grey crescent. If one half does not receive any part of the grey crescent it fails to develop. This shows that the cytoplasm does not merely play a passive part in development, but has the capacity to influence the nucleus. There is an active interaction between the nucleus and the cytoplasm during development.

Cytoplasmic Variation in Different Developmental Stages: Salivary gland chromosomes have numerous bands which represent chromomeres of the many strands of the chromosomes. The bands or chromomeres sometimes swell up to form chromosome puffs or Balbiani rings.

The puffing follows a definite pattern during different stages of development, and represents RNA synthesis activity. Kroeger transplanted nuclei form salivary glands of the prepupa in different early stages of the developing embryo, namely the preblastoderm and the blastoderm. He found that some chromosome puffs disappear while other bands undergo puffing. The new cytoplasmic environment induces changes in the nuçleus. This experiment demonstrates that the cytoplasm varies from one developmental stage to another.

Restriction in Nuclear Potentialities

The work of Briggs and King (1957, 1960) shows that the potentialities of the nucleus become restricted as they pass through successive stages in development. Enucleate host eggs of *Rana pipiens* were prepared by first activating them by pricking with a fine glass needle, and then removing the nucleus. Nuclei from various donor embryos were transplanted into the enucleate host eggs, and further development of the egg was observed.

It was found that when the donor nuclei were from embryos *upto the blastula* stage, the host eggs developed normally. However, when endoderm nuclei obtained from the *late gastrula* were transplanted into enucleate host eggs, most of the eggs did not develop normally. Development usually stopped at the blastula or early gastrula stage. Also, these stages had several abnormalities, mainly in the nervous system and sense organs.

Endoderm nuclei from more advanced stages of development resulted in even more abnormalities of ectodermal structures. Endodermal derivatives like the alimentary canal were not much affected. It was, therefore, concluded that the differentiation capacity of endodermal nuclei is progressively limited. There is restriction of the potentialities of the nucleus at higher stages of development. Another conclusion is that nuclei differ from organ to organ.

Stability of Nuclear Changes: Nuclear changes are stable, irreversible and hereditary is illustrated by the experiments of Fischberg and Blackler (1961). Enucleate host eggs of the frog were supplied by nuclei from a partially developed donor embryo (Fig.). The eggs developed into normal embryos. Nuclei from the blastula stage of these embryos were injected into other enucleate eggs. These eggs also produced a clone of normal embryos. All the nuclei of these embryos have descended from one nucleus.

King and Briggs (1956) have shown that nuclear changes during development are stable. Donor nuclei from the midgut (endoderm) were transplanted into enucleate eggs (Fig.). Various stages, from complete arrest of development to normal embryos, were obtained:

(1) From these stages the nuclei of a blastula were transplanted singly into several enucleate eggs. The abnormalities produced were found to be all alike in the clone produced.

(2) They did not show the variation of the first series. When the process of transplantation was repeated another clone was produced.

(3). Here also, the abnormalities were identical to those of the previous clone. It was therefore concluded that nuclear changes during development are relatively stable.

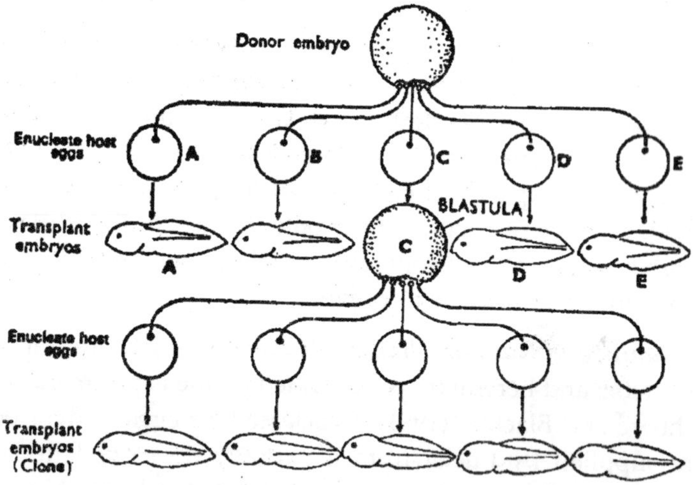

Production of nuclear clones. Nuclei from a donor embryo are injected into enucleate host eggs which develop into transplant embryos. Nuclei from the blastula stage of one of these embryos are injected into another series of enucleate host eggs, which develop into a clone of genetically identical individuals.

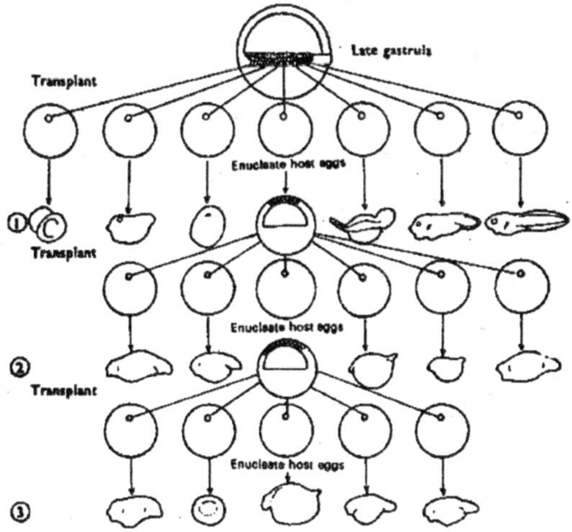

Serial transplantation experiment of King and Briggs (1956).

Nuclear changes are permanent. Moore (1960) studied developmental block in hybrids by back-transfer experiments. Eggs of *Rana sylvatica* were enucleated and fertilized by sperm of Rana *pipiens* (Fig.). The *R. sylvatica* eggs containing the *R. pipiens* nuclei underwent 10 to 12 cleavages, forming a *haploid blastula.* Nuclei from the blastula were transplanted into enucleated *R. pipiens* eggs. Thus the *R. pipiens* nuclei were back in their own *(R. pipiens)* cytoplasm. Development, however, proceeded *only upto the gastrula* stage. This is due to incompatibility between the nucleus and the cytoplasm. It can be concluded that when *R. pipiens* nuclei were in *R. sylvatica* cytoplasm they had undergone a change, and that this change was permanent. Hennen (1963) has confirmed the findings, using diploid instead of haploid nuclei.

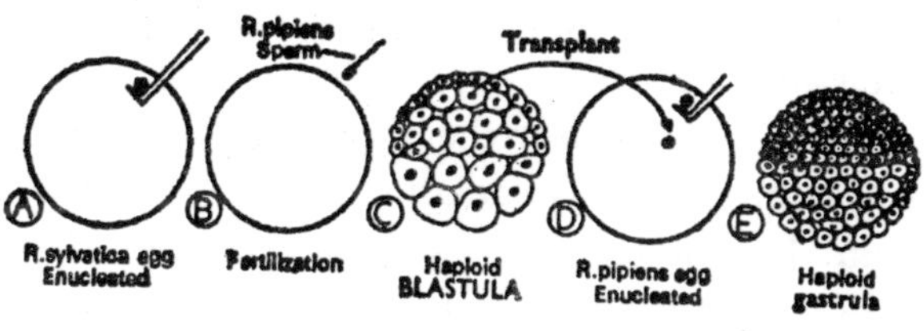

Moore's experiment (1960) on development block in hybrids.

Nuclear changes are not Irreversible: Gurdon and Uehlinger (1966) working on *Xenopus laevis* obtained different results from those of Briggs and King. Nuclei from highly differentiated cells, like those of the intestinal epithelium, were transplanted into enucleated eggs (Fig.). Out of 726 cases, 10 developed into normal tadpoles. This shows that although the capacity to induce normal development decreases with development and differentiation, the changes that take place are not irreversible. Even the nuclei of highly specialised cells contain information required for the formation of a new individual.

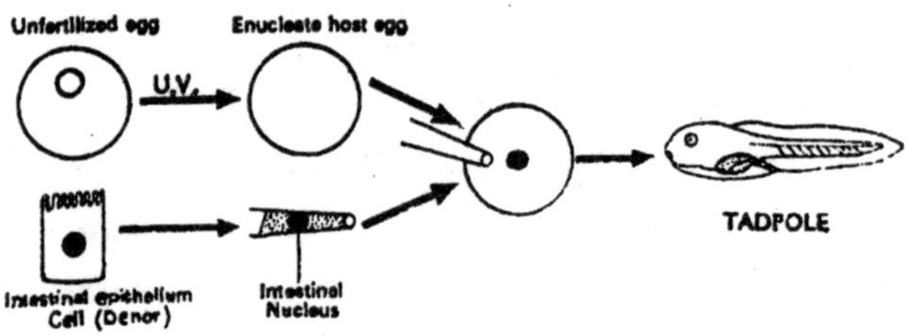

Transplantation of intestinal cell nucleus in Xenopus laevais (Gurdon and Uehlinger, 1966). U.V.=Ultra-Violet radiation.

The results have been explained by Hamburgh (1971) on the basis that some intestinal nuclei had not advanced in differentiation, while others had differentiated. The former initiate normal development while the latter result in abnormalities. Di Berardino and King (1967) have given another explanation. According to them, the donor intestinal nuclei may be from primordial germ cells, which in anurans are located in the endoderm.

Effect on RNA Synthesis: Gurdon and Brown (1965) transplanted nuclei from intestinal cells of gastrulae and larvae into enucleate eggs of *Xenopus laevis*. The nuclei were undergoing RNA synthesis in the intestinal cells, as was shown by their nucleoli. After transplantation, however, RNA synthesis stops within 40 minutes, as is evidenced by the fact that the nucleoli disappear. This demonstrates the influence of the cytoplasm on the nucleus.

Somatic Hybridisation: A flu-like virus, called the *Sendai* virus, causes cells to fuse by modifying the cell surface. Harris (1965) caused fusion between HeLa cells (carcinoma cells) of humans with chicken erythrocytes, by means of the *Sendai* virus (Fig.). The chicken erythrocyte has a nucleus, but it is no longer functional. The cytoplasm of the erythrocyte was washed away by haemolysis. The erythrocyte ghost consisting of a cell membrane and a nucleus was fused with a HeLa cell. The erythrocyte nucleus came to lie in the cytoplasm of the HeLa cell. The nucleus became active and functional, and resumed synthesis of DNA and RNA. This experiment demonstrates nuclear dependence of the cytoplasm.

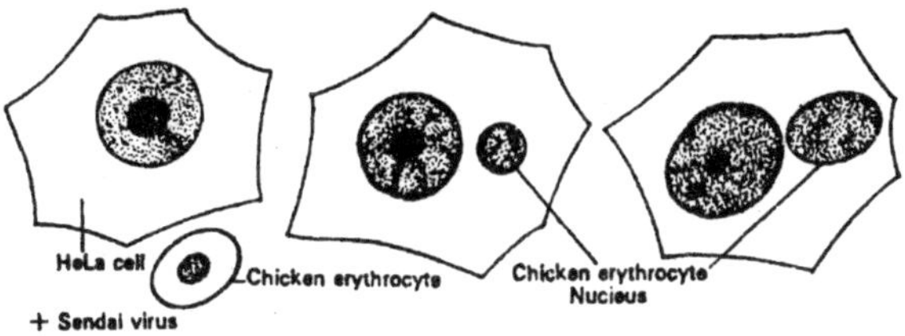

Somatic hybridisation of a HeLa carcinoma cell with chicken erythrocyte with the help of Sendai virus. The chicken erythrocyte nucleus increases in size and becomes active and functional.

Discriminatory Gene Action

As noted previously, the genetic complement of widely different cells of an individual is identical. Each cell contains all the types of genes that are required for the functioning of the organism. Yet each type of cell has a specialised function, and produces only the substances that it requires. This can be explained by the fact that all the genes of a cell do not function at the same time. There is *differential gene action.* Some genes are 'switched on' and function for a time producing a particular protein. They are then 'switched off' and then become dormant. It has been speculated (Moore, 1963; Brachet 1964) that nuclear histones may function as gene inactivators during early embryonic development. Cell differentiation thus results from the fact that different genes are activated at different times. Many genes in a particular cell may not function at all.

Cells are influenced not only by their genes, but also by the by–products of their own metabolism. Thus the cytoplasmic environment provides a feedback mechanism on the activity of the nucleus. Also differentiation of cells may depend upon substances received from neighbouring cells.

Differentiation of nerve cells, for example, depends on an external factor received from certain nearby cells. Because of interaction between the nucleus and the cytoplasm, products of gene action accumulate in the cytoplasm. These bring about changes (differentiation) in cells that were originally similar.

3

Role of Membrane

Plasma membrane encloses the cell and represents its outer living boundary. This membrane was called 'cell membrane' by C. Nageli and C. Cramer in 1855 and 'plasmalemma' by J. Q. Plower in 1931. The terms 'plasma membrane' and 'plasmalemma' are preferred, because the term 'cell membrane' may be confused with 'cell wall' in plants. On the exterior of this membrane, is present an 'extracellular matrix'. Similar cell membranes also separate cell organelles (*e.g.* endoplasmic reticulum, Golgi apparatus, mitochondria, plastids, etc.) from the cytosol, but they will not be called plasma membranes. In all cells, plasma membrane contains proteins, which help in cell recognition, transport of material in either direction or in sensing signals received from outside.

Some of these proteins also help in establishing and maintaining ion gradients across the membranes to facilitate the synthesis of ATP, movement of solutes/ions across the membrane and transmission of signals in all kinds of cells including the nerve and muscle cells. The structure of these membranes in all kind of cells will be briefly discussed in this chapter and the variety of functions (cell sorting, cell-cell adhesion, membrane transport, neurotransmission, vescular transport, etc.) performed by them.

Separation and Chemical Structure

A variety of cells including liver cells, muscles, amoebae, and sea urchin eggs have been used for isolation of plasma membrane. However, plasma membrane of human red blood cells (RBCs) has been studied more extensively than any other membrane for the following reasons: (i) erythrocytes (RBCs) are available in large number from blood banks, (ii) RBCs are relatively uncontaminated by other cell types, (iii) RBCs contain no nuclei or other cell organelles; there are no other membranes other than plasma membrane in these cells, thus avoiding contamination due to other internal membranes; such contamination is a common phenomenon, while isolating plasma membrane from other cell types, where plasma membrane makes only 5% of the cell membrane system; (iv) empty RBC membranes called 'ghosts' can be easily obtained by putting RBCs in a hypotonic salt solution, so that water enters the RBCs, which swell and burst (lyse) releasing their contents and leaving membranes as 'ghosts'. The above process of getting ghosts is described as hemolysis. If hemolysis is mild, permeability function of the membrane can be restored by certain treatments thus giving rise to what are called 'resealed ghosts' (Fig.). But if hemolysis is more drastic, permeability function is permanently lost and resulting membrane is called 'white ghost'. The resealed ghosts can be used for the study of physiological as well as biochemical properties, but white ghosts can be used for the study of biochemical properties only. The membrane ghosts can be studied, while they are still leaky, so that any reagent in which these 'leaky ghosts' are placed, will interact with both sides of the membrane. In the resealed ghosts, however, water soluble reagents can not reach the inner face of the membrane. 'Sealed inside-out ghosts' can also be prepared, so that a reagent will now interact with only the inner face (now facing outside). Tims the 'resealed ghosts' and 'sealed inside-out ghosts' can be used to study separately the external and the internal (cytosolic face) faces of the membrane (Fig.).

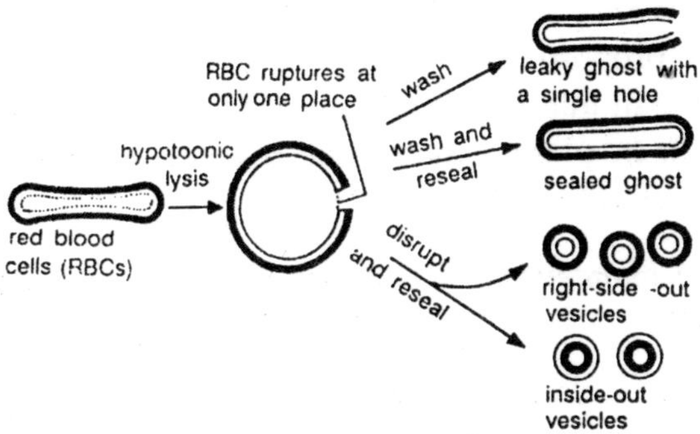

The preparation of unsealed ghosts, sealed ghosts, right-side out vesicles and inside-out vesicles from red blood cells (RBCs).

The chemical constituents of plasma membrane include (i) lipids (28-79%), (ii) proteins (20-70%), (iii) oligosaccharides (only 1-5%) and (iv) water (20% of total weight). Therefore the main constituents of plasma membrane are protein and lipid and their relative proportions greatly vary as shown in Table.

Relative Proportions of Protein and Lipid in Sonic Membranes

Animal and tissue	*Protein (%)*	*Lipid (%)*	*Ratio (protein/lipid)*
Human (myelin)	20	79	0.25
Ral (muscle)	65	35	1.86
Rat (liver)	60	40	1.50
Human (erythrocyte)	60	40	1.50
Rat (liver mitochondria)	70	28	2.50

Lipids as Phospholipids, Glycolipids and Cholesterol: Lipids may account for 25% to 80% of the mass of cell membrane depending upon the tissue and organism involved. In myelin exceptionally, lipids predominate. The main lipid components of membranes are phospholipids, cholesterol, and glycolipids, their relative proportions varying in different cell membranes (Table). While in internal membranes, the lipid is exclusively phospholipid, in plasma membrane it could be glycolipids and/or cholesterol.

Lipid Composition of Different Cell Membranes

Type of lipid	*Liver cells*	*Erythrocytes*	*Myelin*	*Mitochondrion*	*ER*	*E. coli*
1. Phospholipids						
Phosphatidylethanolamine	7	18	15	35	17	70
Phosphatidylserine	4	7	9	2	5	trace
Phosphatidylcholine	24	17	10	39	40	zero
Sphingomyelin	19	18	8	zero	5	zero
2. Chlolesterol	17	23	22	3	6	zero
3. Glycolipids	7	3	28	trace	trace	zero
4. Others	23	13	8	21	27	30

The major proportion of phospholipids is represented by phosphatidyl serine, phosphatidylcholine, and sphingomyclin (Fig.), all of which are neutral phospholipids and tend to pack tightly in membrane bilayer, as will be discussed later in this chapter. Upto 20% of phospholipids are acidic which are negatively charged and are associated with proteins in the membrane due to lipid-protein interactions (*e.g.*, phosphatidylserine). Other phospholipids, such as the inositol phospholipids, are present in small quantities, but are functionally very important particularly in cell signaling. This diversity of lipids in eukaryotic membranes is important, because some membrane bound proteins require specific lipid head-groups to perform their function.

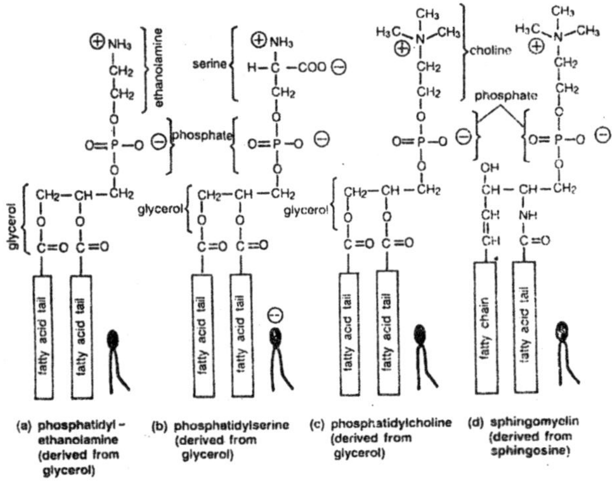

Four representatives with generalised structure of a phospholipid molecule.

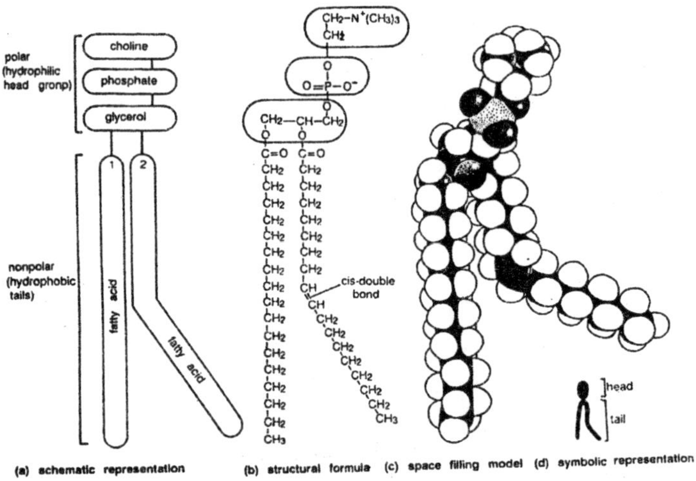

A lipid molecule showing a head and two tails.

Lipids: Lipids are amphipathic and form a bilayer. A lipid molecule is amphipathic and consists of two parts (Fig.), a head (glycerol) which is hydrophilic (water soluble or 'polar') and two tails (fatty acids) which are hydrophobic (water insoluble or 'non-polar'). The lipid molecules make a bilayer,

4.5nm thick, with the tails (non-polar) oriented inwards and perpendicular to the surface of the membrane, so that the tails from two layers of the bilayer will face each other. The external surface of the bilayer which consists of polar moieties (heads) provide a surface for deposition of other components like protein or glycoprotein.

It is the shape and the amphipathic nature of the lipid molecules that make them form lipid bilayers spontaneously in aqueous solution. When lipid molecules are surrounded by water on all sides, they aggregate in such a way that their non-polar or hydrophobic tails are hurried inside and the polar hydrophilic heads are exposed to water. In doing so, depending on the shape of lipid molecules, they may form spherical micelles (when lipids are wedge shaped) with tails inwards, or may form bilayers (when lipids are cylindrical in shape) (Fig).

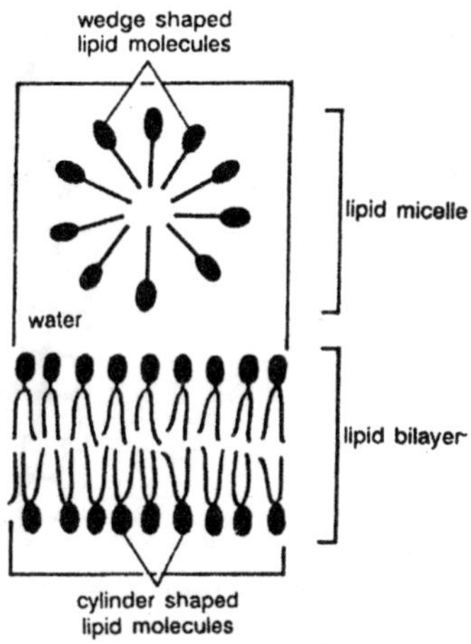

A lipid micelle (formed by wedge shaped lipid molecules) and a lipid bilayer (formed by cylindrical phospholipid molecules), which are formed spontaneously in water (redrawn from Alberts et. al., Molecular Biology of the Cell, 1994).

Lipid Bilayer can be Asymmetrical: Although earlier a symmetry of arrangement of phospholipids in the lipid bilayer was conceived, it was later demonstrated that there is an asymmetry of phospholipids in erythrocyte membrane. There are more choline phospholipids and glycolipids in the outer half of bilayer and more amino phospholipids' in the inner half, lying towards the cytosol.

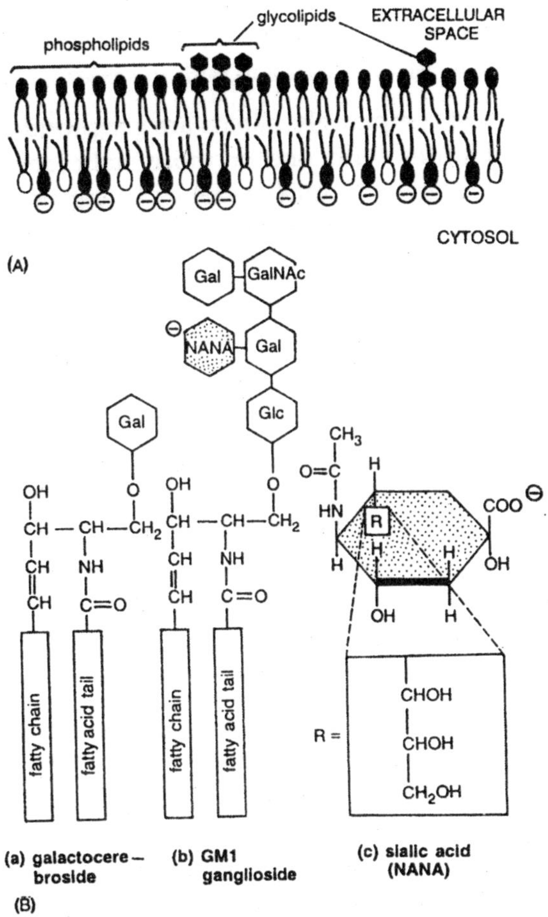

Some examples of glycolipid molecules found in the lipid bilayer; (A) distribution of glycolipids on the non-cytoplasmic cell surface; (B) two types of glycolipids-(a) galactocerebroside and (b) a ganglioside with negatively charged sialic acid residue, whose structure is shown in (c) (redrawn from Alberts et. al., Molecular Biology of the Cell, 1994).

Glycolipids on Plasma Membrane Surface: Glycolipids, forming upto about 5% of lipids in animal cells (28% in myelin; see Table), are invariably found exclusively in the non-cytoplasmic half of the lipid bilayer (Fig.). They form aggregates through hydrogen bonds with one another. The sugar groups are generally added in the lumen of ER and the Golgi apparatus. These sugar groups of glycolipids are generally exposed at the cell surface to allow interaction with the external environment.

The most complex glycolipids are gangliosides containing oligosaccharides with one or more sialic acid (N-acetyl-neuraminic acid or NANA) residues giving negative charge (Fig.). These gangliosides are most abundant in plasma membrane of nerve cells (5-10% of total lipids) and their charge may alter electric fields, across the membrane. In the myelin (providing insulation to nerve cells), as indicated above, glycolipids can be as high as 28%; of total lipids.

The glycolipids also help in cell recognition. For instance, ganglioside GM1 is a cell surface receptor for bacterial toxin causing diarrhoea of cholera. Toxin binds to GM land enters the cells of intestinal epithelium leading to prolonged increase in the concentration of intracellular cyclic AMP, which causes a large efflux of Na^+ and water into the intestine.

Proteins Bound in Membrane

The major functions attributed to plasma membrane are actually performed by membrane proteins, which constitute 20% to 70% of the membrane by mass. Like lipid molecules (glycolipids), proteins also have oligosaccharide chains attached to them (glycoproteins). Thus the surface of the cells facing exterior consists largely of carbohydrates, forming what is described as glycocalyx or cell coat.

The membrane proteins can be found in a variety of forms including the following. (i) Transmembrane proteins extend through the lipid bilayer as a single helix (*e.g.*, glycophorin) or multiple helices, or as barrels (*e.g.*, porin), with a part of their mass on either side of the membrane. When the polypeptide crosses the membrane only once, it is described as 'single pass transmembrane' (*e.g.* glycophorin protein of human RBCs), and when it crosses several times it is called a 'multipass, transmembrane protein' (*e.g.*, band 3 protein of human RBCs). All transmembrane proteins pass all the way across the entire bilayer and there is no established

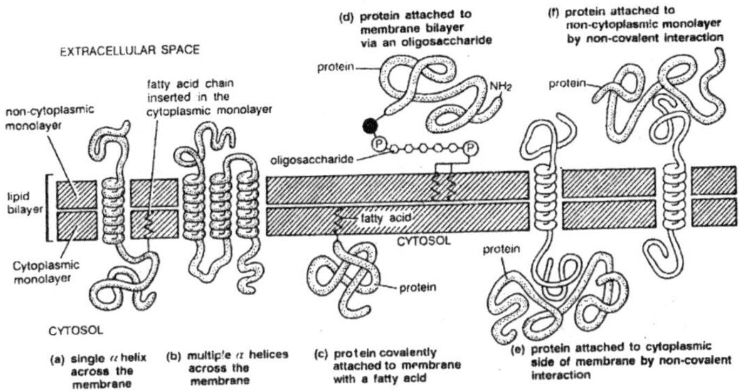

Six different ways (a-f) in which membrane proteins associate with the lipid bilayer (redrawn from Alberts et. al., Molecular Biology of the Cell, 1994).

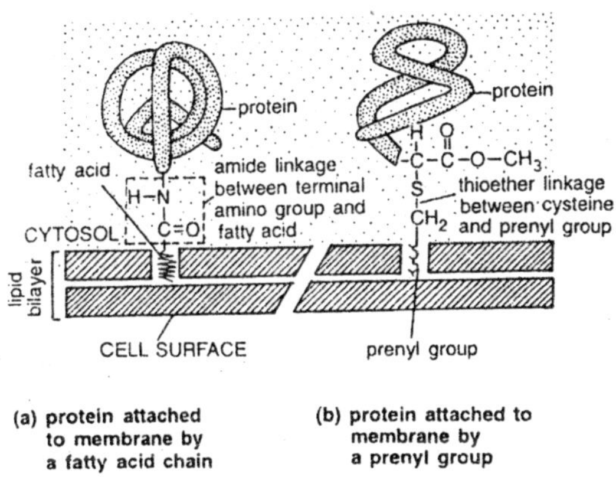

The attachment of extrinsic proteins to plasma membrane with the help of either of the two types of lipid groups - fatty acid or prenyl group (redrawn from Alberts et. al., Molecular Biology of the Cell, 1994).

example of a protein, which is embedded only partly across the lipid bilayer. The transmembrane regions of these proteins are hydrophobic, interacting with hydrophobic tails of lipid molecules. One or both the regions of these proteins lying outside the membrane can be hydrophilic, exposed to water. Hydrophobicity of membrane proteins is increased by covalent attachment of a fatty acid chain that is inserted in the cytoplasmic leaflet of the lipid bilayer (Fig.). (ii) Covalently linked cytosolic extrinsic proteins are located entirely in the cytosol and are attached to membrane by means of covalently attached fatty acid chains or prenyl groups (Fig.). (iii) Covalently linked non-cytosolic extrinsic proteins are found on the external surface of membrane and remain attached, each with the help of an oligosaccharide to the non-cytoplasmic monolayer. (iv) Non-covalently linked extrinsic proteins include those proteins, which are present on either side of the membrane (*e.g.*, spectrin) and are attached to it by non-covalent interactions with other transmembrane proteins. These proteins are sometimes also called 'peripheral membrane proteins', since they can be released from the membrane easily by gentle extraction procedure. Other proteins listed above as (i) to (iii) can not be released easily and are therefore classified as 'integral proteins'.

Segments Spanning the Membrane and those Outside the Membrane: Transmembrane proteins are difficult to crystallise and therefore have not been subjected to x-ray crystallography for a study of their three dimensional structures. However, cloning and sequencing of genes encoding these proteins and the amino-acid sequencing of these proteins have been successfully achieved in many cases giving valuable information, from which the segments spanning the membrane can be predicted. Segments containing 20-30 amino acids residues with a high degree of hydrophobicity (nonpolar side chains give hydrophobicity to an amino acid) are long enough to span the bilayer as a helix and can be identified as a 'hydropathy plot'. Hydropathy plots for 'glycophorin' and 'bacteriorhodopsin', and corresponding explanations are given in Figure. However, for a (3 strand traversing the bilayer, ten or less than ten amino acid residues are needed, so that hydropathy plot technique can not help in this case.

The segments of a transmembrane protein on the cytosolic and non-cytosolic sides of the plasma membrane can be determined in several ways including the following:

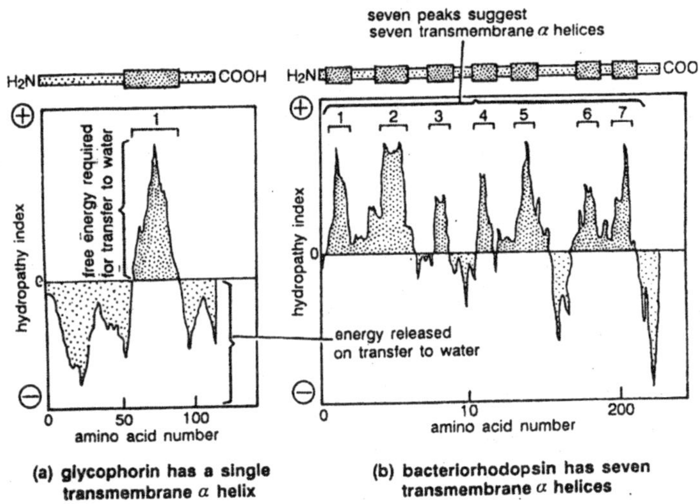

Hydropathy plots of two membrane proteins and their use in locating alpha-helical transmembrane segments (redrawn from Alberts et al, Molecular Biology of the Cell, 1994).

(i) Water soluble (can not enter membrane) reagents, which are radioactive or fluorescent can be used for labelling the segments lying outside the membrane. The membrane may then be solubilised (isolated) and proteins separated by SDS (sodium dodecyl sulphate) PAGE (polyacrylamide gel electrophoresis), so that labelled proteins can be identified. If proteins from intact cells or sealed ghosts are used, libelling will suggest libelling of external (non-cytosolic) segment. Similarly, if sealed inside-out ghosts are labelled, this will suggest libelling of internal (cytosolic) segment and if libelling is obtained in both cases, it suggests the presence of a transmembrane protein,

(ii) In another approach, external or internal surface of membrane may be subjected to protease treatment, and the proteins isolated after treatment may be analysed. If protein is partially digested from both surfaces, it suggests the presence of a transmembrane protein,

(iii) Specific antibodies can also be used to find out the location of that specific part of protein, against which antibodies have been derived.

Glycosylation and Disulphide Bonds on the Non-cytosolic Side of Transmembrane Proteins: Majority of transmembrane proteins are glycosylated on the non-cytosolic side and the sugar is added while the protein is still in the lumen of ER and Golgi. This also explains why glycosylation is available only on non-cytosolic side. The intra-chain disulphide (S-S) bonds between cysteine residues are also formed only on the non-cytosolic side, because the cytosolic side has a strong reducing environment, maintaining these groups in their reduced (-SH) form (Fig.). These disulphide bonds play an important role in stabilising the folded structure of the polypeptide and in making associations with other proteins, etc.

Three Representative Membrane Proteins (Spectrin, Glycophorin and Band 3) from RBCs: Utilising a variety of methods, membrane' proteins of RBCs were separated on SDS-PAGE and 15 major proteins, ranging in molecular weight from 15,000 to 250,000, were detected (Fig.). Of these 15 proteins, three (spectrin, glycophorin and band 3) account for more than 60% (by weight) of total membrane proteins.

These three membrane proteins are arranged in plasma membrane in three different manners and, therefore, will be discussed here as representatives of three major ways, in which the proteins are generally associated in plasma membranes of all kinds of cells.

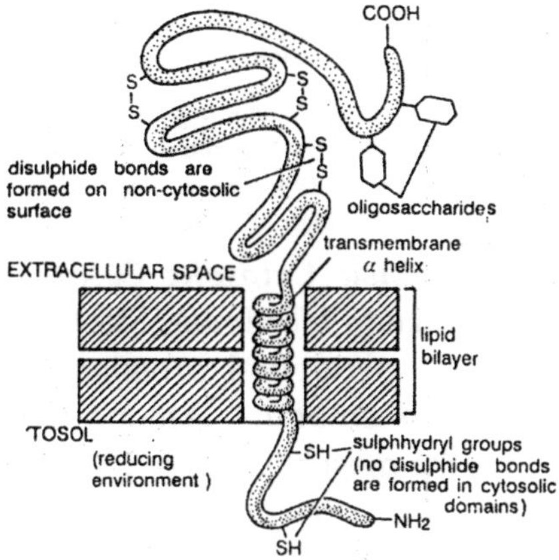

A typical single-pass transmembrane protein; note that disulphide bonds and oligosaccharide chains are found on the extracellular surface, and not on the cytosolic side of the membrane protein (redrawn from Alberts et. al., Molecular Biology of the Cell, 1994).

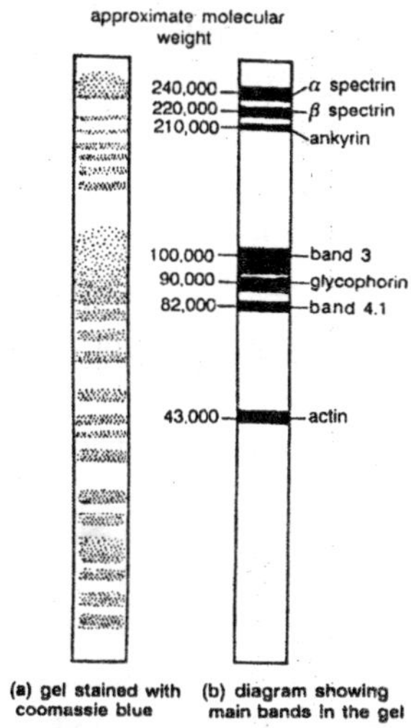

SDS-PAGE patterns of proteins from human red blood cells; note that glycophorin protein (30,000) moves slowly due to large amount of carbohydrate associated with it (redrawn from Alberts et. al., Molecular Biology of the Cell, 1994).

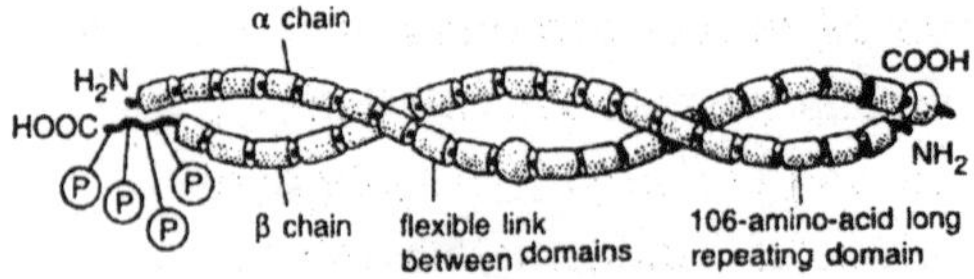

Structure of a spectrin molecule showing alpha and beta chains (each with repeating domains, 106 amino acids long) running antiparallel and intertwined (redrawn from Alberts et. al., Molecular Biology of the Cell, 1994).

Spectrin, an , Extrinsic Cytosolic Cytoskeleton Protein, not Covalently Attached to Membrane: Most of the membrane proteins in RBCs are peripheral proteins associated with cytosolic side of the membrane. Among these peripheral proteins, spectrin is the most abundant (25% of the membrane protein mass; 2.5×10^5 copies per cell). It makes a principal component of cytoskeleton underlying the membrane and thus maintains structural integrity and biconcave shape of the membrane.

Spectrin is a thin, long, flexible, rod shaped heterodimer protein, about 100nm in length. The heterodimer consists of two antiparallel, loosely intertwined flexible α and β chains, non-covalently attached to each other at several points, including both ends. Each of the two (α and β) chains has repeating domains, 106 amino acids long (Fig.). Two heterodimers associate 'head' to 'head' at their phosphorylated heads to form 200nm long tetramers and four to five such tetramers bind short actin filaments with the help of other proteins (including 4.1 protein) to form a 'junctional complex'.

This makes a meshwork on the cytosolic face of the membrane (Fig.), which enables the RBCs to sustain the stress as they pass through narrow capillaries. A deficiency or mutation in spectrin makes a human/mouse anemic, leading to abnormality in shape of RBCs which become spherical instead of concave. Proteins homologous to spectrin, ankyrin and band 4.1 are also present in the nucleated cells, forming cortical cytoskeleton.

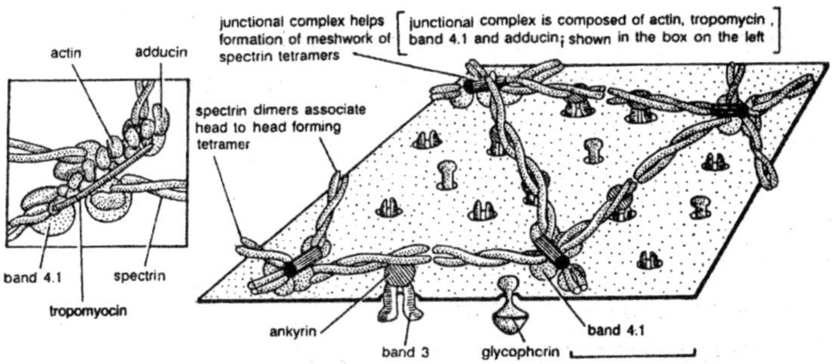

A cytoskeleton on the cytoplasmic side of the membrane in red blood cells; note the network of spectrin dimers, which associate head to head forming tetramers (redrawn from Alberts et. al., Molecular Biology of the Cell, 1994).

Glycophorin, a Single Pass Transmembrane Protein: Glycophorin is a small (131 amino acid residues) single pass transmembrane protein with its hydrophilic carboxy-terminal tail exposed to cytosol, its hydrophobic a-helical segment (23 amino acid residues) spanning the lipid bilayer and its remaining major part on the external surface of the membrane. On the non-cytosolic external surface, glycophorin carries about 100 sugar residues (including 90% of the total negatively charged sialic acid of the membrane) accounting for 60% of the mass of glycophorin, which contains most of the total carbohydrates of the RBCs. Nearly 10 lakh; (1 million) glycophorin molecules are found per RBC, but their function is unknown, their deficiencies causing no disease. Many, cell surface receptors in the nucleated cells belong to the category of 'glycophorin' *i.e.* single pass transmembrane protein, the transmembrane segment being an a (alpha) helix.

Band 3, a Multipass Transmembrane Protein Catalyzing Transport of Anions (Cl^-, HCO_3^-): Band 3 protein derives its name from its position relative to other proteins on the polyacrylamide gel after electrophoresis (Fig.). It is a long (930 amino acid residues) polypeptide arranged as dimers traversing the lipid bilayer as many as 14 times. There are as many as 10^6 molecules of this protein per erythrocyte. The protein band

3 functions as anion transporter and helps RBCs in carrying CO_2 from tissues to the lungs in the form of HCO_3~ ions in exchange of Cr.

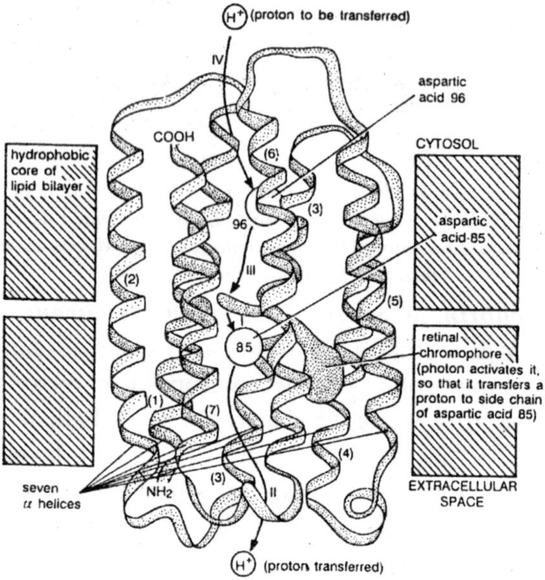

Three-dimensional structure of a bacteriorhodopsin molecule-note the presence of seven transmembrane alpha-helices (1-7) and the path of protons during light activation (redrawn from Alberts et. al., Molecular Biology of the Cell, 1994).

Bacteriorhodopsin (from Bacteria Halobacterium halobium), a Seven a Helices Transmembrane Segments (TMS) Protein, is a Proton Pump: *Halobacterium halobium* represents a class of bacteria, which live in salt-water pools exposed to large amount of sunlight. They have evolved a variety of light activated proteins including bacteriorhodopsin, which is a light activated proton pump. Bacteriorhodopsin molecule contains a light absorbing group or chromophore (called retinal), which gives the protein its purple colour. This retinal is related to vitamin A and is identical to chromophore found in the rhodopsin of vertebrate eye. The retinal is linked to a lysine side chain of the protein. Due to activation by a photon of light, the chromophore changes its shape and causes a series of changes in bacteriorhodopsin protein leading to transfer of one H^+ ion from the inside to the outside of the cell. In bright light, several hundred protons can be pumped every second by one bacteriorhodopsin molecule. This establishes a proton gradient across the membrane facilitating the production of ATP by another protein, thus providing energy to the bacterial cell.

Bacteriorhodopsin is a multipass transmembrane protein having seven transmembrane α helices, which are closely packed, each helix containing about 25 amino acids (Fig.). The light receptor rhodopsin in vertebrates and many cell surface receptor proteins resemble bacteriorhodopsin, in having seven transmembrane α helices and therefore sometimes described as seven sisters proteins.

Porins (Transmembrane Proteins) Cross the Membrane as β Barrel: Although generally, in the transmembrane proteins, the segments traversing the membrane are α helices, they can also be present as β sheets (β barrel). Porins represent one such protein found in the outer membrane (which surrounds plasma membrane) of many bacteria like *E. coli*, and allow selected hydrophilic solutes (upto 600 daltons) to pass across this outer lipid bilayer. Proteins in the outer membrane of mitochondria and chloroplasts also resemble porins in having β sheet instead of α-helix, as their transmembrane segments. In 1990, three dimensional structure of a porin from *Rhodobacter capsulatus* was determined by x-ray crystallography. It is a trimer, each monomer forming a β barrel, and forms a pore while traversing the lipid bilayer. The β barrel is formed from a 16-stranded antiparallel β sheet, curved to form a cylindrical structure. Polar side chains line the aqueous channel and the nonpolar side chains project outside to interact with the surface of the hydrophobic lipid bilayer.

Protein Complexes in Membranes: Sometimes, several proteins associate together in the membrane forming protein complexes performing a variety of complex functions. One such complex is the 'photosynthetic reaction centre' that was studied in detail in bacteria and its atomic structure published in 1985. This was the first transmembrane protein to be crystallised and studied by X-ray crystallography and its structure is shown in Figure. The structure consists of four subunits L, M, H, and a cytochrome. The subunits L and M, each consisting of five α helices, make the core of the reaction centre and contain electron carrier coenzymes. Such protein complexes are formed by a variety of proteins which harvest energy and transduce signals from the outside world into intracellular pathway.

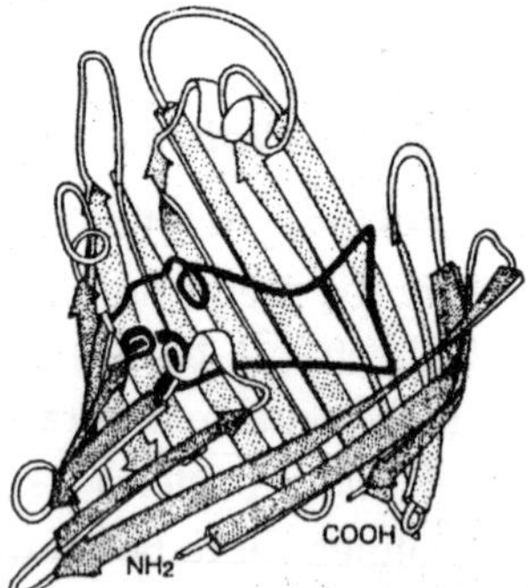

(a) a porin protein consisting of 16 stranded antiparallel transmembrane β barrel

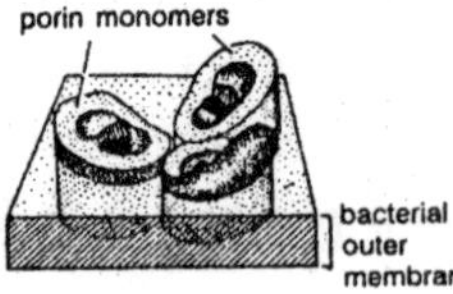

(b) three monomers associate to form a trimer in porin protein

Three dimensional structure of a porin trimer of Rhodobacter capsulatus: (a) 16 stranded antiparallel transmembrane beta (β) barrel; (b) association of three monomers, each having a channel with a protruded loop of a polypeptide, narrowing the lumen through which diffusion of solutes occurs (redrawn from Alberts et. al., Molecular Biology of the Cell, 1994).

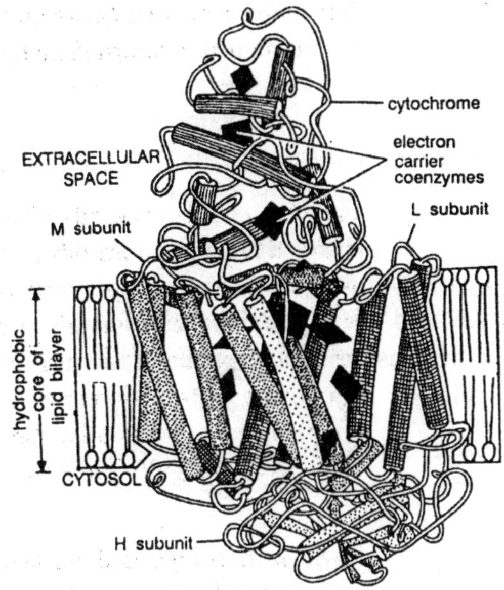

Three dimensional structure of the photosynthetic reaction centre of the bacterium Rhodnpseudomonus viridis (redrawn from Alberts et. al., Molecular Biology of the Cell. 1994).

Specific Proteins for Specific Membrane Domains: Although proteins are mobile within the lipid bilayer, there

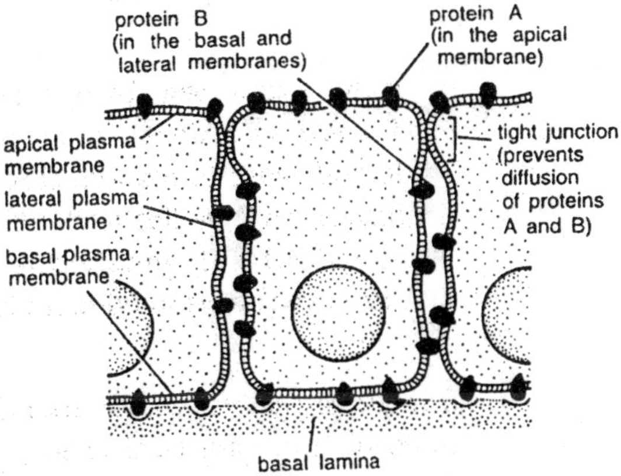

A few epithelial cells showing restricted distribution of plasma membrane proteins to basal and apical regions of the cell (redrawn from Alberts et. al., Molecular Biology of the Cell, 1994).

are mechanisms which allow confinement of specific proteins in specific membrane domains. In cells lining the gut and kidney tubules, there are specific proteins confined to the apical domain and to the basolateral domain of the cell (Fig.). There are also mechanisms for the transport of these specific proteins to specific domains within the cell.

Cell Coat or Glycocalyx (Rich in Sugar Residues): As discussed earlier, most of the lipids in the outer monolayer of lipid bilayer and the non-cytosolic external segments of the extrinsic as well as intrinsic proteins of the plasma membrane, are glycosylated.

They are, therefore, described as glycolipids and glycoproteins, respectively. This is true of both animal and plant cells. The sugar residues in extracellular matrix (ECM) are also found as polysaccharide chains of proteoglycan molecules.

All these sugar rich molecules make a sugar rich zone on the surface of plasma membrane, which is described as cell coat or glycocalyx (Fig.) and can be visualised by stains like ruthenium red or by marker tagged lectins which specifically bind to carbohydrates. The function of the cell coat can be varied including protection, cell recognition, cell-cell adhesion, inflammatory responses, etc.

CAMs (Cadherins and Selections) and Integrins as Membrane Proteins: A variety of membrane proteins present in or on the plasma membrane are now known and only few have been described in this chapter as a representative sample, particularly including those which have been studied in detail. There are a variety of other proteins including a variety of 'cell adhesion molecules' or 'CAMs' like 'cadherins' which are Ca^{++} dependent CAMs, 'integrins' found in extracellular matrix or ECM and functioning as receptors and 'selections' which mediate inflammatory responses.

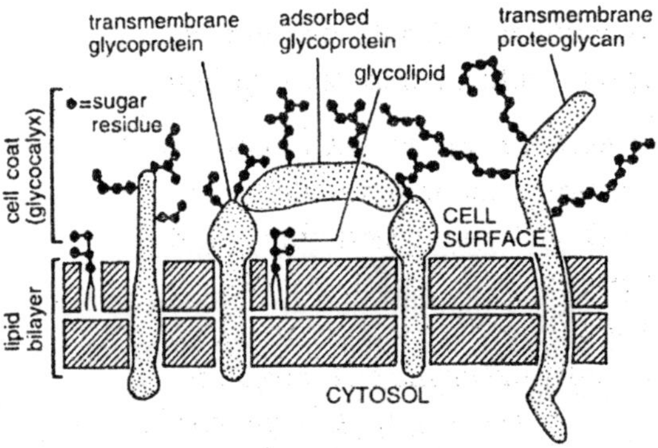

Structure of a cell coat or glycocalyx formed due to sugar rich molecules on the surface of plasma membrane (redrawn from Alberts el al., Molecular Biology of the Cell, 1994).

Abstract of Membrane

(Plasma Membrane-Cytoskeleton Interaction)

These extrinsic proteins make a boundary between the cytoskeleton and the plasma membrane. They control cell shape, delimit specialised membrane domains and help in cell adhesions (attachment with other cells and to the substratum). The meshwork consisting of these boundary proteins, which are responsible for association of plasma membrane with underlying cytoskeleton, is described as 'membrane skeleton'. For erythrocytes, the components of this membrane skeleton were shown earlier in Figure, where a meshwork consisting of spectrin, actin and other proteins is attached to plasma membrane through 'ankyrin' and protein '4.1'. The 'membrane skeleton' also has proteins (*e.g.* adducin, tropomyosin, damatin or 4.9, tropomodulin), which do not bind directly to the membrane, but add to the stability of membrane skeleton. Similar 'membrane skeletons' have been studied in 'platelets' (anucleate blood components) and in multinucleated cells of 'striated muscles'. The defects in the membrane skeleton of these cells are responsible for a variety of hereditary diseases in human beings, which explains the significance of these studies (*e.g.* 'Bernard Soulier syndrome', a bleeding disorder, 'Duchenne and Becker muscular dystrophies').

Organisation of Lipids and Proteins (Models for Structure of Membrane)

Artificial Membrane Systems: As discussed earlier in this chapter, biological membranes are known to be the result of lipid-protein interactions. Their arrangement can be ascertained through artificial models prepared through monolayer films. Fatty acids, phospholipids, cholesterol and cholesterol esters can be packed in single layers and their arrangements can then be studied.

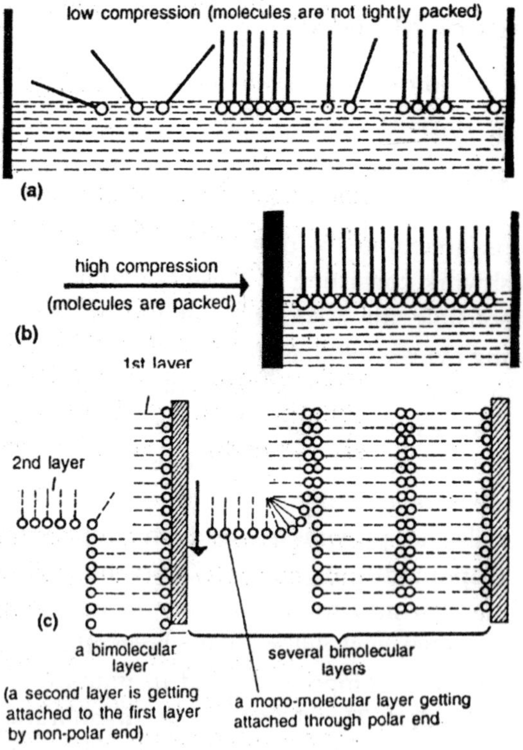

Steps involved in the production of artificial membrane system (redrawn from De Roberts et. al., Cell Biology. 6th ed)

The film balance devised by Langmuir in 1917 was used for making monolayer films. The instrument consists of a shallow trough filled with water on which lipid substance can be spread. A barrier can be pushed across the trough to compress the film (Fig.). Upon evaporation of solvent, a film (one molecule thick) is formed. At first, some molecules are not well aligned due to ample space but as the barrier is pushed across the trough, the surface area is reduced and the molecules are compressed to give a packed film. The molecules under this condition exert a balanced pressure which can be measured by film balance.

The monolayer thus obtained, by successive dippings can give rise to bimolecular layers. Thus, lipid bilayers can also be produced artificially which will have biophysical properties comparable to some biological membranes except that they do not show selectivity for the passage of various ions. Other properties of biological membranes may be acquired by lipid bilayers due to incorporation of certain polypeptides and proteins. A variety of other models of membrane structures have been prepared including lipid-water system which help considerably in the study of properties and structure of biological membranes.

Historical Models for Structure of Plasma Membrane: Different models for explaining the structure of plasma membrane have been put forward from time to time depending upon the information available at a particular time. Most of these models are only of historical importance now, since the fluid mosaic model, discussed later in this chapter, is now universally accepted. Some of these historical models will be briefly discussed.

Lipid and Lipid Bilayer Models (by Overton; Gorter and Grendel): Before the isolation of plasma membranes, only indirect information was available to explain the structure of plasma membrane. Overton in 1902 postulated that plasma membrane is composed of a thin layer of lipid, because it was observed that substances soluble in lipid could selectively pass through the membranes. Subsequently Gorter and Grendel in 1926 suggested that plasma membrane is composed of double layer of lipid molecules, because they found that the lipid extracted from erythrocyte membranes was twice the amount expected if a single layer was present throughout the surface area of these cells (hardly any membranes other than surface membranes are found in erythrocytes). These experiments and ideas of Gorter and Grendel laid the foundation of future models of membrane structure.

Protein-lipid Bilayer-protein (Unit Membrane) Model (by Davson Danielli and Robertson): The initial lipid bilayer model of Gorter and Grendel had to be modified, when surface tension measurements made on the membranes, suggested the presence of proteins. It was observed that surface tension of cells is much lower than what one would expect if only lipids were involved. It could also be demonstrated that if protein is added to model lipid water system, surface tension is lowered. This gave an indirect evidence that proteins may be involved. Davson and Danielli, therefore, proposed that plasma membrane contained a lipid bilayer with protein on both surfaces. Initially they supposed that proteins existed as covalently bonded globular structures bound to the polar ends of lipids. Subsequently they developed the paucimolecular model in which the protein appears to be smeared over the hydrophilic ends of the lipid bilayer (Fig.). This model remained popular for many years.

With the availability of electron microscope later, fine structure of plasma membrane could be studied. Definite plasma membrane of 6nm to 10nm (10nm=100 Å; 1nm=10^{-6} mm) thickness was observed on surface of all cells, and plasma membranes of two adjacent cells were found to be separated by a space, 1-15nm wide. It was also observed that the plasma membrane of most of the cells appeared to be three layered. Two outer dense layers were about 2.0nm thick and the middle layer about 3.5nm.

The early ideas of Gorter and Grendel and those of Davson and Danielli were first formalised by Robertson in 1959 in the form of his unit membrane concept (Fig.). This concept of unit membrane with three layers (two protein layers and one lipid bilayer) only supported the concept proposed earlier by Davson and Danielli. In this unit membrane the less dense middle layer corresponded to hydrocarbon chains of lipids. Thickness of unit membrane (10nm) was found to be greater in plasma membrane than in intracellular membranes of endoplasmic reticulum or Golgi complex.

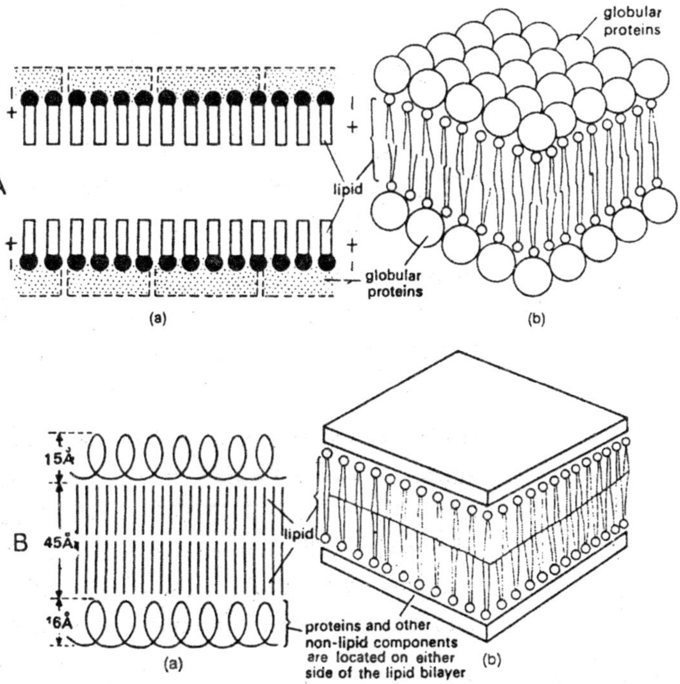

Model of plasma membrane as proposed by (A) Davson and Danielli, (B) Robertson: In each case, (a) a view of vertical section and (b) three dimensional view, (note the smear like protein layer on either side of lipid bilayer).

Universally Accepted Fluid Mosaic Model for Plasma Membrane: Our present knowledge of plasma membrane is based on integration of data from chemical analysis and those from the study of biophysical properties with the help of a variety of techniques. They have contributed to a better understanding of how the main components are integrated in plasma membrane. In this connection, following four major techniques/discoveries are important,

(i) The freeze fracture technique, used for a study membrane structure, was discussed in and is illustrated. Freeze-fractured electron microscope, revealed the presence of bums and depressions (7-8nm in diameter) which are randomly distributed. These were later shown to be intramembrane protein particles, which traverse the bilayer (as shown earlier),

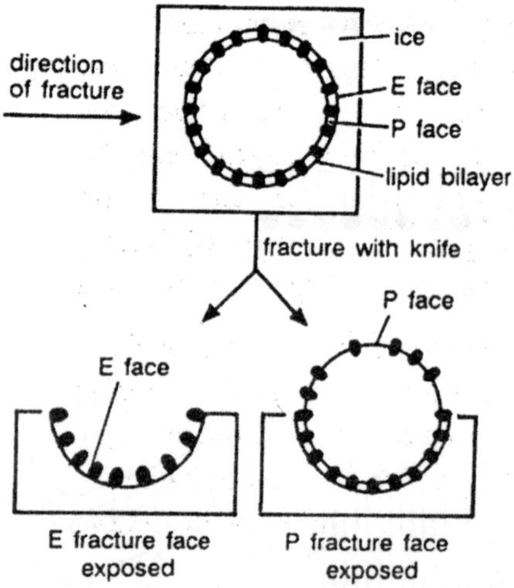

Freeze-fracture electron microscopy. The drawing shows how the technique provides images of the hydrophobic interior of the cytoplasmic (or protoplasmic) half of the bilayer (called the P face) and the external half of the bilayer (called the E face). After the fracturing process shown here, the exposed fracture faces are shadowed with platinum and carbon, the organic material is digested away, and the resulting platinum replica is examined in the electron microscope.

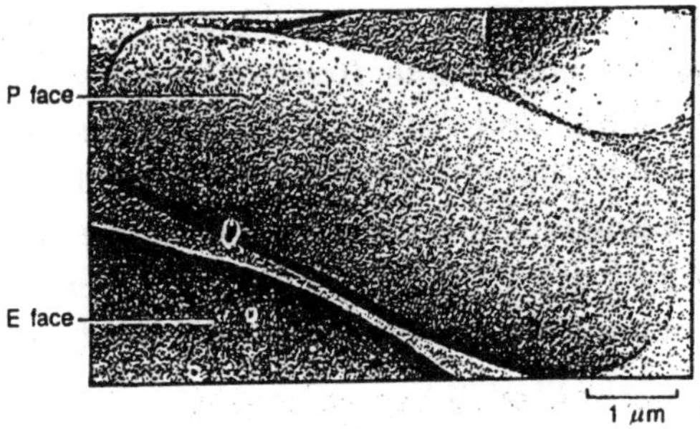

Freeze-fracture electron micrograph of a human red blood cell (from alberts et. al., Cell and Molecular Biology of the Cell, 1994).

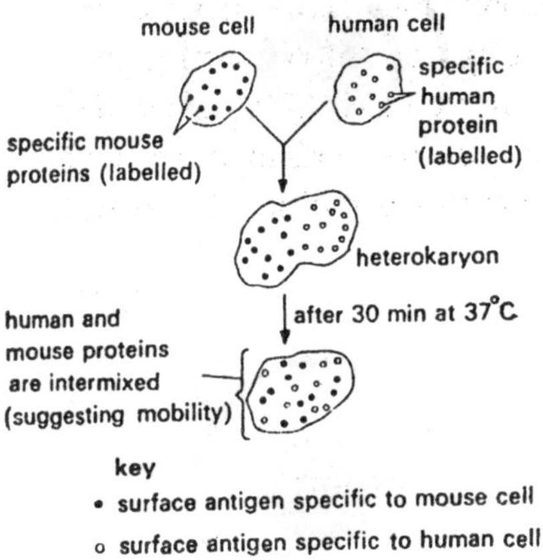

Diagrammatic representation of the rapid intermixing of cell surface antigens, as observed by Frye and Edidin in their experiment.

(ii) Frye and Edidin (1970) labelled selectively the species specific proteins of human and mouse cells and then fused these cells of the two species to make a heterokaryon. After incubating the heterokaryons for 30-35 minutes at 37°C, human and mouse proteins in these heterokaryons were seen intermixing (as demonstrated by using specific antibodies), so that human and mouse proteins became randomly distributed suggesting that membrane proteins are mobile in the plane of the membrane (Fig.).

(iii) Further evidence about mobility of proteins within the lipid bilayer came from the processes described as patching and capping. It was observed that when ligands like antibodies have more than one sites for binding the specific proteins on the cell surface, the proteins tend to aggregate into clusters through cross-linking. This indicates that proteins diffuse laterally in the bilayer (Fig.).

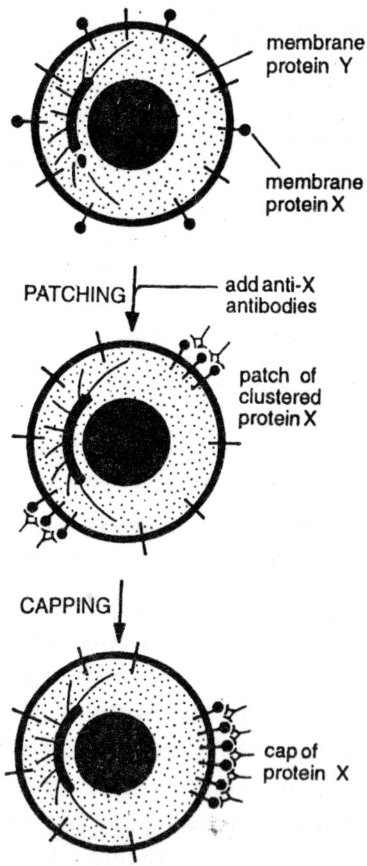

Antibody-induced patching and capping of a cell surface protein on a white blood cells (redrawn from Alberts et. al., Molecular Biology of the Cell, 1994).

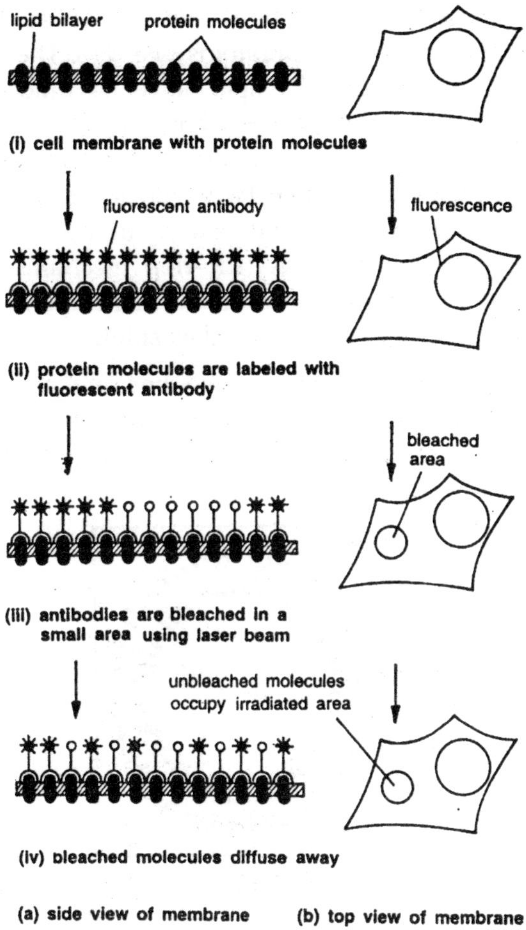

Measuring the rate of lateral diffusion of a membrane protein by FRAP technique: (a) side view; (b) top view (redrawn from Alberts et. al., Molecular Biology of the Cell, 1994).

(iv) Fluorescence recovery after photobleaching (FRAP) has also been used for measuring rates of lateral diffusion of proteins. A cell surface protein of interest is marked with a fluorescent ligand (*e.g.*, antibody). The ligand is bleached in a small area by a laser beam and the time taken for bleached and unbleached fluorescent ligands to diffuse and mix is measured. The rates of diffusion of proteins vary but are 1/10th or 1/100th of the rate of diffusion for phospholipids (see Fig.). The evidences as above suggested that lipid bilayer has fluid properties enabling membrane proteins to diffuse rapidly. Rotational diffusion (about its axis) and lateral diffusion of proteins is possible. However no evidence of flip-flop mechanism as suggested for lipids has been available for proteins (flip-flop mechanism means exchange of molecules from one monolayer, with those in the monolayer on the other side).

In early 1970s, evidence also became available to suggest that not only proteins, but individual lipid molecules are also able to diffuse freely within the lipid bilayers. This

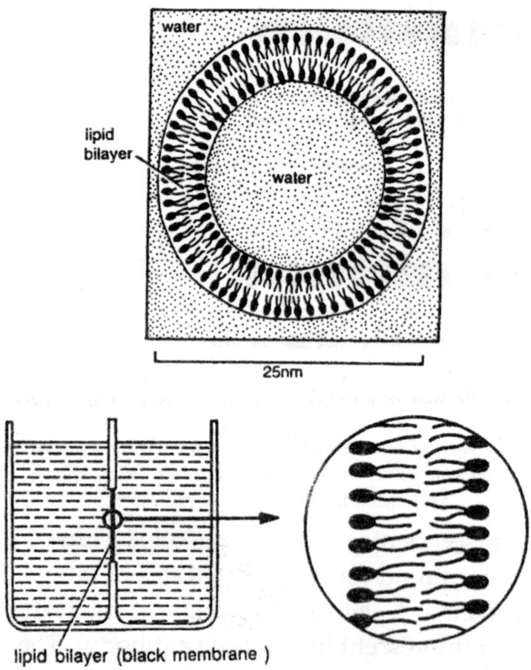

A cross-sectional view of a synthetic lipid bilayer, called a black membrane, used to measure the permeability of synthetic membranes.

was demonstrated in synthetic as well as isolated biological membranes obtained from mycoplasmas, bacteria and red blood cells. Initially, this was demonstrated in the following two types of synthetic lipid bilayers:

(i) liposomes which are spherical vesicles varying from 25nm to 1/ μ m (1000nm) in diameter (Fig.) and

(ii) black membranes formed across a hole in a partition between two aqueous compartments (Fig.).

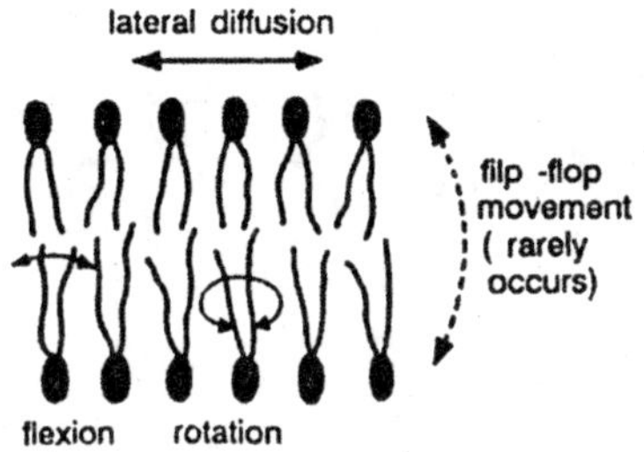

Different types of movements for phospholipid molecules in a lipid bilayer.

The motion of individual lipid molecules could be measured by 'spin libelling' its polar head group with the help of groups like nitroxyl group (>N-O) containing an unpaired electron. The spin of unpaired electron creates a paramagnetic signal, that can be detected by electron spin resonance (ESR) spectroscopy. The motion and orientation of a spin labelled lipid can be deduced from the ESR spectrum. These studies involving spin libelling followed by ESR spectroscopy suggested that phospholipid molecules in synthetic bilayers very rarely migrate (less than once a month for any molecule) from the monolayer on one side to the monolayer on the other side, a phenomenon described as 'flip-flop' (see above and note that membrane proteins can not flip flop). The lipid molecules can also rotate or readily exchange places within the same monolayer (10^7 times in a second) with a diffusion coefficient (D) of about 10^{-8} cm^2/sec, so that a lipid molecule could diffuse the length of a large bacterial cell (~2 μ m) in about one second. Even when the lipid molecule is static, the hydrocarbon chains are flexible. Similar results were obtained from isolated biological membranes, except that in the natural membranes, the presence of 'phospholipid translocators' was demonstrated, which catalyze the flip-flop of specific phospholipids from one monolayer (where they are synthesised) to the opposite monolayer. Different types of movements of phospholipid molecules in a lipid bilayer are shown in Figure.

On the basis of experiments described above, the fluid-mosaic model was proposed by S.J. Singer and G.L. Nicolson.

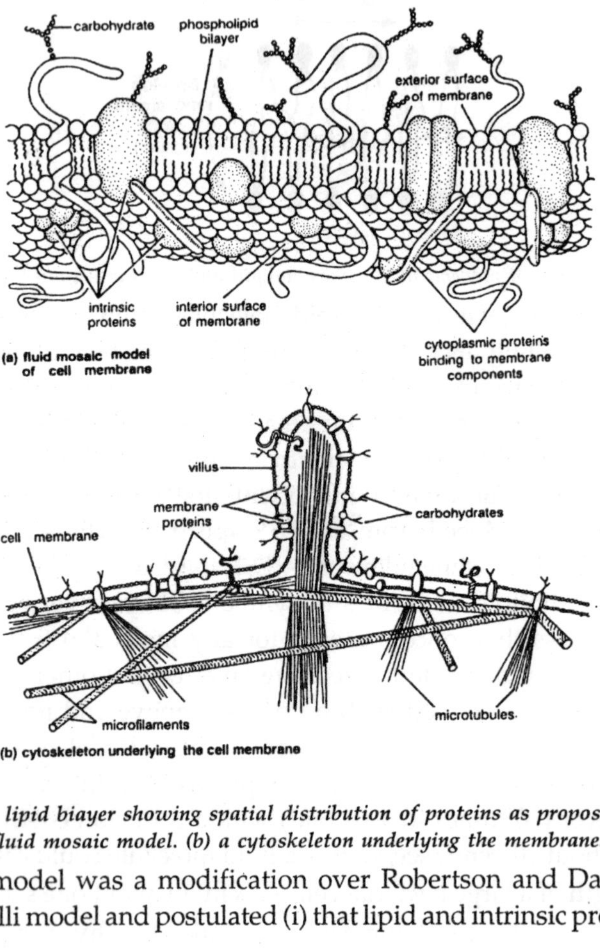

(a) A lipid biayer showing spatial distribution of proteins as proposed in fluid mosaic model. (b) a cytoskeleton underlying the membrane.

This model was a modification over Robertson and Davson-Danielli model and postulated (i) that lipid and intrinsic proteins are present in a mosaic arrangement and (ii) that biological membranes are semi-fluid so that the lipids as well as intrinsic proteins are able to make movements within the bilayer. This concept of fluidity in this model implies that components of membrane *i.e.*, lipids, proteins and oligosaccharides are held in their positions by means of noncovalent interactions. This derives support from the fact that components can be dispersed by solvents or detergents without breaking any bonds.

The fluid mosaic model and the cytoskeleton underlying the cell membrane are depicted in Figure. It can be seen that intrinsic proteins are intercalated to greater or lesser extent into a continuous lipid bilayer.

Such proteins may be in contact with an aqueous solvent on both sides of the membrane. The fluid mosaic model has received support from most of the later work done on membrane systems, and has become the basis of our understanding of the role of membranes in the cell. It is almost certain that this model, with modification described below, will remain acceptable for many years.

Modification of Fluid Mosaic Model: The fluid mosaic model, described above, envisaged that the cell membrane is 'a two dimensional oriented solution of integral proteins in the viscous phospholipid bilayer'. This model suggested a random two dimensional diffusion of membrane components.

However, on the basis of recent work, now we know that although lipids and a fraction of the labelled protein population appear to diffuse freely, movement of other proteins is much more complicated than originally envisioned in the fluid mosaic model. One big surprise was that a substantial fraction of the proteins is confined, at least transiently, to small domains in the membrane of a cell. Another surprise was that a few membrane proteins undergo rapid, forward-directed transport towards the cell edge, perhaps propelled by cytoskeleton motors.

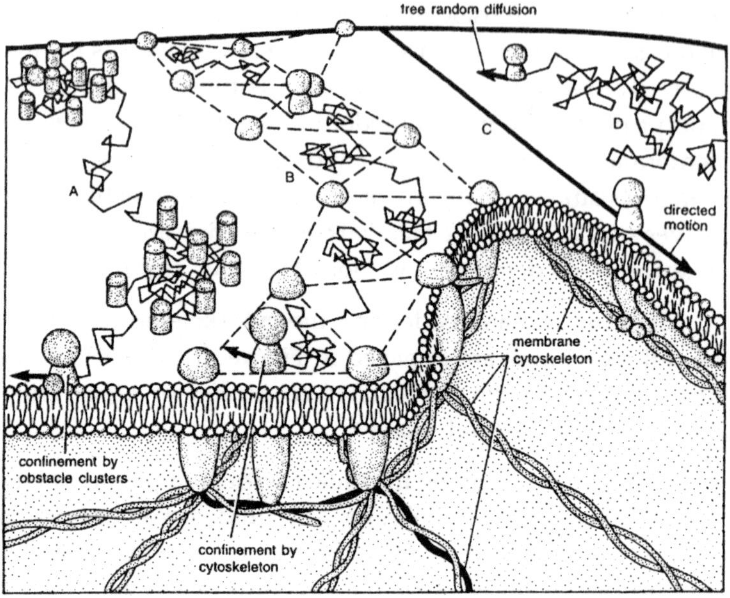

A modified version of fluid mosaic model envisaging mix of dynamic activities including confinement of proteins in specific domains due to obstacles (A) or cytoskeleton (B), highly directed movements (C); or the free random diffusion (D).

The transient confinement of integral proteins has been seen most clearly for (i) certain cell adhesion molecules (CAMs) including cadherins and neural cell adhesion molecules (N-CAMs), and for (ii) receptors for nutrient and growth factors. The domains, where proteins get confined are 300-600 nm in diameter and the confinement lasts for 3-30 seconds. Such confinement of proteins has been explained recently by a 'membrane skeleton fence' model (Kusumi *et. al.*, 1993) according to which, a spectrin-like mesh-work on the cytoplasmic side of the membrane sterically confines transiently some membrane-spanning proteins.

The above features of cell membrane, demanding revision of our original concept of fluid mosaic model, were revealed through the use of atleast three new techniques: (i) fluorescence recovery after photobleaching (FRAP), (ii) single particle tracking (SPT) and (iii) optical laser trap (OLT). The details of these techniques are beyond the scope of this book. However, it is certain that the plasma membrane is now known to be, an intriguing mix of dynamic activities, in which its components may randomly diffuse (as proposed in fluid mosaic model), or be confined transiently to small domains or experience highly directed movements (Fig.). These features cause considerable lateral heterogeneity in the membrane.

Fluidity of Bilayer Depends on its Composition (Hydrocarbon Chains and Cholesterol): Fluidity of lipid bilayer depends on its temperature and composition. It may undergo a phase transition from liquid to a gel state at a characteristic freezing temperature, which is dependent on its composition. This temperature is lower (meaning that membrane is difficult to freeze) if hydrocarbon chains are either short (short chains can not easily interact) or have double bonds (cis-double bonds produce kinks making it difficult for chains to pack together). Bacteria, yeast and other cold blooded animals adjust lipid composition to maintain fluidity of membrane even at low temperature.

Phase transitions are also affected by cholesterol, which can sometimes reach a level of one molecule for each phospholipid molecule. Since the hydroxyl group of cholesterol is close to polar head, and its plate like steroid rings interact with the adjoining region of hydrocarbon chain, it decreases mobility of hydrocarbon chains of phospholipids. This leads to decrease in permeability of membrane and also inhibits phase transition, when present in high concentration, although cholesterol otherwise tends to make lipid bilayers less fluid.

4

Structure of Membrane

All cells are bounded by a thin membrane called the *plasmalemma*. This membrane is not visible under the light microscope. The structure seen under the light microscope is the *cell membrane*. This consists of the plasmalemma along with surrounding *cell cement*. In the broad sense the term 'cell membrane' also includes the limiting membranes of cell organelles like mitochondria and lysosomes, and other membranes like those of the nuclear envelope, the endoplasmic reticulum and the Golgi complex. These membranes, however, resemble the plasmalemma in having no cell cement. The plasma membrane may be protected by other coverings.

The plasma membrane of the egg is surrounded by the *vitelline membrane* and the *jelly layer*, both of which are secreted by the ovary. In some tissues the cell cement fills the gap between adjacent cells. Fusion of the cell cement forms a supporting layer, the *basement membrane*, for a sheet of cells.

Chemical Composition of Cell Membranes

Membranes from different sources vary in their composition. They essentially consist of *lipoproteins* which are special non-bonded combinations of *lipids* with *proteins.* In general, membranes contain about 60% protein and 40% carbohydrate by dry weight. *Carbohydrate* is usually present to the extent of 1-10% of the total dry weight in *glycoproteins* and *glycolipids.* In membranes of some cell organelles the nucleic acids DNA and RNA have also been reported, but are most likely contaminations.

The Proteins

Membranes contain three different classes of proteins, *structural proteins, enzymes* and *carrier proteins. Structural proteins* form the 'backbone' of the cell membrane. They have little catalytic activity and are extremely lipophilic. Their amino acid composition is nearly the same. The plasma membrane consists largely of structural proteins. The average molecular weight of structural proteins is 3×10^4. *Enzymes* form the major component of many membranes and are catalytic proteins. The endoplasmic reticulum, mitochondria, and plasma membrane contain many enzymes. The structure of the enzymes varies from membrane to membrane. *Carrier proteins* or permeases transport substances cross the membrane against the concentration gradient. The molecular weight of structural and carrier proteins are rather similar.

The amount of protein varies in different cell membranes. Myelin contains only 20% protein, plasma membranes about 50% and the inner mitochondrial membrane 75%.

The plasma membrane proteins fall in two main categories, *intrinsic* or *integral* proteins and *extrinsic* or *peripheral* proteins. The former are firmly associated with the membrane, while the latter have a weaker association and are bound by electrostatic interaction. Human erythrocyte glycoproteins consist of three chemically distinct regions: (1) an *N-terminal part* external to the membrane and containing all the carbohydrate, (2) a middle *hydrophobic region* located within the membrane and (3) a hydrophilic *C-terminal portion,* rich in protein but lacking carbohydrate, on the internal side of the membrane. The middle intramembranous part appears to be intimately associated with the membrane phospholipids.

The glycoprotein of human erythrocyte membrane has a polypeptide backbone to which are attached two types of oligosaccharide chains, a *straight chain* and a longer *branched one* at about 10 sites (Fig.).

Polypeptides of Human RBC Membrane

The red cell membrane consists of a *lipid matrix* with which are associated membrane *proteins.* The membrane lipids are organised in a closely packed bilayer and show mobility. The proteins of the membrane can be classified into two main types, *extrinsic* and *intrinsic* proteins (Fig.).

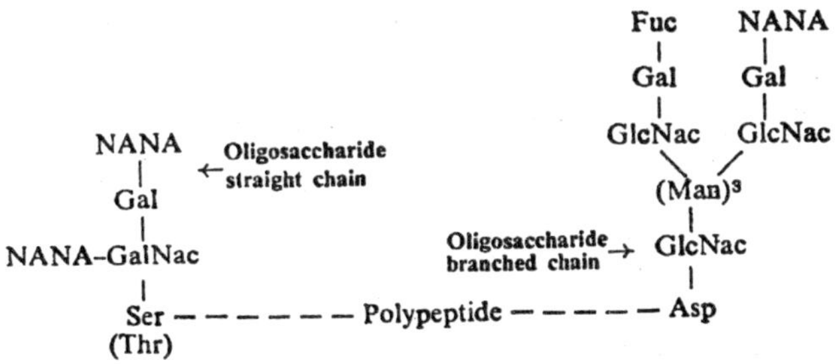

Structure of human RBC glycoprotein (MW 50,000, 60% carbohydrate, 40% protein).

NANA.	N-acetyl neuraminic acid.	Fuc. Fucose.
Gal.	Galactose.	GlcNac. N-acetyl glucose.
GalNac.	N-acetyl galactose.	Man. Mannose.
Ser.	Serine.	Asp. Aspartic acid.

The *extrinsic* or *peripheral* proteins are readily dissociated from the membrane, and can be isolated by relatively simple means like manipulation of ionic strength or pH. They are believed to be associated with the polar heads of the lipid molecules. The *polar amino acids* are thought to be on the outer surface of the protein molecule and the *non-polar* acids in the interior.

The *intrinsic* or *integral* membrane proteins are tightly bound to the lipid bilayer. They dissociate from the membrane with difficulty, requiring more drastic treatment, such as the use of detergents. The intrinsic proteins are believed to have *non-polar amino acid* residues in the interior of the molecule as well as the surface of the molecule in contact with the membrane lipid. They thus have a higher percentage of non-polar amino acids. Some intrinsic proteins may partially penetrate either surface of the lipid bilayer, while others may span the entire membrane, protruding at both ends.

By using *sodium dodecyl sulphate* (SDS)-gel electrophoresis several bands are obtained. These have been designated as bands 1, 2, 3, 4.1, 4.2, 5, 6 and 7. Many of the major bands on the electropherogram probably correspond to single polypeptide chains, or to a predominant class of polypeptides. In addition there are a number of minor species of polypeptides that are not detectable by this process. Application of periodic acid-Schiff's reagent (PAS) to SDS gels of total membrane proteins results in four bands, PAS-1, 2, 3 and 4, corresponding to *glycopeptides*. The location and structure of different polypeptides and glycopeptides will now be considered.

Membrane Proteins-lying Outside: The extrinsic membrane proteins include band 1, 2, 4, 5 and 6 polypeptides.

Bands 1 and 2 (Spectrum): The polypeptide chains of the spectrum polymers (bands 1 and 2) are located along the inner surface of the membrane. They are thought to be close to glycopeptides. The polypeptides have been considered to be two closely opposed single chains. (MW values of bands 1 and 2 are between 225,000 and 250,000). Some workers have suggested that they might be aggregates of smaller molecular weight polypeptides. Spectrum polymers are very similar to the polypeptide of the muscle protein *myosin*.

Band 4 is often split into bands 4.1 and 4.2. It is not known whether the polypeptides of band 4 are one or several different polypeptides. They are located on the inner side of the membrane and might be associated with band 3 polypeptide.

Band 5 (Actin or Actin-like Protein): Band 5 polypeptide (MW 45,000) is believed to be *actin* or *actin-like.* It is probably located near the spectrum polymers. There is some reason for considering band 1, 2 and 5 proteins as representing an *actomyosin-like complex.* This complex is considered to form the *cytoskeleton or contractile apparatus* of the cell membrane (*"membrane muscles'"*). It is thought to maintain membrane shape and to be responsible for the endocytosis reaction.

Band 6: Polypeptide has been identified as the monomeric form of the enzyme *glyceraldehyde-3-phosphate dehydrogenase.* It may be located near the band 3 polypeptide.

Entire Membrane Proteins: The integral membrane proteins include bands 3, 7 and PAS-1, 2, 3 and 4. In addition there are minor proteins like *acetylcholinesterase (AChe), ATPase* and some uncharacterised *glycopeptides.*

Band 3 polypeptide represents a subunit of the presumed *anion channel.* It apparently has a molecular weight of about 90,000 and appears to exist as a disulphide-linked dimeric form that extends across the lipid bilayer. Parts of the polypeptide chain extend outside and parts extend into the cytosol. It contains about 5-8% carbohydrate on a dry weight basis. The carbohydrate *(oligosaccharide)* is composed of *mannnose, galactose* and *N-acetylglucosamine* in the ratio of about 1: 2: 2. Traces of *fucose* and *glucose* are also frequently found. Band 3 protein has been implicated in anion, phosphate and glucose transport.

Band 7: The arrangement of band 7 protein in the membrane is not clear, but there are indications that it is inside the lipid bilayer.

PAS-1 and PAS-2 (glycophorin A) are believed to be the interconvertible forms of the same polypeptide chain. These sialoglycopeptides appear to exist in a dimeric form that extends across the lipid bilayer. PAS-1 appears to be the dimeric form of PAS-2.

The sialoglycopeptide *glycophorin A* is the basic subunit of the PAS-1 dimer and represents about 75% of the total sialoglycopeptides of the red cell membrane. The glycophorin A molecule has MN blood group activity. The complete amino acid sequence of glycophorin A has been determined. It consists of a single polypeptide chain of 131 amino acids to which are linked 16 *oligosaccharide side chains.*

Of these 15 chains are attached to either *seryl* or *threonyl* residues by *O-glycosidic bonds.* One chain is attached to an *asparagine* residue (number 26) by *N-glycosidic bonds.*

All the oligosaccharide chains are attached to the amino acids within one-third the length of the chain from the N-terminal. Many of the approximately 20 non-polar acids making up the part of the polypeptide chain within the lipid bilayer are *hydrophobic.* The amino acids near the C-terminal are acidic. This part of the chain is therefore well adapted to bind to basic peptides or cations.

PAS-3 glycopeptide is similar to glycophorin A in its overall carbohydrate composition, but the polypeptide components are apparently different. PAS-3 has a sugar rich segment, probably near the N-terminal, and a hydrophobic segment within the lipid bilayer. It, however, appears to lack the C-terminal segment present on the inner side of the lipid bilayer in glycophorin A.

The polypeptide is thus inserted into the lipid bilayer, but does not appear to pass through. Such proteins might be less tightly bound to the membrane than the integral proteins which pass through the membrane. A, I and S blood group activities have been suggested in a sialoglycopeptide which is comparable to PAS-3.

PAS-4 band is found between PAS-1 and PAS-2 in most sialoglycoprotein preparations. There is some evidence to indicate that it may be a modified form of either PAS-3 or glycophorin-A. The glycopeptides have been associated with ABH blood group activity. However, it has also been suggested that ABH activity is confined to *glycolipids.* Thus the possibility of glycolipid contamination cannot be ruled out in the reported presence of ABH activity in glycopeptides.

Minor Glycopeptides: In addition to the major proteins and sialoglycopeptides a large number of minor glycopeptides are probably present in the human red cell membrane. It is speculated that they are loosely associated with the membrane and are thus of the semi-integral type. *Acetylcholinesterase* (AChe) is a minor (from the molecular weight point of view) integral protein which appears to be attached to the external surface of the membrane. *ATPase,* another minor integral protein, is probably located on the inner surface of the membrane.

THE LIPIDS

The lipids of the cell membrane are *polar lipids* which contain *hydrophilic heads* and *hydrophobic tails.* The hydrophobic and hydrophilic regions may be bridged by a *glycerol* moiety (Fig.), a *sphingenine* derivative or homologue, or a *sterol.* In *glycerol* derivatives the primary hydroxy group of glycerol carries the *hydrophilic head* grouping. To the two other hydroxy groups are esterified *long-chain fatty acids* which form the hydrophobic *tails.* The tails can also contain long-chain *fatty aldehyde* and *alcohol* molecules.

Sphingenine derivatives also have the *hydrophobic head* attached to the primary hydroxy group. One of the two long aliphatic chains is built into the structure. The other is attached to the *amino group* by an *amide linkage.*

Lipid Factors of Membranes: The three main lipid constituents of cell membranes are *phospholipids, glycolipids* and *sterols* (Fig.). Phospholipids contain a *phosphate* moiety in the hydrophilic head. They can be distinguished into *glycerophospholipids* with a *glycerol* backbone and *sphingophospholipids* based on *4-sphingenine (sphingosine).*

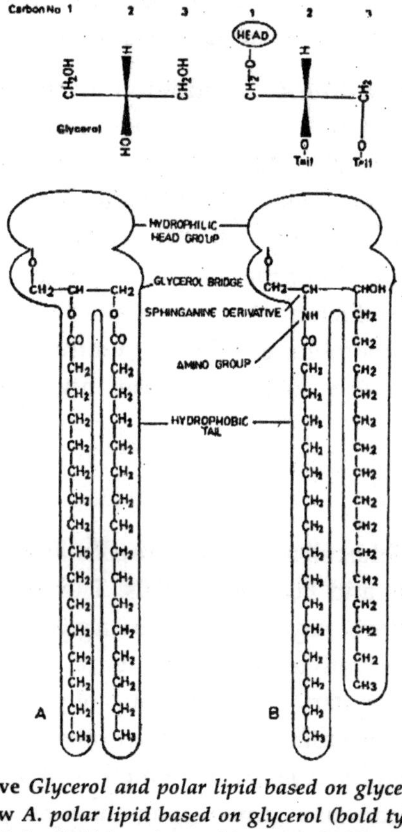

Above ***Glycerol and polar lipid based on glycerol.***
Below ***A. polar lipid based on glycerol (bold type).***
B. Polar lipid based on sphinganine (bold type).

A. Glycerophospholipids. The parent compound is *phosphatidic acid* (PA).

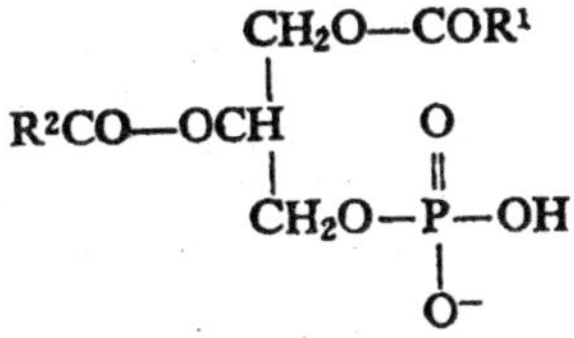

Phosphatidic acid (PA)

1. *Phosphatidyl serine (PA-serine)*

   —$CH_2CH\ (NH_2)\ COOH$

2. *Phosphatidyl ethanolamine (PA-ethanolamine, cephalin)*

   —CH_2—CH_2-NH_3+

3. *Phosphatidyl choline (PA-choline,* lecithin)

   -CH_2-CH_2-N+$(CH_3)_3$

4. *Phosphatidyl glycerol* (PA-glycerol)

   —CH_2—CHOH-CH_2OH

5. *Diphosphatidyl glycerol* (PA-glycerol-PA, cardiolipiu)

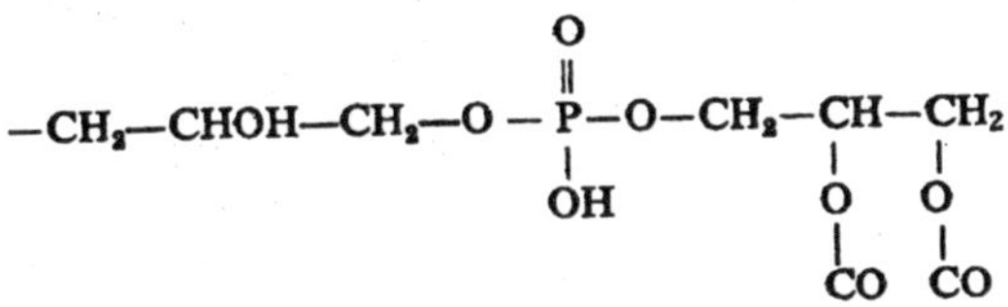

Long aliphatic chains

6. *Plasmalogens* have an ether-linked *vinyl side chain* in position 1 instead of an esterified fatty acyl chain of other glycerophospholipids.

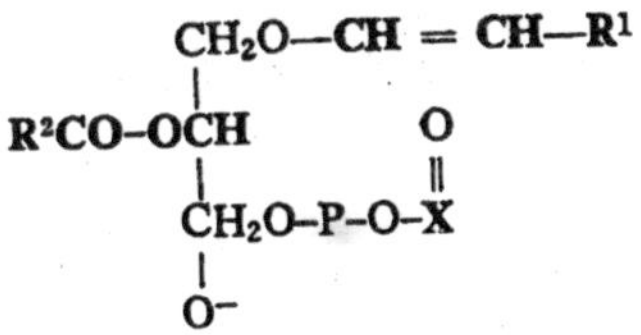

Plasmaloge.

Choline plasmalogen (X = choline) is abundant in heart muscle.

Ethanolamine plasmogen (X = ethanolamine). Relatively high concentrations are present in myelin of nervous tissue and lesser amounts in heart muscle.

Sphingophospholipids: The central compound is *4~sphingenine (sphingosine),* a derivative of *sphingenine.*

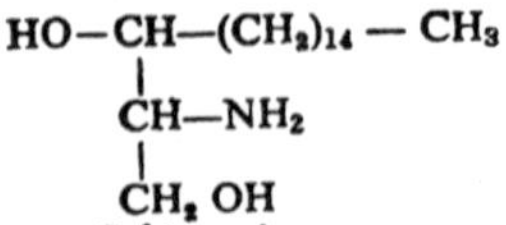

Sphinganine

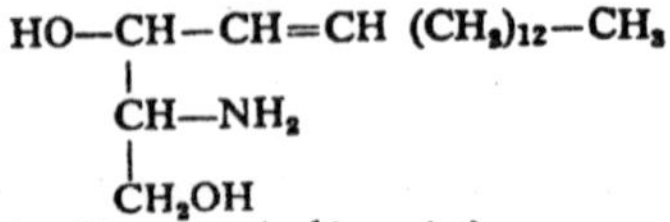

4-sphingenine (sphingosine)

1. 4-D-hydroxysphinganine (phytosphingosine)is the main sphing ophospholipid of plants.

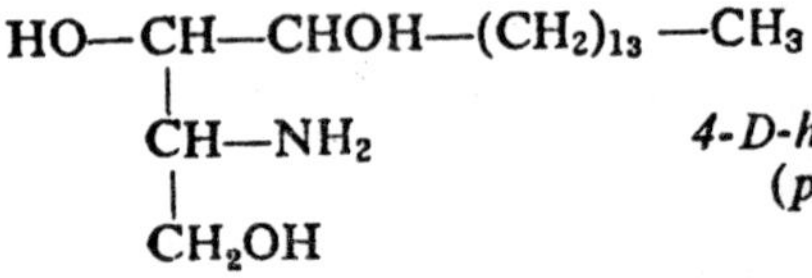

4-D-hydroxysphinganine (phyiospingosine)

2. Sphingomyelin (ceramide-P-choline) is similar to phosphatidyl choline except that the glycerol moiety is replaced by *4-sphingenine.* One fatty acid chain is linked to 4-sphingenine by an *amide bond.*

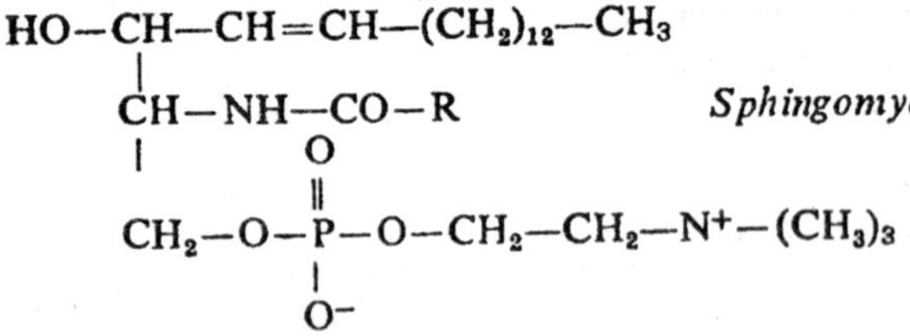

Sphingomyelin

Glycolipids contain one or more monosaccharide residues and are based on *4-sphingenine (sphingosine)* or *ceramide.* A ceramide is a sphingosine to which a *fatty acid* is linked by an *amide bond.*

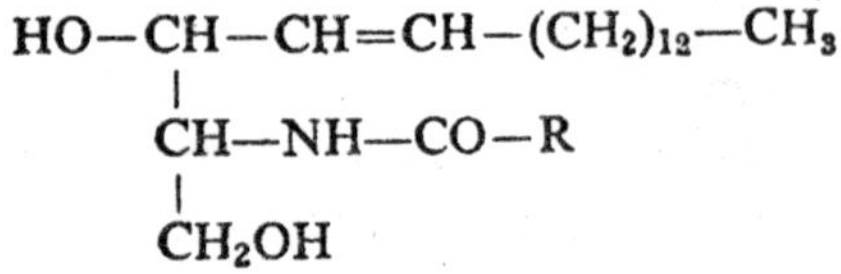

Ceramide

1. Cerebrosides (ceramide-sugar) contain a single monosaccharide unit which is usually *galactose (monogalactosyl ceramide),* although *glucose (monoglycosyl ceramide)* or other sugars may also be found.

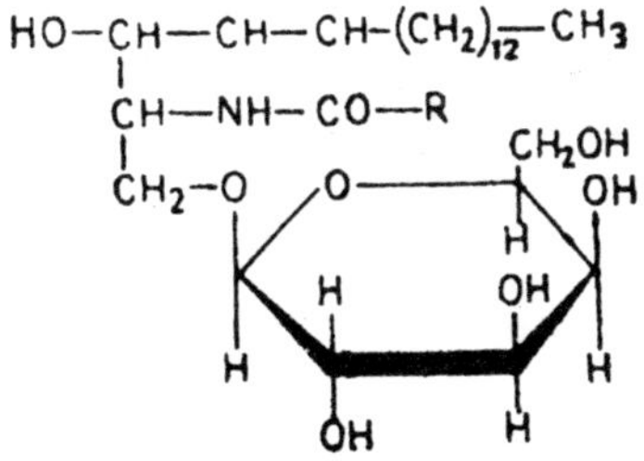

Monogalactosyl ceramide

Sulphatides are sulphuric acid esters of cerebrosides with a sulphate group attached to position 3 of the monosaccharide.

2. *Gangliosides* (ceramide-sugars) are glycosphingolipids containing *sialic acid.* They are tetraglycosyl ceramides to which are attached 1-3 *sialic acid (N-acetyl-neuraminic acid;* NANA) residues.

Galactose—N-acetylgalactosamine—Galactose—Glucose

Sialic acid (on Galactose); **Sialic acid — Sialic acid** (on Galactose); **Ceramide** (on Glucose)

Sterols are steroid alcohols which contain a cyclopentanoperhydrophenanthrene nucleus:

1. *Cholesterol* is the most abundant sterol in animal tissue. It is usually a minor component in cell membranes of higher plants.
2. *Phytosterols* (plant sterols) are the major sterol components of plant cell membranes. They include *sitosterol* and *stigmasterol.*
3. Ergosterol is a major sterol of the membranes of eukaryotic micro-organisms.

Membrane Lipid Division

1. Neutral fats are largely absent from cell membranes. Neutral fats such as *triglycerides* are found mainly in the cytoplasm and represent the major form of storage lipids.

2. Glycerphospholipids are the principal constituents of bacterial membranes. Sphingolipids and cholesterol are absent. In animal cell membranes *glycerophospholipids* and *sphingophospholipids* comprise the *polar lipids,* while the principal *non-polar* membrane lipids are neutral *sterols.*

3. Use of chemical markers has shown that phospholipids are asymmetrically arranged in human erythrocyte membranes. The outer membrane leaflet contains the *zwitterionic* phospholipids *sphingomyelin* and *phosphatidyl choline,* while the inner membrane leaflet contains *phosphatidyl ethanolamine, phosphatidyl serine* and, when present, *phosphatidyl inositol.* The head groups of phospholipids in the inner membrane leaflet are largely *anionic.*

4. In rat liver membranes phospholipids comprise about 60% of the lipids in plasma membranes and Golgi membranes, about 80% in the rough endoplasmic and nuclear membranes, and about 90% in mitochondrial membranes.

5. Phosphatidyl choline *(lecithin)* and *phosphatidyl ethanolamine (cephalin)* are the most abundant glycerophospholipids in higher plants and animals. Cephalin is the main phospholipid of bacteria: lecithin is rarely present.

6. Phosphatidyl glycerol is present is small amounts in animal mitochondrial membranes. In plant membranes it constitutes 20-30% of phospholipids, and in chloroplasts 40-60%. The amount of phosphatidyl glycerol varies in bacterial membranes, being as high as 70% of the membrane phospholipid in Gram positive bacteria. Phosphatidyl glycerol is a precursor of *diphosphatidyl glycerol (cardiolipin)* which is found in mitochondria, chloroplasts and bacteria.

7. Choline plasmalogen is abundant in heart muscle. *Ethanolamine plasmalogen* is present in relatively high concentration in myelin and in lesser amount in heart muscle. In bacteria plasmalogens are confined to anaerobes.
8. The membranes of eukaryote cell organelles contain *sterols* in varying amounts. The plasma membrane is comparatively very much richer in *cholesterol.*
9. Cholesterol: phospholipid ratio. In human erythrocyte membranes the outer membrane leaflet is richer in *cholesterol* than the inner leaflet. In myelin outer membrane leaflet the cholesterol: phospholipid ratio is equimolar, while in the inner leaflet the ratio is 3:7.
10. Liver plasma membranes have a low phosphatidyl choline (lecithin) content and high phosphatidyl serine, sphingomyelin and cholesterol content.
11. Cholesterol controls the fluidity of fatty acid chains of phospholipids. It enhances the stability of phospholipid bilayers and also reduces their permeability.

Design of Membrance

In an attempt to explain the physical and biological features of cell membranes two main categories of hypotheses have been proposed, the *bilayer models* and the *micellar* or *subunit models.* In the *bilayer models* the protein and lipid constituting the membrane are believed to occur in layers. In the *micellar model* the membrane is believed to consist of a number of similar units.

Design of Bilayer

Lipid Membrane: In 1895 Overton found that fat-soluble substances passed easily through the cell membrane. He therefore concluded that the cell membrane contained lipids. Later workers like Hober (1910) and Fricke (1925) found that the intact cell had low electrical conductivity, indicating a lipid layer. The existence of a lipid layer was confirmed on the basis of experiments on wetting the cell surface with oil (Dawson and Belkiri; 1929; Mudd and Mudd, 1931). A drop of oil placed in contact with the cell spreads over and adheres to the cell surface.

Gorter and Grendel (1925) were the first to suggest a possible structure of the cell membrane. They studied erythrocytes are found that the surface membrane was composed of a double layer of lipid molecules (Fig.). The polar groups of these molecules were situated on the outside of these layers.

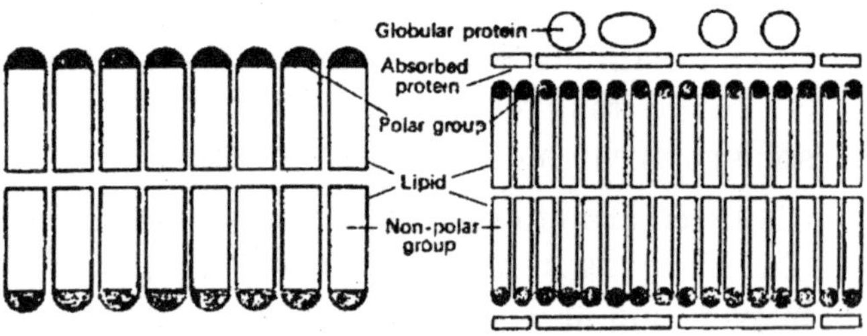

The lipid membrane
The Danielli-Davson
of Gorter and Grendel (1925).
trilaminar sandwich model of
the cell membrane.

Protein-lipid-protein (sandwich models)

Danielli Davson Design

By studying the surface tension of cells (Harvey and Cole, 1931; Danielli and Harvey, 1935) the existence of protein was indicated. This led Davson and Danielli (1935) to propose a lipoprotein model of the cell membrane. According to this model the bimolecular lipid layer is similar to that proposed by Gorter and Grendel.

It consists of two layers of molecules with their polar regions on the outer side. Globular proteins are thought to be associated with the polar groups of the lipid (Fig.).

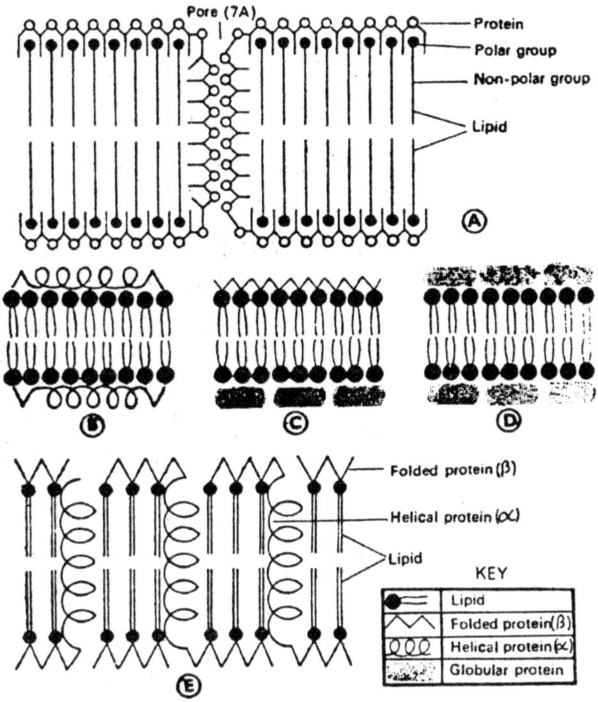

(A) The cell membrane with protein lined pores (Danielli, 1954).
(B-E) Other postulated arrangement of proteins.

This basic model has been modified several times. Danielli (1938) suggested that the proteins are of two types: tangentially arranged proteins in contact with the lipid, and globular proteins on the outer surface. In another variation (Davson and Danielli, 1943; Danielli, 1954) the proteins are considered to be in the form of a folded *B* chain (Fig.A). Protein-lined *polar pores* of about 7A diameter are present in the membrane. These pores are very small and cannot be seen under the electron microscope.

They probably permit the passage of small ions and water molecules. In still other variations the proteins are thought to be in the coiled a form on both sides of the lipid layer (Fig.B) or are thought to be asymmetrical, with a folded *B*-chain on one side and globular proteins on the other (Fig.C).

Models with globular protein on both surfaces (Fig.D) or with folded protein on both surfaces and helical proteins extending into the pores (Fig.E) are also visualised.

Lipids in the Membrane: The lipids in the membrane consist mainly of phospholipids, with their non-polar groups near each other and their polar groups directed outwards. The lipid layer in many cases consists of a phospholipid *lecithin,* alternating with a steroid molecule *cholesterol* (Fig. D). The *lecithin* molecule consists of two lipid chains of glycerol and a polar head containing *phosphate* and *choline.* According to Finean (1953) the head is bent around like a walking stick, and forms a bond with *cholesterol* which lies parallel to the lipid chain (Fig.A). According to another interpretation (Vandenheuvel, 1963) the second lipid chain, which is unsaturated at the ninth carbon atom curls around the end of cholesterol (Fig.B). Thus both hydrocarbon chains lie close to cholesterol. Other arrangements of the lipid have been suggested. It has been found that phospholipid molecules with cholesterol form globular units or *micelles* in water. In these micelles the hydrophobic groups are packed inside, and the hydrophilic groups point outwards (Fig.).

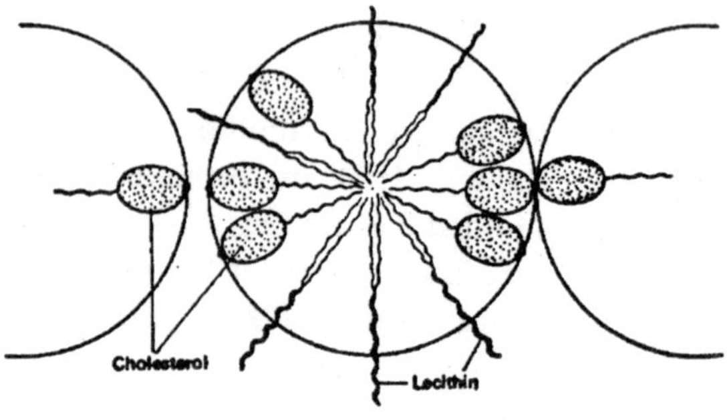

Globular units or micelles.

Single Membrane

In the early 1950s Robertson examined the structure of different membranes of the cell. In 1953 he put forward his *unit membrane* model. The basic unit membrane structure was considered to be general for a wide variety of plant and animal cells. Membranes of cell organelles like mitochondria and lysosomes, and other cell membranes like those of the Golgi complex, the nuclear envelope and the endoplasmic reticulum were thought to have the unit membrane structure, indicating its cellular universality.

Under the electron microscope, after osmium fixation, the cell membrane appears like two dense osmiophilic bands separated by a clear zone. The unit membrane is considered to be trilaminar, with a bimolecular lipid layer between two protein layers (Fig.). Each dense band is made up of protein (20A) and the polar groups of the lipids (5A), and is thus 25A thick. The clear zone is 25A thick and consists of the bimolecular lipid layer without the polar groups. Thus the unit membrane is 75A thick, with a 35A lipid layer between two protein layers, each 20A in thickness.

In this respect it resembles the Danielli-Davson model. It, however differs from the Danielli-Davson model in that the protein is asymmetrical. On the outer surface is *mucoprotein,* while on the inner surface is *non-mucoid protein.* Work in the mid-1960s cast serious doubt on the universality of the unit membrane concept. The Danielli-Davson model and Robertson's unit membrane model are both based on the structure of myelin which is a non-typical membrane. It is now believed that the arrangement of lipids and proteins may vary in different membranes.

Artificial membranes have been prepared, consisting of bimolecular lipid layers with proteins adsorbed on both sides of the lipid. On osmium fixation and observation under the electron microscope these membranes appear as two dark bands 25-30A thick, with a clear space of 20-25A between them. The appearance of these artificial membranes is thus very similar to that of plasma membranes.

Unit membranes vary a little in total thickness. Sometimes the membrane is asymmetric, the outer side being thicker and denser than the inner one.

The plasmalemma surrounding the cell is thicker at the free surfaces of cells than where it is in contact with other cells. Also the plasmalemma is thicker than the unit membranes of the endoplasmic reticulum.

The Greater Membrane Model

This model resembles the trilaminar model in that a lipid layer is sandwiched between two layers of "structural proteins. Robertson, however, believed that the inner and outer surfaces of the membrane were different.

The internal surface of the membrane was thought to be covered with *unconjugated protein,* and the outer surface with *glycoprotein,* which is superimposed on the structural protein. Attached to the glycoprotein are *oligosaccharide side chains* with negatively charged *sialic acid* terminals. Thus the membrane is asymmetrical and has structural polarity.

Kavanau's Lipid Pillar Design

This is a modification of the Danielli-Davson model. The lipid layer exists in two forms. Under certain conditions it is in the form of *pillars,* while in others it is in the form of *flattened discs.*

The space between the pillars forms pores for the passage of ions. The membrane with pillar structure is thicker than the membrane with the disc structure.

The interior of each pillar is formed of the nonpolar tails of the phospholipids, while the surface is formed of the polar heads. Protein layers are present on both sides of the membrane. This model cannot explain active transport or the differential permeability of Na and K ions.

III. Models in which the Proteins are Considered to Penetrate the Lipid Layer.

According to some workers the proteins are not found on the outside of the lipid layer as in the Danielli-Davson model, but are considered to partially or fully penetrate the lipid layer. This model can explain the low surface tension of biological membranes just as well as the protein-lipid-protein models.

1. *Benson's Model (Fig.):* Benson (1966) proposed a model on the basis of a study of chloroplast membranes. The membrane lipids and protein have a hydrophobic association. The lipid tails are bound by hydrophobic regions with complementary hydrophobic regions within the interior of proteins. The charged polar heads of the phospholipids lie on the surface of the membrane and are capable of binding ions. Flexion of contractile proteins facilitates ion transport.
2. *Lenard and Singer's Model (1966):* According to this model one-third to one-fourth of the protein's are in *helical conformation* while the rest most likely form *random coils.* In the earlier membrane models proteins were supposed to be in extended β-configuration.
3. *Mosaic Membrane Concept*: Baum (1967) considered the back bone of the membrane to be consisting of cuboidal units, 80A in diameter. Each unit of protein is toast shaped, and is covered on both sides and along the edges by phospholipids. The heads of the phospholipids stick out while their hydrophobic tails form complexes with the hydrophobic surface of the protein. In mitochondrial membranes the stalk and head are attached to the backbone.
4. *The fluid-mosaic Model of Singer and Nicolson (1972):* The essential feature of the fluid-mosaic model is that biological membranes are considered to be quasi-fluid

structures in which the lipids and integral proteins are arranged in a mosaic manner.

The fluid-mosaic model of Singer and Nicolson (1972) is now widely accepted as best explaining the properties of the cell membrane (Fig.). This model assumes that there is a continuous bilayer of *phospholipid* molecules in which are embedded *globular proteins.* The proteins have been compared to icebergs floating in a sea of the phospholipid bilayer. Thus biological membranes are considered to be *quasi-fluid* structures in which lipids and integral proteins are arranged in a *mosaic* manner. While the Danielli-Davson model assumes *hydrophilic bonding* between lipids and proteins, the Singer-Nicolson model considers the lipid-protein association to be *hydrophobic.* The fluidity of the membrane is the result of this hydrophobic interaction. It should be noted that the phospholipids and many intrinsic proteins are *amphipatic* molecules, *i.e.* both hydrophilic and hydrophobic groups occur within the same molecule.

The globular proteins of the membrane are considered to be of two different types *extrinsic (peripheral)* proteins and *intrinsic (integral)* proteins. The peripheral proteins are soluble and readily dissociate from the membrane. They are entirely outside the lipid bilayer. The integral proteins are relatively insoluble and dissociate with difficulty. Some may partially penetrate either surface of the lipid bilayer, while others penetrate right through. The latter are in contact with the aqueous solvent on both sides of the membrane. The integral proteins are amphipatic. Their hydrophilic polar heads protrude from the surface of the membrane, while the non-polar regions are embedded in the interior of the membrane. The integral proteins are capable of lateral diffusion in the lipid bilayer.

When phospholipids are dispersed in water they form a lipid bilayer. The polar heads of the lipid molecules project into the aqueous phase. The hydrophobic chains aggregate together. Studies with nuclear magnetic resonance (n.m.r.) and electron spin resonance (e.s.r.) techniques indicate that the lipid bilayer has many dynamic motional properties.

(i) Firstly, it is possible that there is rapid internal motion involving flexing within each lipid molecule.

(ii) Secondly, a rapid lateral diffusion of the lipids is possible.

(iii) Thirdly, a slow 'flip-flop' motion, *i.e.* a transfer of lipid molecules from one side of the bilayer to the other, is also possible.

(iv) Lastly, the lipid molecules might rotate about their axes. Because of the rapid movement of the lipid and protein molecules the Singer-Nicolson membrane is considered to be highly fluid. This contrasts with the static picture of the membrane in the Danielli-Davson model. The proteins of the membrane are concerned with the enzymatic activity of the membrane, with transport of molecules, and with a receptor function. The lipid bilayer provides the permeability barrier.

Micellar Design

Corpascular nature of membrane structure and the repeating unit concept.

Fernandez-Moran (1962) and Sjostrand (1963) considered the membrane to consist of *globular units* or elementary particles. The globules, 40A-70A in diameter, form repeating units which are closely packed together. All membranes, however, do not have this structure. It is possible that both the unit membrane and the globular form are present in the cell. Under certain environmental or metabolic conditions one form may give rise to the other. Some workers consider the corpuscular nature to be an artifact. On the other hand Sjostrand and Barajas (1968) hold that the typical triple nature may be the result of denaturation.

According to Green (see Green, 1970) the cell membranes consist of fused *repeating units* (Fig.). Two types of membranes are distinguished, *monopartite* and *multipartite*. In *monopartite* membranes the repeating units do not have any projections. Examples of such membranes are the outer membrane of the mitochondrion and the plasma membrane of erythrocytes. In *multiparite* membranes the repeating units have projections. Each repeating unit is divisible into a *basepiece*, a *stalk* and a *headpiece*. The monopartite repeating units correspond to the basepieces of the multipartite units.

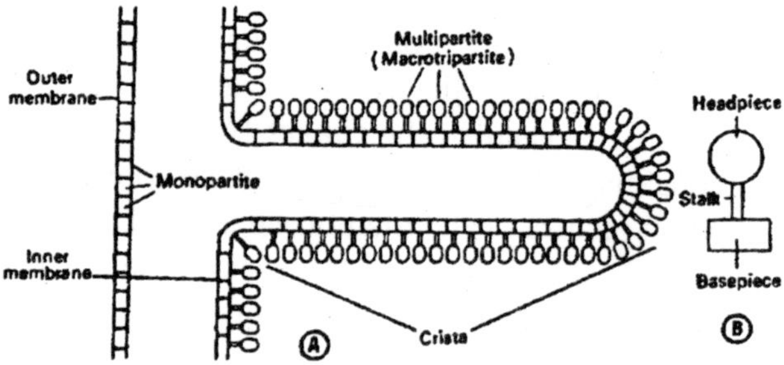

Green's repeating unit model (A) Crista of mitochondrion. (B) Multipartite repeating unit.

Multipartite repeating units include *macrotripartite* and *microtripartite* units. The macrotripartite repeating units are larger than the microtripartite repeating units. They are found in membranes in which electron transfer is coupled to synthesis of ATP, *e.g.* the inner membrane of the mitochondrion. Membranes having microtripartite repeating units have the capacity to carry out ATP-energised active transport.

The membrane of the sarcoplasmic reticulum, which transports Ca^{++}, the plasma membrane of R.B.C. which transports K^+ and Na^+, and the microvilli which transport sugars and amino acids, all have microtripartite repeating units. In macrotripartite membranes ATPase function is localised in the headpieces, while in microtripartite membranes, it is localised in the basepieces. In microtripartite repeating units the headpiece and stalk are more firmly attached to the basepiece than in the macrotripartite repeating unit.

The Bilayer and the Micellar Hypotheses—A Summation: Electron microscope studies have provided support for both the bilayer structure and the micellar (subunit) structure. Electron micrographs have clearly revealed the three layers of the unit membrane. On the other hand studies of the chloroplast and inner mitochondrial membranes show the presence of subunits in the form of repeating globules.

It cannot be said definitely which of the two cases represent the natural condition. Distortions resulting from preparation techniques could apply to either case. A possible explanation is that different membranes may show different types of structure, or that there may be transformation between the bilayer and the micellar states (Fig.).

The membranes of the mitochondria and chloroplasts appear to be constructed of a bilayer backbone on which is imposed a subunit structure.

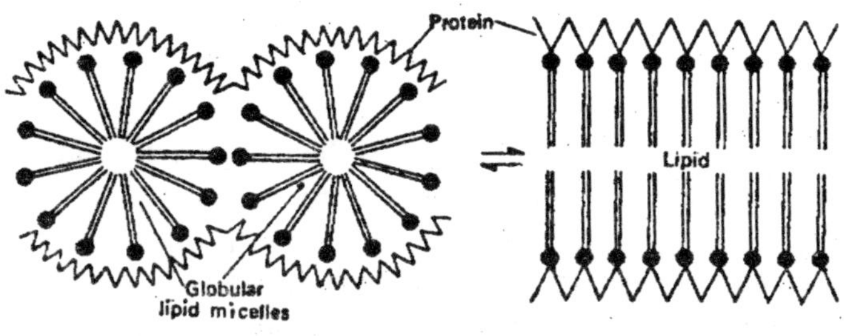

Transformation between micellar and bilayer states of the cell membrane.

Role of the Cell Membrane

In this Section the term 'cell membrane' is being used in the broad sense to include the membranes of various cell organelles, in addition to the plasma membrane which bounds the cell surface. Many metabolic processes occur within components of the intracellular membrane system.

The Conveyance

The Concentration Gradient, Osmosis: A membrane which allows the passage of a solvent but not of a solute is called a *semipermeable membrane.* A membrane which permits one substance to pass through more easily than another is said to be *selectively permeable.* A selectively permeable membrane allows the passage of both solvent and solute. Cell membranes are selectively permeable rather than semipermeable.

Molecules diffuse from a region of greater concentration to a region of lesser concentration. The difference in the levels of the two concentrations is called the *concentration gradient. Osmosis* is the diffusion of water (or a solvent) across a membrane in response to the concentration gradient. Many *artificial membranes* have been used as analogues to the plasmalemma in biological study. The common membranes are the *copper ferrocyanide* membrane and the *cellophane dialysis* tubing. *Natural membranes* like the outer membrane of the intestine of the ox, and the epidermis from the scale of an onion, are also used.

The cell is surrounded by fluids which may be *isotonic, hypertonic* or *hypotonic* to the fluids of the cell, An *isotonic* fluid has the same osmotic pressure as that of the cell fluids, *i.e.* the concentration gradient is zero. Water moves both in and out of the cell, but there is no net gain or loss. The osmotic pressure of a *hypertonic* fluid is greater than that of the cell fluids because of a higher concentration of dissolved substances. Water moves from inside the cell to outside resulting in shrinkage of the cell. A *hypertonic* fluid has a lesser osmotic pressure than the cell fluids because of a smaller proportion of dissolved substances. Cells placed in a hypotonic solution increase in volume because of inward diffusion of water.

If a sea-urchin egg is placed in diluted sea water, which is *hypotonic* to the cell fluids, then it swells, If placed in sea water which is concentrated by evaporation *(hypertonic)*, then it shrinks.

In normal sea water *(isotonic)* the egg neither swells nor shrinks. Similarly erythrocytes shrink if placed in a hypertonic salt solution (1.25%), and swell in a hypotonic solution (0.66%). There is no change in an isotonic solution (0.95%).

The plasma membrane acts as a barrier which, however, permits the movement of certain substances into and out of the cell. Thus the membrane regulates the passage of certain nutrient molecules into the cell and the removal of waste products from the cell.

Transport of molecules across the membrane may be *active* or *passive*. Both active and passive transport involve *selectivity*. Some molecules cross the membrane more easily than others. A *carrier molecule* may also be involved in both systems.

The passage of molecules through the membrane from a high-concentration to a low concentration region is called *passive transport*. Transfer of molecules takes place *along* the concentration gradient, and *no energy is required*.

In *active transport* molecules usually move from regions of low concentration, to regions of high concentration, *i.e. against* the concentration gradient. Active transport *requires energy*, and is dependent upon ATP supply in many cases. If the giant axon of the squid is treated with cyanide, ATP synthesis stops and transport of Na^+ ions across the membrane is affected. Intracellular injections of ATP restores extrusion of N^+ ions.

Transport of metabolites across biomembranes takes place in at least four ways:

Passive Transport —	(i)	Simple diffusion
	(ii)	Facilitated diffusion
Active transport —	(iii)	Simple active transport
	(iv)	Group translocation

Simple Diffusion: Transport of metabolites across the membrane along the concentration gradient and without the use of a carrier molecule is called simple diffusion. Movement of substances takes place from a high concentration to a low concentration region and the concentration gradient disappears as diffussion occurs. Simple diffusion does not involve any stereo-specificity (*i.e.* both L and D isomers move across at equal rates), and is a slow process. Consequently it is not believed to be an important mechanism for transport across cell membranes.

In the *Danielli-Davson model* it was assumed that passage of substances took place through small (7A) rigid protein-lined *pores* in membrane (Fig.). According to the *Singer-Nicolson fluid mosaic model* the pores may not be stable, but may be constantly appearing and disappearing *(statistical pore concept).* They are believed to be formed by the appearance of gaps in the highly fluid lipid bilayer because of random movement of membrane phospholipids. Small polar molecules could cross the membrane through the gaps (pores) which arise in a random manner and are transitory.

Facilitated diffusion resembles simple diffusion in that it does not require energy and takes place along the concentration gradient. It, however, differs in certain respects. Firstly, the process is *stereospecific, i.e.* only one of the two possible isomers, L and D, is transported. Secondly, it shows *saturation kinetics.* Increase in the concentration of the substance to be transported results in an increase in the rate of transfer up to an asymptotic value. Thirdly, a *carrier* is required for transport across the membrane.

The carriers are proteins with a relatively low molecular weight (9,000 to 40,000). Experimental evidence indicates that the proteins are highly selective. Carrier proteins specific for individual sugars and amino acids, phosphate, Ca,$^{++}$ Ma^{+} and K^{+} have been isolated. The carrier protein molecules are presumed to move to and fro across the membrane by *thermal diffusion.* The metabolite binds to the carrier protein at the outer surface of the membrane to form a *carrier-metabolite complex.* This diffuses along the concentration gradient, *i.e.* from high concentration to low concentration regions. The metabolite is set free at the inner surface of the membrane because of the relatively low concentration of metabolite on the inner side of the membrane. Transportation of metabolite continues as long as there is a concentration gradient. The entry of glucose into erythrocytes is an example of faciliatated transport.

Active transport appears to be of two general types, *primary active transport* and *secondary active* transport.

Primary active transport is directly related with chemical energy (ATP) or electric energy (electron flow). Examples of primary active transport are Na^+, K^+ *translocating ATPase in mammals* and *proton translocating ATPase of bacteria.*

The existence of *sodium and potassium pumps* has been demonstrated in many eukaryote cells. Na^+ is pumped out of the cell by the sodium pump and K^+ is pumped into the cell by a coupled process. The two pumps apparently operate simultaneously, and in the absence of either Na^+ or K^+ movement of both Na^+ and K^+ stops.

In 1954 an enzyme was discovered which functions as the monovalent ion pump. This enzyme, called *ATPase,* was found to be an integral plasma protein. Na^+, K^+ ATPases have been found in a wide variety of tissues and there is evidence indicating that the *ATPase is the ion pump.* ATPase is inhibited by a group of compounds called *cardiac glycosides* (*e.g. ouabain).* The enzyme consists of two polypetide chains, a large (MW 135,000) subunit which penetrates the membrane and a small (MW 30,000-40,000) subunit. Na^+, K^+-ATPase spans the membrane and has functional sites on both surfaces of the membrane.

It has been suggested that the essential part of the ion transport ATPase process is *cyclic phosphorylation-dephosphorylation* initiated by Na^+ and K^+ respectively. Na^+ and ATP bind to specific sites of the ATPase complex. Bound Na^+ is required for *phosphorylation* of the larger subunit of ATPase. Phosphorylation of ATPase probably leads to a major conformational change resulting in a reorientation of the enzyme within the membrane, causing Na^+ to pass through the membrane.

Similarly protein dephosphorylation may be brought about by bound K^+, resulting in reversion to original conformation and K^+ transport.

According to another view such large conformational changes in ATPase may not be taking place. Ion translocation is probably carried out by *minor conformational changes* in ATPase resulting from its phosphorylation and dephosphorylation.

It has been suggested that ATPase has a *channel* through its centre through which ion transport takes place.Secondary active transport depends upon chemiosmotic energy (membrane potential and/or ion gradients). Examples of secondary active transport are the *glucose* transport system of the intestinal epithelium of mammals and the *lactose* permease system in *E.coli*.

The free surface of the intestinal epithelium has numerous *microvilli* which are formed by projections of the *brush border membrane.* Primary active transport results in the Na^+ being pumped out of the cell and K^+ being pumped into the cell. The electrochemical sodium ion gradient can be then utilised for *secondary active transport of glucose* into the cell against the concentration gradient. Thus there is glucose-Na^+ cotransport catalysed by a glucose carrier. Such sodium-dependent transport has been observed for various amino acids and sugars in different vertebrates and for amino acids in bacteria.

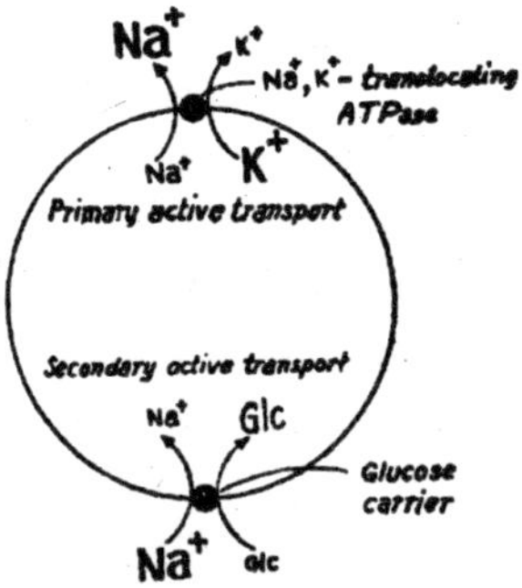

Schematic representation of active transport in intestinal cell. Na^+, K^+ active transport at the top, and glucose-Na^+ cotransport at the bottom.

The sodium pump maintains a higher concentration of Na^+ outside the cell than on the inner side. This results in a tendency for Na^+ to enter the cell. This it does in the form of a carrier-sugar or carrier-amino acid complex.

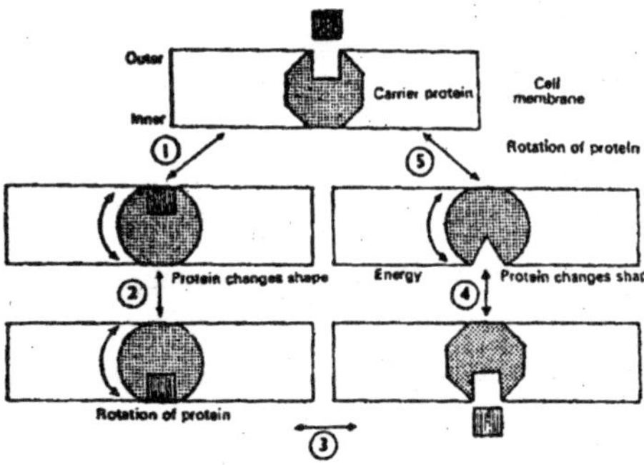

The revolving door model of active transport.

Jacques Monod and his associates studied the transport of *lactose* (milk sugar) across the cell membrane of the bacterium *E. coli.* This bacterium accumulates lactose 500-1,000 times against the concentration gradient. A 'revolving door' model of active transport has been proposed to explain the passage of lactose through the cell membrane. The carrier, a protein, is visualised as a revolving (rotating) door in the cell membrane (Fig.). The carrier protein has a slot, which normally faces outside, into which fits the substance to be transported.

The carrier protein is believed to undergo a change in shape (conformational change) when the substance enters the slot, and thereby rotates so that the slot comes on the inside. The substance is released into the cell, and the protein now returns to its original immobile form. Energy is now required to change the shape of the carrier protein, as a result of which it again rotates, so that the slot again faces outside.

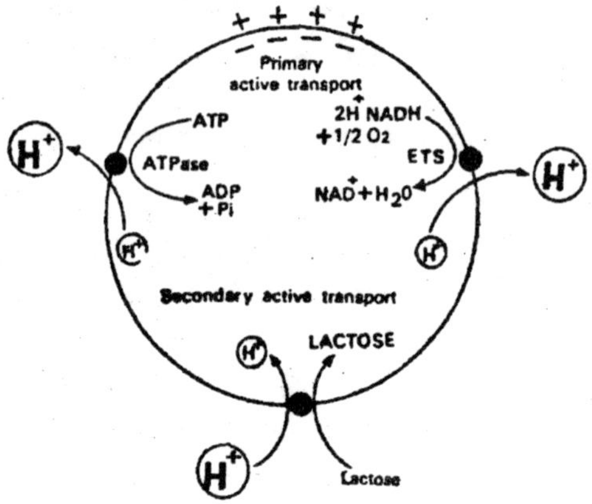

Diagram of active transport in a bacterial cell

Lactose transport in bacterial cells may be explained as follows (Fig.). As a result of *primary active transport* protons are pumped out through either the proton-translocating ATPase or a component of the electron transport (ETS). This sets up a proton gradient with higher concentration of protons outside the cell. This results in a tendency for protons to enter the cell. Lactose entry is now coupled to proton entry *(secondary active transport).*

It will be seen that there are four possible types of carrier models for transport:

1. Facilitated *diffusion* of the mobile carrier molecule across the membrane.
2. Ion translocation through a channel in ATPase by *minor conformational changes* in the ATPase molecule.

3. *Major conformational change* in the carrier when it attaches to the particular molecule that it normally transports.
4. *Rotation* of a carrier molecule, the diameter of which is approximately that of the membrane *(revolving door model).*

That carrier proteins are involved in certain types of transport mechanisms is well established. However, the exact mechanism by which carriers transport, substances across the membrane whether by diffusion, minor conformational changes or by rotation is not known. Large conformational changes like diffusion and rotation are probably not responsible for transport because hydrolysis of ATP and ion transport are tightly coupled processes (see Saier and Stiles, 1975). Ion translocation possibly takes place through the channel in ATPase as a result of minor conformational changes.

Group Translocation: In this process the substrate is altered by the enzyme that catalyses membrane transport. Transport of a variety of sugars like *glucose, fructose* and *mannitol* takes place across bacterial membranes through the *phosphotransferase system* (PTS). The sugar is released inside the membrane as a phosphorylated derivative *(sugar phosphate)* which cannot go back through the membrane. An advantage of this system is that the sugar phosphate released can directly be utilised for metabolic activity. The PTS always uses *phosphoenol pyruvate* (PEP) as the energy form (Fig.). Important components of the PTS are *two enzymes* (I and II) and a *heat stable protein* (HPr).

PEP is first dephosphorylated to *pyruvate* and the phosphate group released is taken up by *enzyme I*, a cytosol enzyme.

$$\text{PEP+Enzyme I} \xrightarrow{Mg^{++}} \text{Enzyme I} \sim \text{P+Pyruvate}$$

Enzyme I then transfers the phosphate group to the heat stable protein (HPr).

$$\text{Enzyme I} \sim \text{P+HPr} \longrightarrow \text{HPr} \sim \text{P+Enzyme I}$$

HPr is a small (MW 10,000) *histidine-containing protein* also found in the cytosol. Both enzyme I and HPr are general phosphate carrier proteins and do not show any specificity. They do not bind sugars and are hence not carrier proteins.

Enzyme II is actually an enzyme complex containing enzymes Ha and IIb, Mg^{++} and *phosphatidyl glycerol*. Enzyme IIa is *sugar-specific, i.e.* it carries only a specific type of sugar. The cell synthesises the enzyme specific for the type of sugar in which it is growing. Enzyme II is located in the cell membrane, probably in the outer region. It catalyses the transfer of the phosphate group from HPr to the sugar. Unlike enzyme I which is phosphorylated, enzyme II does not itself undergo phosporylation, but only catalyses the phosphorylation of sugar.

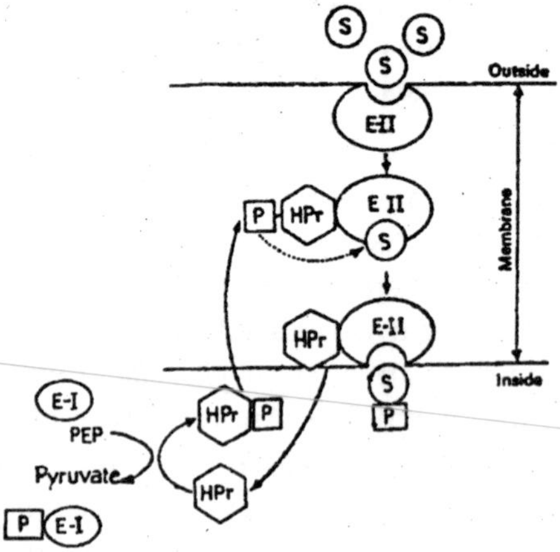

PEP-Phosphotransferase system. PEP.-Phosphoenol pyruvate. Hpr.-Heat resistant protein. S. Sugar, P-Phosphate. E-I-Enzyme I. E-II-Enzyme II complex.

$$HPr \sim P+Sugar \xrightarrow{EnzII} Sugar\text{-}6\text{-}phosphate+HPr$$

It is assumed that enzyme II undergoes a conformational change, thus bringing the sugar phosphate on the inner side of the membrane. The sugar phosphate is then released into the cell. HPr is then rephosphorylated by enzyme I through dephosphorylation of PEP to pyruvate.

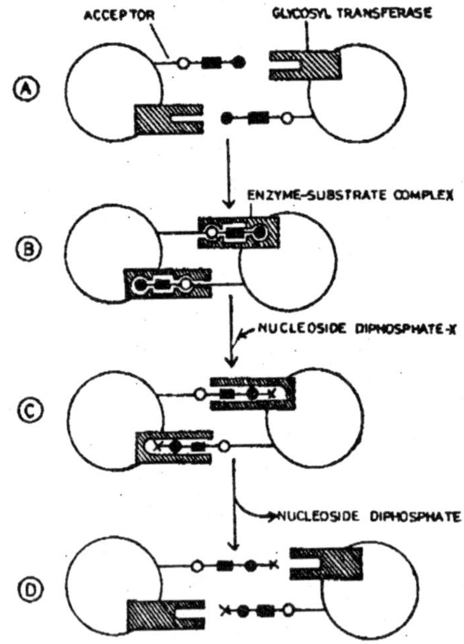

Model for the role of glycosyl transferases in cellular adhesion.

A. *Two cells, each carrying glycosyl transferases and acceptor molecules (oligosaccharides).*

B. *The cells come together forming enzyme-substrate complexes.*

C. *One more monosaccharide residue (X) added.*

D. *The enzyme-substrate complex dissociates and the cells separate.*

Cell Recognition and Combination

Mammalian leucocytes recognise foreign cells like bacteria and engulf them by phagocytosis, but leave other cell types in the blood alone. Similarly macrophages of the spleen can differentiate between healthy and worn out erythrocytes and destroy the latter by phagocytosis. The sites for cell recognition are known to lie on the surface of the plasma membrane. The amino sugar *sialic acid* in possibly involved in cell recognition and adhesion.

Roseman (1970) has proposed a theory for cellular adhesion. According to this theory the cell surface carries both *glycosyl transferases* and *glycosyl acceptor* molecules, which are oligosaccharides made up of monosaccharide units (Fig.).

The transferase of one cell binds with a specific receptor molecule of a neighbouring cell in an enzyme-substrate reaction. Addition of a monosacharide sugar residue to the acceptor chain is believed to bring its elongation. This results in the dissociation of the enzyme-substrate complex, and separation of the cells.

Antigen Distinctness

The glycoproteins on the surface of the cell membrane determine the antigen specificities of the cell. The different blood group systems are all based on the antigenic properties of erythrocytic cell membranes. The ABH blood group system is based on the relationships between antigens on R.B.C. and antibodies in blood serum. The antigenic determinants on the surface of erythrocytes are mainly *glycolipids.* Those of soluble blood group substances are *glycoproteins.* Both M and N antigens are carried by the major *sialoglycoprotein* of the erythrocyte membrane.

A major problem in the transplantation of organs from one human being to another is tissue rejection. Transplants between genetically similar individuals are accepted, while those between genetically different individuals are rejected. This rejection is due to the immune response of the host. Recognition of foreign material depends upon specific antigens *(histocompatibility antigens)* on the cell membrane of implanted cells.

The plasma membrane glycoproteins carry these antigens. If the recognition sites on the cell membranes of the cells of organs could be modified, then tissue rejection would not take place and successful organ transplantation could be carried out.

Hormone Receiver

It is known that hormones control the metabolism of cells. The cell membrane contains receptors which recognise specific hormones and convey the information in the latter to the interior of the cell. This stimulates a change in the metabolism of the cell. Studies have been carried out on membrane-bound hormone receptors of several hormones, including glucagon, insulin, adrenocorticotropic hormone (ACTH), angiotensin, growth hormone (GH), thyrotropin-releasing hormone (TRH), follicle-stimulating hormone (FSH), luteinising hormone-releasing hormone (HRH), human chorionic gonadotropin (HCG) and luteinising hormone (LH), vasopressin, oxytocin, parathyroid hormone (PTH), calcitonin, prostaglandins E (PGE), thyroid-stimulating hormone (TSH), prolactin, somatomedin, nerve growth factor (NGF), epidermal growth factor (EGF) and vasoactive intestinal polypeptide (VIP).

Location of Hormone Receptors: Hormone receptors are most commonly located in the plasma membrane, possibly on the outer surface of the membrane. The receptors for steroid hormones are, however, located in the cytoplasm. These hormones penetrate the plasma membrane and bind to the cytoplasmic receptors. The hormone-receptor complex travels to the nucleus where it influences the expression of genes.

Receptor Action: Membrane receptors have two essential functions, recognition of specific hormones and initiation of changes in the metabolism of the cell.

The first step in membrane receptor action is the recognition and binding of the hormone to the receptor (Fig.). Only a specific hormone can bind to a receptor site. This specificity is probably due to the complementary structures of the hormone and the receptor ('lock and key'). It is assumed that the binding of the hormone (H) to the receptor (R) results in the formation of a hormone-receptor complex (HR).

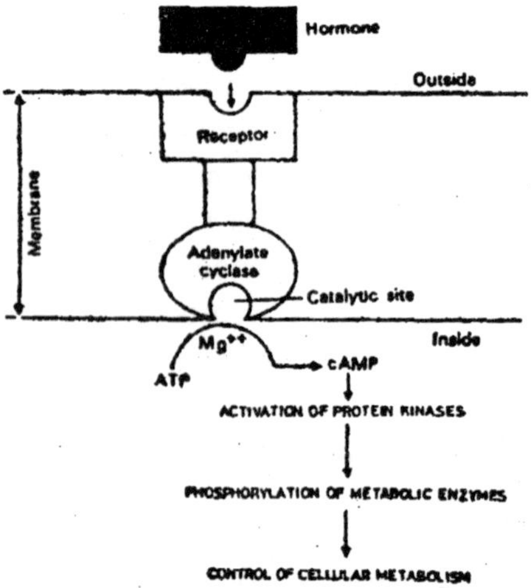

Receptor-adenylate cyclase action.

Hormone-receptor binding results in the activation of *adenylate cyclase,* a membrane-bound enzyme. This enzyme is believed to be located at the inner surface of the plasma membrane and contains binding sites for ATP and Mg ions. Activation of adenylate cyclase results in the generation of cyclic AMP (adenosine monophosphate) from ATP. Cyclic AMP (cAMP) activates *protein kinases* which phosphorylate a variety of *metabolic enzymes.*

Depending upon the type of enzyme, phosphorylation may either increase or decrease the catalytic activity of the enzyme, and hence control cellular metabolism. Cyclic AMP thus acts as a *second messenger,* conveying information carried by the hormone *(first messenger)* from the plasma membrane to the interior of the cell. The receptor may be coupled to the enzyme by an intermediate *coupler,* possibly phospholipids.

Adenylate cyclase may be stimulated by many different hormones. For example, the adenylate cyclase of the fat cell is regulated by seven different hormones and inhibited by three. It is difficult to imagine 10 separate receptors having physical association with adenylate cyclase. In the model proposed by Cautrecasas (1974) this difficulty has been resolved (Fig.). According to this model, the receptor by itself does not have an affinity for adenylate cyclase. However, the hormone-receptor complex formed by association of the hormone with the receptor has great affinity for the enzyme. The HR complexes are supposed to diffuse, laterally till they collide at random with adenylate cyclase and bind with it. This brings about a modification in the catalytic site of the enzyme, resulting in the generation of cAMP.

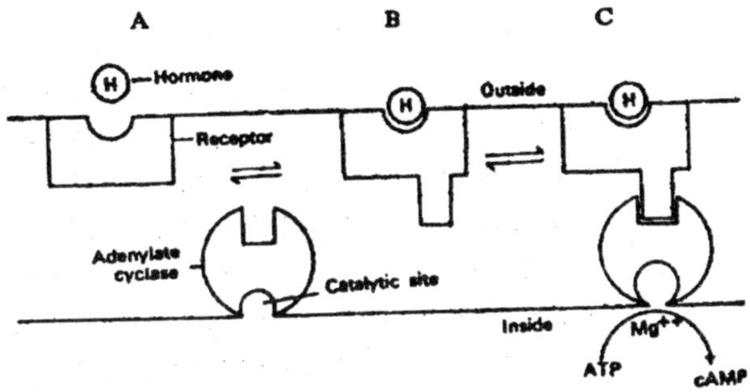

Cautrecasas model (1974) of receptor action.

A. *Hormone binds to receptor.*
B. *The hormone-receptor complex formed has high affinity for adenylate cyclase.*
C. *The hormone-receptor complex may colloid with adenylate cyclase by lateral diffusion and bind with it. The catalytic site of adenylate cyclase is modified, resulting in the generation of cAMP.*

Secretion: Polypeptide chains are synthesised by ribosomes and released into the lumen of ER cisternae (Fig.). Secretory protein is next transported to the Golgi complex where it may undergo modification (*e.g.* glycosylation in case of glycoproteins). Secretory vesicles released from the Golgi complex move to the periphery of the cell and fuse with the plasma membrane. This fusion apparently depends upon the interaction between the integral proteins of the plasma membrane and the secretory vesicle. Release of secretory products therefore ultimately takes place through the plasma membrane.

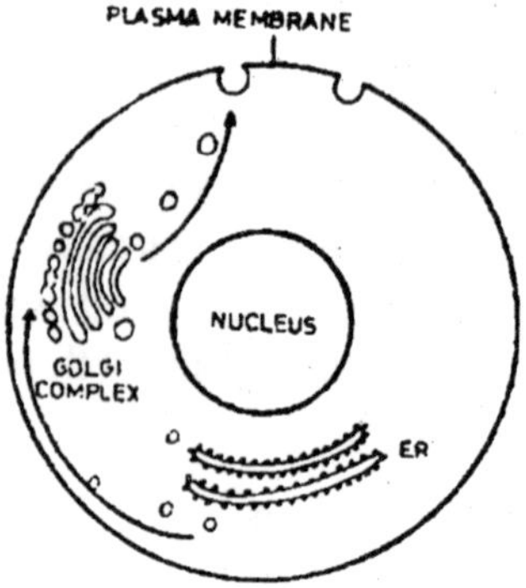

Role of plasma membrane in secretion.

Oxidative Phosphorylation: The inner membrane of the mitochondria and the plasma membrane of bacteria contain the *electron transport chain* which plays an important part in cell respiration. This chain consists of a series of components which can transfer electrons. Electrons from substrates pass down the chain resulting in reduction and oxidation of each component. During this process there is a decrease in free energy, about half of which is utilised for the synthesis of ATP. This process is called *oxidative phosphorylation.*

Endocytosis vs. Exocytosis: An important activity of the plasma membrane of certain cell types is *endocytosis.* Endocytosis is the process by which material is transported into cells by formation of vesicles. The term includes two essentially similar processes, *phagocytosis* (cell eating) and *pinocytosis* (cell drinking). Phagocytosis is the bulk injection of solid food into the cell, while pinocytosis refers to the injection of fluid material. The reverse process by which membrane lined material is removed from the cell is called *exocytosis.*

Phagocytosis involves folding of the plasma membrane around the material that is being engulfed and the subsequent formation of an intracellular vesicle *(phagosome).* The phagosome fuses with a *primary lysosome* to form a *secondary lysosome* in which the food material is digested by enzymes. Phagocytosis is found in many Protozoa, where it serves for the nutrition of the cell. In the Metazoa it is a method of defense against foreign bodies like bacteria, dust and various colloids, *e.g.* in scavenging white blood cells. Residual undigested material is egested by *exocytosis.* Ingestion of small colloidal particles is sometimes called *ultraphagocytosis.* Phagocytosis is found in the granular WBC and in cells of the reticulo-endothelial system (histocytes, reticular cells, endothelial cell).

Pinocytosis is the intake of fluid material into the cell by the formation of *pinocytic vesicles* or *pinosomes.* The fluid may contain organic molecules or other nutrient material in solution. Experiments using labelled proteins have shown that the amoeba ingests ('drinks') about one-third its volume of protein solution during the feeding period. The protein apparently acts as a stimulus to pinocytosis.

If an amoeba is placed in water, or in water to which carbohydrate has been added, no pinocytosis takes place. However, if placed in water to which proteins, certain amino acids or ions are added, pinocytosis begins. Pinocytosis provides the cell with additional interior interface where active and passive transport can be carried out. It is therefore a process which supports transport of materials into the cell. Both phagocytosis and pinocytosis are active mechanisms which require energy. This is shown by the fact that glycogen breakdown, glucose uptake and oxygen consumption all increase during phagocytosis by leucocytes.

Exocytosis is a process which is essentially the reverse of endocytosis. The membrane of a cell vesicle fuses with the plasma membrane and releases its contents outside the cell. Exocytosis serves as a means of extruding undigested material from the cell. It is also the principal mechanism by which hormones and other substances are secreted from the cell.

Chemoreception: Molecules associated with the cell membrane respond to a variety of stimuli. Chemoreception or the response to chemical stimuli is shown by a variety of organism ranging from bacteria to mammals. The bacterium *E. coli* has chemical receptors, which appear to be proteins, involved in membrane transport in its membrane. Bacteria and Protozoa are attracted to compound like amino acids, sugars, and organic acids, and repelled by hydrophobic compounds, phenolic compounds and acids.

The chemical receptors in the membrane of bacteria appear to be transport proteins in some cases. Thus the sugar transporting *phosphotransferase system* also appears to be associated with chemotactic response. Blocking any one component of the phosphotransferase system blocks both sugar transport and chemotaxis. This suggests that passage of sugar through the membrane is required before a substrate elicits a chemotactic response. In mammals, binding proteins associated with the cell membranes are believed to serve as chemical receptors for taste and smell.

It is believed that in man a different receptor protein recognises each of the four distinct taste qualities: sour, sweet, bitter, and salty. A protein which binds to sweet compounds has actually been isolated. Specific receptor proteins have also been postulated for membranes of olfactory receptor cells.

Act of Transmitting

The transmission of nerve impulses takes place at the surface membrane of nerve cells.

Junctional Intricate

Usually there is a uniform intercellular gap of 100-200A separating adjacent cells. Sometimes, however, contact between cells results in a modification of the cell membrane. There are specialised regions in which there is firmer intercellular attachment. One type of contact found is some epithelial cells is called the *junctional complex*. Such a type of contact has been observed in the intestinal epithelium of the hamster (Fawcett, 1966) and in the gastric mucosa of the bat, among other examples.

In epithelial cells four types of junctional differentiation of cell membranes are present.

1. The *tight junction* or *zonula occludens.*
2. The *belt desmosome* or *intermediary junction (zonula adherens).*
3. The *spot desmosome* or *macula adherens.*
4. The *gap junction* or *nexus.*

The zonula occludens or occlusion zone (tight junction) (Fig.).

Sometimes also called *the terminal bar*, it is found near the free surface of cells. The 'terminal bar' of light microscopists includes both the tight junction and the zonula adherens.

In the region of the tight junction the plasma membranes of two adjacent cells are fused at a series of points containing *sealing strands* which form lines of attachment. The sealing strands are composed of rows of integral membrane proteins, each row being contributed by one plasma membrane. The strands block the passage of substances between cells. They are connected to a network of fine *cytoplasmic filaments* which reinforce the junction. The tightness of the junction depends upon the number of sealing strands, and the extent to which they are interconnected to from a network.

Tight junctions prevent the free passage of substances across the epithelium. Thus nutrients absorbed across epithelial cells at the expense of energy are prevented from leaking back into the lumen of the intestine through spaces between the cells.

Tight junctions are also apparently essential for normal embryonic development, and are found as early as in the two-cell stage.

Cells adhere to each other by means of junctions called *desmosomes.* These are of two main types, *belt desmosomes* and *spot desmosomes.* The belt desmosome (zonula adherens, intermediary junction) is found just below the tight junction. It is in the form of a band on the inner side of the cell membrane of epithelial cells.

The intercellular space in the junctional zone is filled with fine filaments. The filaments associated with the belt desmosome are 70A in diameter and appear to contain *actin.* Since actin is also found in muscle cells, it has been suggested that the filaments are contractile. These filaments might help to close gaps in the epithelium resulting from death and sloughing away of cells, and may be responsible for movement and changes in shape of epithelial cells in the developing embryo during organ formation. Associated with the belt desmosome is the *adherens web (terminal web)* which is formed by separation of the *core microfilaments* supporting the microvilli.

Spot desmosomes (maculae adherens) are disc-shaped points of contact between the plasma membranes of adjacent cells (Fig.). Here the intercellular gap is about 300-500A. The spot desmosome consists of a disc-shaped plaque (0.5 μm diameter) on the cytoplasmic surface of each cell membrane. Non-contractile 100A filaments called *tonofilaments,* which form the structural framework of the cytoplasm, are attached to the plaques. Thin filaments *(transmembrane linkers)* arising from the plaques fill the intercellular gap between the membranes. The filaments are bisected by a dense line called the *central stratum.*

Hemidesmosomes: In the basal region of some epithelial cells only half desmosomes may be present. Such structures are called *hemidesmosomes.* They serve as anchoring sites for bundles of tonofilaments, and also for joining the cell membrane of epithelial cells to the underlying basement membrane. Gap junctions are patch-like areas of close intercellular contact. The intercellular space is narrow (about 30A) in the region of the gap junction. The gap junction consists of a disc-shaped area on each cell membrane containing several hollow, cylindrical particles (Fig.).

The particles are about 70A in diameter, and form intercellular pipes through which exchange of certain substances between two adjacent cells takes place. The channels in the particles are about 20A in diameter and permit the passage of molecules of molecular weight up to 1,000 daltons, including ions, most sugars, amino acids, nucleotides, vitamins, steroid hormones and cyclic AMP. Thus a cell can utilise such substances from adjacent cells to which it is connected. Such a connecting system is important for cells, especially in the cells of embryos before establishment of the circulatory system. Calcium ions regulate the permeability of gap junction channels. Injection of calcium ions into a cell results in the uncoupling of the cell from adjacent cells. When the calcium level returns to normal the channels again become functional.

The sensitivity of gap junctions to calcium ions appears to be an essential factor in tissue repair after injury. When a cell is injured there is an inflow of calcium ions from the surrounding fluid. This causes the gap junctions of the cell to close, probably by collapse of channel elements. Thus loss of nutrients from undamaged adjacent cells is prevented. As the wound closes, cells make contact with other normal undamaged cells, and new functional gap junctions are formed within 30 minutes. In electrically excitable tissue,gap junctions permit transmission of electrical activity without the necessity of a neurotransmitter. In such cases they are known as *electrotonic synapses*. The contraction of the muscle cells of the heart and of smooth muscles is synchronised by gap junctions.

5

Shifting Membrane

In all living organisms, it is vitally important that cells and cell organelles should allow transport of a variety of substances into and outside of these structures. Such a transport is important so that the cells may respond rapidly to stimuli (*e.g.*, sights, sounds, smells). The substances transported may include a variety of micromolecules like nutrient molecules, metabolites, and a variety of ions (Na^+, K^+, Ca^{++}, Cr, H^+) (Table). These substances which need to be transported may be small hydrophobic or nonpolar (soluble in oil *i.e.*, in lipid membrane) or may be polar molecules (water soluble). They pass at a high speed through the hydrophobic, impermeable plasma membrane, mainly consisting of lipid molecules (Fig.).

The transport of large uncharged polar molecules and charged molecules (ions) is facilitated by regulated pores/ channels and by the transport proteins or pumps found in the membrane. Cells can also transfer macromolecules and even large particles across their membranes through processes described as exocytosis and endocytosis, which are facilitated by the formation of vesicles. This chapter includes only membrane transport which may or may not make use of carrier/

Different Types of Molecules and their Possible Transport through Plasma Membrane.

Type of molecules	*Examples of molecules*	*Transport through plasma membrane*
1. Hydrophobic (nonpolar) molecules	O_2 (32), CO_2 (44) N_2 (28), Benzene (78)	Rapidly diffuse
2. Uncharged small polar molecules	H_2O(18), C_2H_5OH(46), urea (60), glycerol (92)	Rapidly diffuse
3. Uncharged large polar molecules	glucose (180), sucrose (342)	Hardly diffuse at all; move through pores using carrier proteins
4. Charged molecules (ions-hydrated *i.e.* polar)	H^+, Na^+, K^+, Ca^{2+}, Mg^{2+}, Cl^-,HCO^-_3, PO^{3-}_4	Do not diffuse except using ion channels or active transport

* molecular mass (in kilodaltons) of each molecule shown in parenthesis.

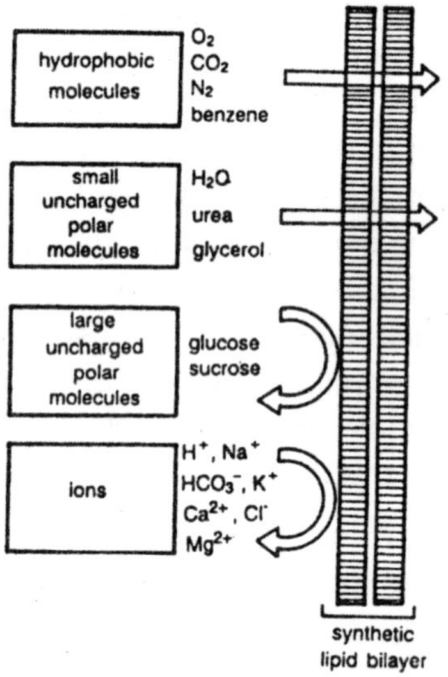

Relative permeability of a synthetic lipid bilalyer to different classes of molecules (redrawn from Alberts et. al., Molecular Biology of the Cell, 1994).

channel proteins. The two main classes of membrane proteins include 'carrier proteins' and 'channel proteins'. The carrier proteins have parts which move during transfer of specific molecules across the membrane and the channel proteins form a narrow hydrophilic pore permitting passive movement of small inorganic ions. Thus, the transport proteins, whenever utilised may either merely provide a path or may actually take part in the transport event. The membrane transport can be broadly classified into (i) passive transport including 'passive diffusion' and 'facilitated diffusion' and (ii) active transport (Fig.).

Another subject involving membrane transport is the response of cells to external and internal stimuli, which involves muscle movement and very rapid intercellular communications. These communications make use of receptor proteins in the membranes of excitable cells (nerve cells or neurons) and involve regular transport of ions and other substances called neurotransmitters.

However, this transport of ions and neurotransmitters is restricted to nerve cells, or neurons and therefore deserve a separate treatment. Therefore, in this chapter, there are two parts, the first part dealing with the membrane transport involving transport of all kind of ions and other substances

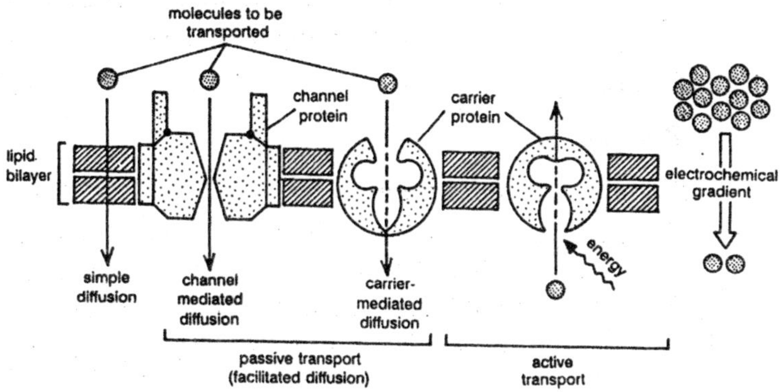

Comparison of passive transport along an electrochemical gradient with active transport against an electrochemical gradient (redrawn from Alberts et. al., Molecular Biology of the Cell- 1994).

across the membranes of all kinds of cells and the second part dealing with the neurotransmission involving transport of ions and neurotransmitters across the membranes of only nerve cells or neurons.

General Membrane Conveyance

Passive Transport: Passive Diffusion Transport of Small Suncharged Molecules: In passive diffusion, the substance moves from a higher concentration to a lower concentration, generally without the help of any special transport system, until the concentration of the substance on both sides of the membrane becomes the same (carrier proteins may also be rarely involved in passive transport; *e.g.*, passive glucose transporters are known for mammalian cells). The free energy or chemical potential difference (ΔG) and the rate of flow (J_c) for an uncharged molecule are given by

$$\Delta G = G_2 - G_1 = RT\, l_n \frac{[C_2]}{[C_1]}$$

$$J_c = -P\{[C_2]-[C_1]\}$$

where, $[C_2]$ and $[C_1]$ = concentrations of two sides

$[C_2] - [C_1]$ = concentration gradient

G_2 and G_1 = potentials on two sides

R = gas constant (2cal deg^{-1} $mole^{-1}$);

T = absolute temperature

P = permeability coefficient (cm/sec)

P is a constant describing, how readily the molecule leaves the water solvent and crosses the hydrophobic barrier of plasma membrane (Fig.). It depends on three parameters K, D and X as follows:

$$P = \frac{KD}{X}$$

K = partition coefficient

$$= \left(\frac{\text{solubility of molecule in hydrophobic solvent}}{\text{solubility of molecule in water}} \right)$$

D = diffusion coefficient (rate of diffusion)

X = thickness of membrane

Transport of Charged Molecules: For a charged molecule, the situation becomes more complicated, since the movement depends on electrochemical potential. If z is the charge on transported molecule, F is Faraday's Constant (charge on one mole of electrons = 96,485 coulombs per mole) and V is the electric potential difference (voltage difference) on the two faces of a membrane, then the electrochemical potential (ΔG) is given by the following equation:

$$\Delta G = G_2 - G_1 = RT \; l_n \frac{[C_2]}{[C_1]} + zFV$$

$$V = V_2 - V_1$$

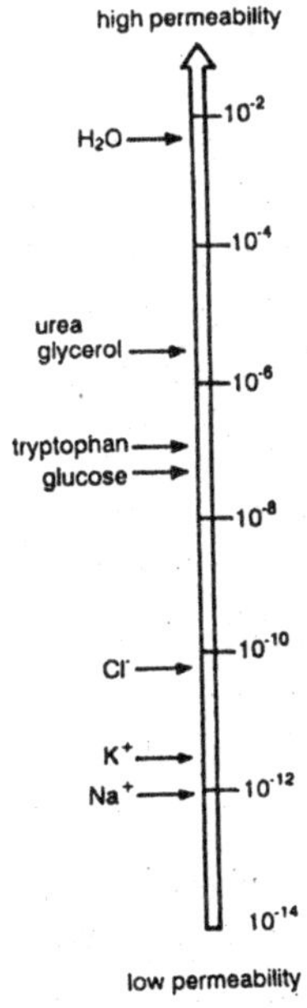

Permeability coefficients (cm/sec) for the passage of various molecules through synthetic lipid bilayers (redrawn from Alberts et. al., Molecular Biology of the Cell, 1994).

The term zFV accounts for the movement of a charge across a potential difference (due to ions), which depends on z and V (F being a constt.). If side 2 has a higher potential (V_2) than side 1 (V_1), V is positive, so that for a negatively charged ion (z = –1), the term zFV is negative and will reduce AG. However, if the net value on the right side of the equation is negative the ion will move spontaneously from side 1 to side 2 and if positive it will move from side 2 to side 1.

Passive Transport—Transport of Ions Across an Ion Gradient Ion Channels: Ion fluxes across cellular membranes mediate a variety of essential biological processes including the following: cell volume regulation, swimming behaviour in unicellular organisms like paramecium, movement of stomatal pores, leaf closing response of mimosa plant, muscle contraction, exocrine cell secretion, excitation of neurons for signal transmission, etc.

In many cases, these biological processes depend on fluxes of specific ions, that are stimulated and regulated by intracellular and extracellular signals. These ion fluxes, as will be discussed later in this chapter, may be facilitated by active transport involving proteins like ATPase, rhodopsin or may also involve passive processes like symport or antiport involving facilitated diffusion.

Besides these processes involving transport of ions through active transport, ion fluxes are also facilitated by another diverse family of integral membrane proteins called ion channels (each ion channel is a single channel protein), which have been the subject of active research for several decades now. These ion channels, present in all eukaryotes from protists and fungi to plants and animals, possess specific properties to perform specific functions, so that they differ from simple aqueous pores in (i) ion selectivity (flow of only specific ions is permitted), (ii) activation gating (channel's opening is regulated) and (iii) inactivation gating (channel's closing is regulated).

Channel proteins are also involved in the formation of gap junctions which are large pores between two adjacent cells.

Ion channels were actually discovered nearly 50 years ago and their electrical function was demonstrated by a variety of very sophisticated methods. However, till recently nothing was known about the structure and function of ion channels at the molecular level. Now, genes for a number of ion channels have been cloned and shown to express in systems, which can be used for a study of their function at the electrophysiological level. These studies made available the following information: (i) pictures of molecular architecture of proteins, which make these ion channels; (ii) views of membrane topology of the constituent subunits of these ion channels; (iii) the identity of regions of protein sequences that participate in specific channel functions.

Ion channels are hydrophilic pores formed by 'channel proteins' which differ from 'carrier proteins' or 'pumps' generally involved only in active transport of substances across plasma membrane. It is estimated that more than one million ions can pass through one channel per second, a rate which is 1000 times greater than the fastest rate of transport mediated by any carrier protein (for a Na^+ channel, it is estimated that more than 8000 Na^+ ions pass each millisecond, when the channel is open). Another difference is that ion channels can not be coupled to an energy source to carry out active transport.

Therefore, ion channels mediate only passive transport (downhill) to allow diffusion of ions (*e.g.*, Na^+, K^+, Ca^{++}, Cl") down their electrochemical gradients across a plasma membrane, although this movement of ions is regulated in a very sophisticated manner. These ion channels (specially Na^+ and K^+ ion channels) are specially used in the nerve cells for receiving, conducting and transmitting signals in the form of an 'action potential'. However, action potential in some muscles, eggs and endocrine cells depends on voltage gated Ca^{++}

channels. Voltage-gated Na^+, K^+ and Ca^{++} channels are also found in some cell types that are electrically not excitable.

More than 100 types of ion channels have already been described and new ion channels are still being described. Ion channels can be divided into distinct families and subfamilies, so that in different species, ion channels belonging to the same family have structural similarity, and in a given species ion channels belonging to different families differ in structure and function. Following distinct families of ion channels are known— (i), voltage-gated channels; (ii) mechanical-gated channels; (iii) ligand-gated channels (Table).

Of these, only two types of ion channels are known to be involved in neuronal excitability: (i) voltage-gated channels activated by change in voltage due to transport of K^+, Na^+ and Ca^{++}, (ii) ligand- gated channels activated by neurotransmitters like acetylcholine, serotonin, glutamate and gamma-amino butyric acid (GABA).

Each of these two types of ion channels is formed either of a more or less cylindrically symmetric aggregate of multiple subunits or of tandem-repeated homologous domains within a single polypeptide. The ion conduction pore is located on axis of the symmetry, although these pores may not have the kind of rotational symmetry, earlier envisaged.

Voltage gated Na^+, K^+ and Ca^{++} channels have been shown to have a surprisingly high degree of similarity in amino acid sequence suggesting their common evolutionary origin, although each of them has structural and functional diversity. A four fold symmetry has been suggested for each of the voltage activated K^+, Na^+ and Ca^{++} ion channels.

For instance in voltage activated K^+ channels, four aromatic residues, one from each subunit, take part in making a pore blocking site for tetraethyl-ammonium, so that all the four simultaneously interact with K^+ ions with precisely

Some Families and Subfamilies of Ion Channels.

Family of channel	Subfamilies of channels	Excitatory/inhibatory
1. Voltage-gated cation channels	Na^+ channels K^+ channels (including delayed and early) Ca++ channls	Excitatory
2. Mechanical-gated channels	—	—
3. Ligand gated ion channels		
(a) Neurotransraitter-gated channels		
(i) Cation channels	Acetylcholine-gated Na channels (acetylcholine receptor) Serotonin-gated Na^+ channels Glutamate-gated Na^+ channels	Excitatory
(ii) Anion channels	GABA gated Cl^- channels Glycine gated Cl^- channels	Inhubitory
(b) Ion-gated channels Ca^{2+} activated K^+ channels	—	—
(c) Nucleotide-gated channels	—	—

equal energetic contributions. Each subunit (600 amino acids long) is a polypeptide with six transmembrane α helices and two β strands (between helices 5 and 6) lining the pore (Fig.).

In voltage-gated Na^+ and Ca^{++} channels, each of the four subunits is a single large polypeptide chain. Similarly, a five fold symmetry has been suggested for the conduction pore of ion channels activated by neurotransmitters (ligands) like acetylcholine, glutamate and GABA. For instance, it has been shown that each of the five subunits (α,α,β,γ,δ) of nicotinic acetylcholine receptor channel (Fig.) has residues (at corresponding equivalent position), which have equal electrostatic influence on ion conductance.

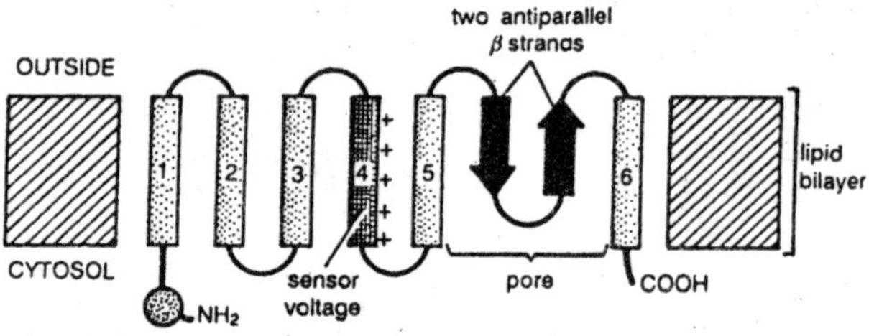

(a) six helices of a polypeptide chain making one subunit of a voltage-gated K^+ channel

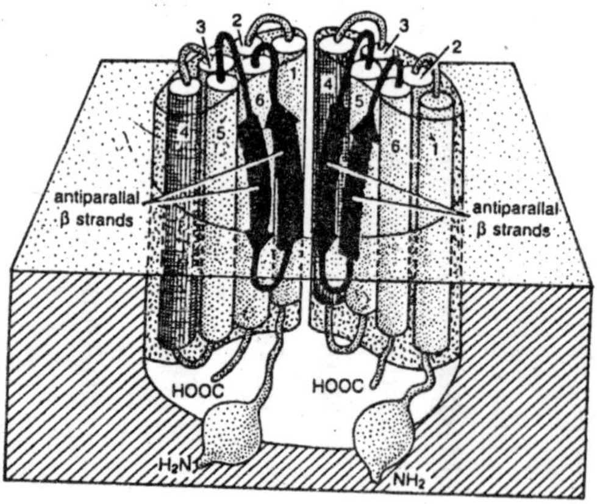

(b) a voltage-gated K^+ channel (only two of the four subunits are shown)

Structure of a voltage-gated K^+ channel having six alpha-helices and two antiparallel beta-strands (redrawn from Alberts et. al., Molecular Biology of the Cell, 1994).

It has also been shown that the linings of both kinds of ion channels, 'those having four fold symmetry and those having five fold symmetry (Fig.) are formed by a sequence of 20-25 residues repeated in each subunit of the channel.

Perhaps the most common ion channels are K^+ ion channels found in plasma membrane of all animal cells. Some of the K^+ ion channels are open even in unstimulated cells and are thus called 'K^+ leaky channels'. This term actually covers a variety of K^+ ion channels but they share the property of making plasma membrane more permeable to K^+ ions than to other ions like Na^+ions. Therefore, they play a critical role in maintaining the 'membrane potential', which is the voltage difference between the two faces of a plasma membrane.

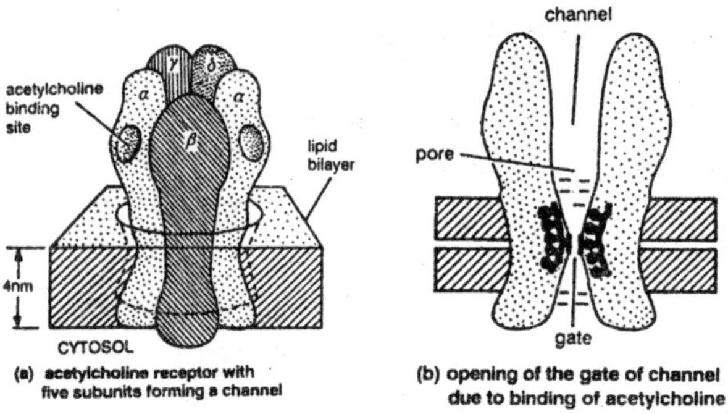

Structure of acetylcholine receptor having five subunits forming the channel, which opens on binding of acetylcholine (redrawn from Alberts et. al., Molecular Biology of the Cell. 1994).

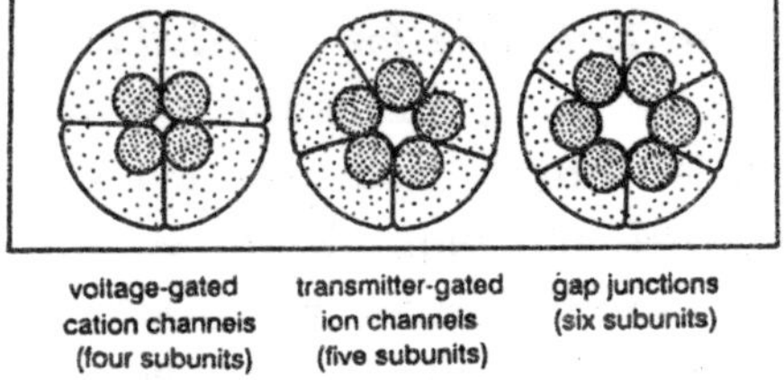

Three classes of channels; note the difference in number of protein subunits and pore diameter (redrawn from Alberts et. al., Molecular Biology of the Cell, 1994).

This membrane potential is also generated by active transport involving electrogenic H^+ pumps located in the mitochondrial inner membrane. Similar electrogenic pumps generate membrane potential in plants and fungi. The membrane potential in typical animal cells is, however, largely maintained by passive ion movement (involving ion channels like K^+ leaky channels).

Intracellular concentration of Na^+ ions is low and is balanced by high concentration of K^+ ions, so that the positive charge carried by cations becomes equal to the negative charge carried by anions within a cell. K^+ ions move across the membrane not only due to K^+ leaky channels, but also due to 'Na$^+$, K^+-ATPase pump'.

However, higher concentration of K^+ ions inside the cell creates a concentration gradient for K^+ ions forcing K^+ ions to leave the cell, but the electrical force due to anions forces K^+ ions to stay within the cell. At a particular K^+ ion concentration, therefore, no efflux of K^+ ions will take place, despite a steep concentration gradient.

The membrane potential, at which the electrical force due to anions balances the force due to cations concentration gradient (in other words, when electrochemical gradient for different ions is zero) is described as resting membrane potential, at which there will be no net flow of ions across the plasma membrane.

Patch Clamp Technique for the Study of Ion Channels: During the last 20 years, the nature and behaviour of ion channels was also directly studied in living systems, by the technique of 'patch clamping' developed and used by two neuroscientists, Erwin Neher and Bert Sakmann (both winners of 1991 Nobel Prize in Physiology/Medicine).

They used a tiny 1-micron-wide pipette (hooked upto a set of electronic equipments to measure voltage difference or ion flow) and applied it to a patch of membrane of the muscle cells to measure the current flow through the transmembrane ion channel of a single activated acetylcholine receptor (a ligand gated channel).

The 'patch clamp' technique was refined by creating a 'gigaseal' through the use of 'freshly made fire polished pipettes', which did not allow any leakage between pipette and the cell surface (Fig.).

Ever since this technique of 'patch clamp' was developed and refined, it has been used for studying the electrical activity of (i) nerve cells as well as non-neuronal cells of mammalian brain (to know clues about memory), and that of (ii) secretory cells (to know the chloride channel defect in cystic fibrosis). The technique has also been used to fill a cell with a known substance (salts, nucleotides, ion indicators or signaling molecules) to answer questions about the signaling pathways in cell membranes.

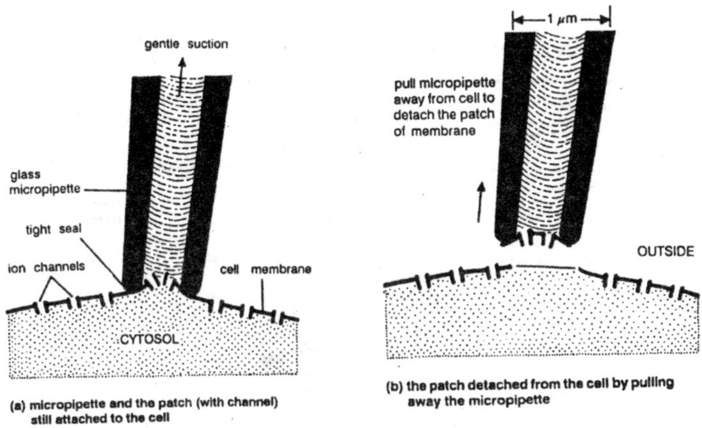

The technique of patch-clamp recording; patch is the portion of membrane covering the tip of micropipette and clump is the electronic device maintaining (or clamping) the membrane potential at a set value, while recording-ionic current through channels (redrawn from Alberts et. al., Molecular Biology of the Cell, 1994).

'Ionophores' as Tools to Increase Permeability of Membranes: Ionophores are small hydrophobic molecules that dissolve in plasma membranes and thus increase their permeability to specific ions. Microorganisms use them as weapons for competition or for preying, but biologists use them in studies for membranes.

They shield the charge of transported ion, so that it can penetrate the hydrophobic lipid bilayer and allow movement of ions along the electrochemical gradient (no energy is used, so that it is a passive transport system, comparable to ion channels).

Examples of ionophores include valinomycin (a mobile ion carrier, which transports K^+), A23187 (a mobile ion carrier, which transports bivalent cations like Ca^{++} and Mg^{++}) and gramicidin A (it is an ion channel, only 15 amino acids long, assisting the transport of monovalent cations along the gradient).

Some Carrier Proteins involved in Passive/Active Transport.

Family of transporter	Examples	Transport system
1. Sugar transport (uniporter)	Glucose transporter	Facilitated diffusion
2. Cation transporting ATPases	(i) Na^+, K^+ – ATPases (ii) Ca^{++} – ATPases (iii) H^+, K^+ — ATPases	Active transport
3. ABC transporters (ATPases)	(i) Multidrug resistance (MDR) ATPase (mammalian cells) (ii) Periplasmic-substrate-binding-protein dependent ATPase (bacteria) (iii) Chloroquine resistance ATPase *(Plasmodium falciparum)* (iv) Mating pheromone exporter (yeast) (v) Cystic fibrosis transmembrane regulator (CFTR) protein	Active transport
4. Symporters (Na^+ driven)	(i) Na^+ – glucose symporter (intestine) (ii) Na^+ – proline symporter (bacteria) (iii) Na^+ – HCO_3^- symporter (glial cells)	Active transport
5. Antiporters		
Cation antiporters	(i) Na^+ – H^+ exchanger	Facilitated diffusion
Anion antiporters	(ii) Cl^- – HCO_3^- exchanger (erythrocytes)	
Cation/anion antiporters	(iii) Na^+ dependent Cl^- – HCO_3^- exchanger	

Passive Transport: Facilitated Diffusion: Transport rates of many ions and small molecules across the plasma membrane need to be much higher than anticipated from passive diffusion, to sustain vital life processes. On actual measurements also, these rates were found to be higher in many cases. For example, in human red blood cells (RBCs), these rates for chloride ions and glucose were 106 to 107 times larger than those across simple bilayer membrane and have been attributed to specific carrier proteins, which facilitate diffusion (Table).

The carrier proteins are found in all natural membranes including those found in RBCs and have the following two features in common; (i) they facilitate movement of solutes in thermodynamically favoured direction (AG) and (ii) they display affinity and specificity for the solute to be transported. Consequently, facilitated diffusion rates reach a saturation point (V_{max}) with increase in the concentration of solute, so that when velocity (V) of flow is plotted against the solute concentrations, the graph takes the shape of a rectangular hyperbola, unlike a linear graph obtained in the case of simple passive diffusion (Fig.).

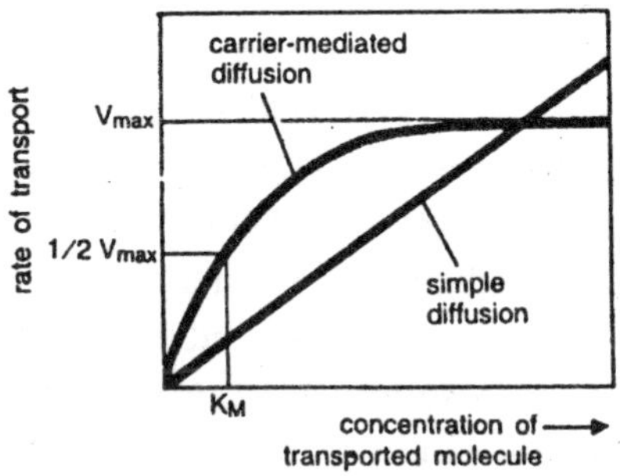

A comparison of the kinetics of simple diffusion and carrier mediated diffusion.

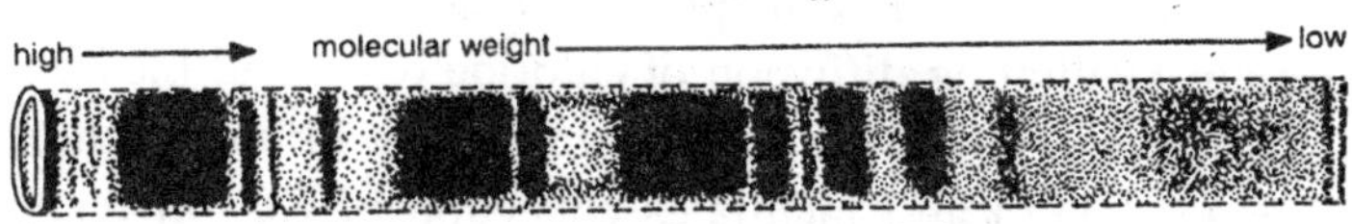

(a) SDS gel electrophoresis of erythrocyte membrane proteins

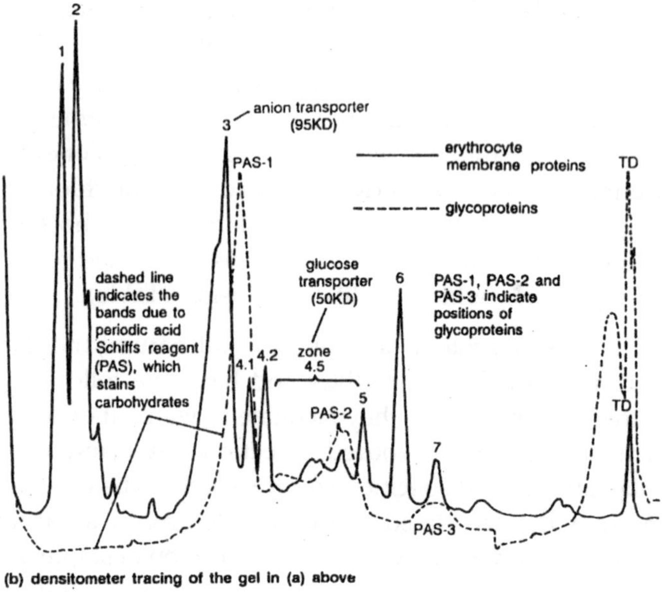

Arrangement of glucose transport protein in the erythrocyte membrane (redrawn from Garrett and Grisham, 1995).

The facilitated diffusion may be exemplified by the example of glucose and anion transporters of erythrocytes (Fig.). The glucose transporter of erythrocytes is a protein of 50kD molecular mass and a typical erythrocyte contains 500,000 molecules of this protein, which in its active form is a trimer, with its both C and N terminal ends located on the cytoplasmic side. The reduced ability of insulin to stimulate glucose transport in diabetic patients is due to reduced expression of some of these glucose transport proteins meant for facilitated diffusion (glucose can be transported in other cells by passive transport as well as active transport).

Similarly, anion transporter of erythrocytes is a 95kD protein facilitating diffusion of chloride (Cl^-) and bicarbonate (HCO^-_3) ions. The protein is known to have 14 transmembrane segments (Fig.) and facilitates collection of CO_2 in respiring tissues by Cl^-—HCO_3 exchange. This CO_2 is later taken by the blood to the lungs, where bicarbonate diffuses out of RBCs in exchange of Cl^-.

Carrier proteins are mainly involved in facilitated diffusion and active transport, although rarely they may also take part in passive diffusion. These carrier proteins may be classified as follows (Fig.):

(i) uniporters, when a single solute is transported from one side of the membrane to the other;

(ii) symporters, when transfer of one solute depends on the simultaneous or sequential transfer of a second solute in the same direction, and

(iii) antiporters, where transfer of one solute depends on the simultaneous or sequential transfer of a second solute, but in the opposite direction. For instance, glucose transport from high concentration to low concentration in facilitated diffusion (as discussed above for erythrocytes) is mediated by uniporters, but the glucose transport from low to high concentration (as happens in intestine and kidney cells) involves symport with the transport of Na^+ ions. The anion transporter discussed above belongs to the category of antiporters, where Cl^- and HCO_3^- move in opposite directions.

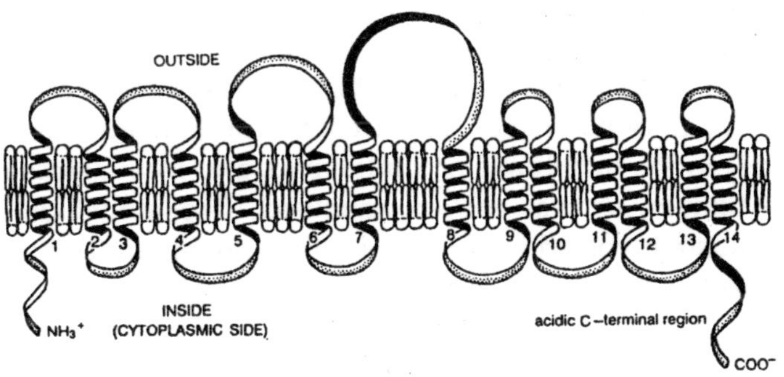

Arrangement of anion transport protein in the membrane (redrawn from Garrett and Grisham, 1995).

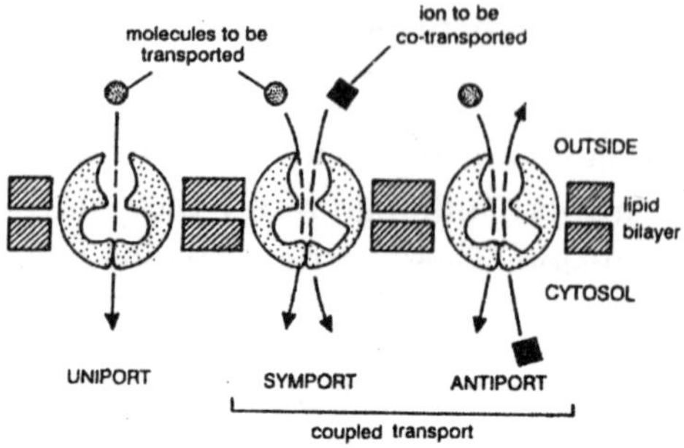

Three years of carrier mediated transport(uniport symport and antiport (redrawn from Alberts et. al., Molecular Biology of the Cell, 1994).

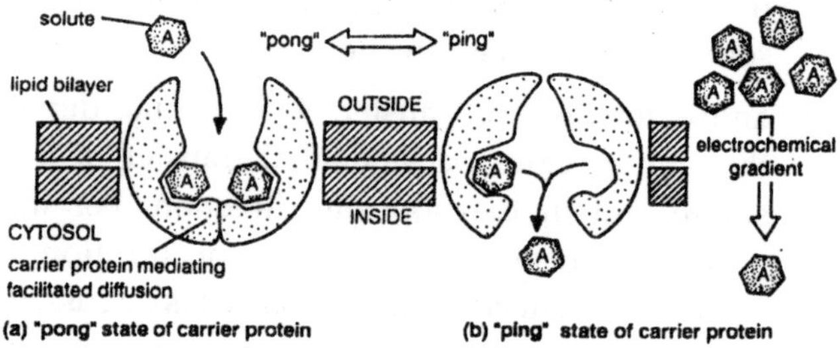

Reversible conformational change from 'pong' to 'ping' state in carrier protein to mediate facilitated diffusion of a solute along the electrochemical gradient (redrawn from Alberts et. al., Molecular Biology of the Cell, 1994)

The above transport involves a reversible conformational change in carrier proteins, so that the solute binding site of carrier protein is alternately exposed first on one side of the membrane and then on the other side. Since most of these carrier proteins are now known to be multipass transmembrane proteins, it is not likely that a carrier protein tumbles (or rotates) in the membrane or shuttle back and forth across the lipid bilayer, as was earlier visualised. The model of the mechanism involved in the use of carrier protein in facilitated diffusion is shown in Figure.

Active Transport: When a molecule moves from lower concentration to higher concentration, as is often required in the cells, energy input is required and the transport is described as 'active transport'. Mostly, the energy is derived from ATP, but rarely also from light (*e.g.* in bacteriorhodopsin protein in *Halobacterium halobium* during photosynthesis) or from ion gradients (*e.g.*, electron or proton transport). In all these cases, energy from chemical reaction (ATP hydrolysis) or from light is utilised for mechanical work (transport). Active transport is always mediated by carrier proteins or pumps, although passive transport may or may not involve carrier proteins. Ion channels are never involved in active transport; they are involved in passive transport only.

ATP Driven Active Transport Systems: Hydrolysis of ATP is coupled with the following transport systems (i) Na^+, K^+ transport (sodium pump), (ii) Ca^{++} transport, (iii) H^+, K^+ transport, (iv) ABC transporter superfamily, (v) Osteoclast proton pumps.

Na^+, K^+-ATPase System (Sodium Pump): All animal cells actively throw out Na^+ ions and take in K^+ ions, the two processes being facilitated by an integral protein called 'Na^+, K^+-ATPase' or 'sodium pump', which operates as an antiporter. This pump is also exploited to drive transport of sugars and amino acids and operates then as a 'Na^+-sugar' or 'Na^+-amino acid' symporter (Table). In most cells, Na^+ concentration is 5-15mM and K^+ concentration is 100-140mM, the reverse being the situation in extracellular space (Na^+, 100-140mM and K^+, 5-15mM) (Table). It is necessary, because K^+ is needed for many functions, for which Na^+ is inhibitory. This includes the following functions:

(i) Na^+, K^+ and Cl^- and other ion gradients help neurons to communicate,

(ii) they also regulate cell volume and cell shape,

(iii) they help in transport of amino acids, sugars, nucleotides and other substances. In fact upto 20-40% of total metabolic energy of the cell is consumed in the maintenance of these ion gradients and this energy consumption reaches 70% in the neural tissues.

A Comparison of Ion Concentration within and Outside a Typical Mammalian Cell (Modified from Alberts et. al., 1994).

	Type of ions	Concentrations (mM)	
		within the cell	*outside the cell*
1.	Cations		
	Na^+	5-15	100-140
	K^+	100-140	5-15
	Mg^{++}	0.5	1-2 (10^{-3}M)
	Ca^{++}	10^{-4}(10^{-7}M)	1-2 (10^{-3}M)
	H^+	7×10^{-5} (10^{-72}M or pH 7.2)	4×10^{-5} (10^{-74}M or pH 7.4)
2.	Anions		
	Cl^-	5-15	110

Other anions, whose concentrations are not given here include HCO^-_3, PO_4^{3-}.

Each ATPase molecule, that is dependent on Na^+ and K^+ consists of (i) a subunit (120kD), consisting of 10 transmembrane helices and two large cytoplasmic domains, and (ii) a β subunit (35kD), consisting of one transmembrane segment and a large extracellular domain.

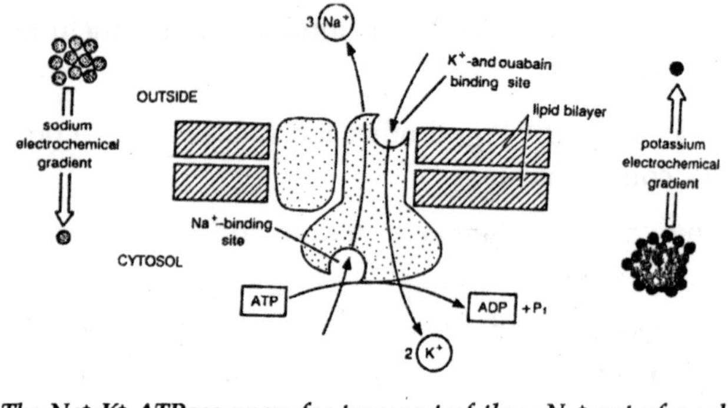

The Na^+-K^+ ATPase pump for transport of three Na^+ out of a cell for every two K^+ into a cell against their gradients (redrawn from Alberts et. al., Molecular Biology of the Cell, 1994).

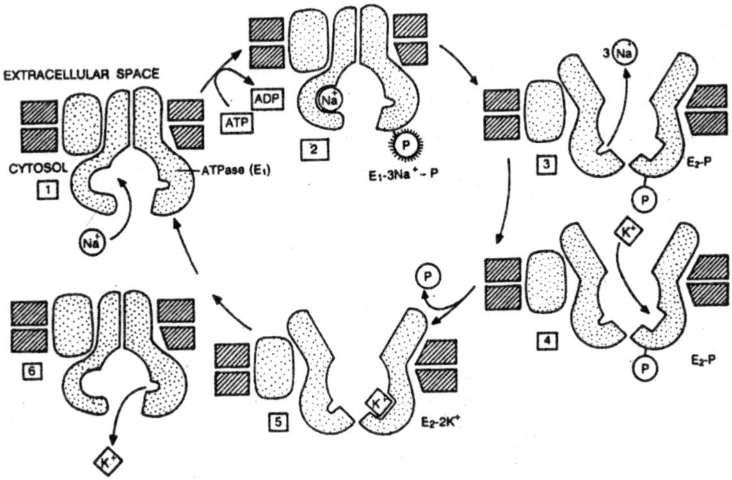

A model for the pumping cycle of Na⁺-K⁺ATPase involving reversible Na⁺ dependent phosphorylation and K⁺ dependent dephosphorylation of ATPase (redrawn from Alberts et. al., Molecular Biology of the Cell, 1994).

The ATPase hydrolyses ATP on the cytoplasmic side of the membrane, so that three Na^+ ions are transported out of the cell and two K^+ ions are transported into the cell for each ATP molecule hydrolysed. Since this involves net movement of one positive charge outward per cycle, the sodium pump is described as electrogenic in nature. The enzyme ATPase exists in two forms: (i) E_1 form has affinity for Na^+ and ATP; it gets readily phosphorylated in the presence of Mg^{++} to form E_1–P carrying three occluded Na^+ ions. E_1–P changes to E_2-P, which has low affinity for Na^+ ions, but high affinity for K^+ ions. This E_2-P form releases $3Na^+$ and binds $2K^+$ ions on the outside of the cell giving rise to $E_2 — 2K^+$. (Fig.) which releases $2K^+$ in the interior of the cell. The net process, thus, can be written as follows:

$$ATP + H_2O + 3Na^+(\text{inside}) + 2K^+(\text{outside}) \longrightarrow$$
$$ADP + Pi + H_2O + 3Na^+ (\text{outside}) + 2K^+ (\text{inside})$$

It has been shown that Na^+, K^+-ATPase, in its E_2-P state is used by cardiac glycosides (*e.g.*, animal steroids like ouabain, which inhibits Na^+, K^+-ATPase) for binding, and thus forms a stable E_2-P-(cardiac glycoside) complex. This inhibits the function of Na^+, K^+-ATPase resulting in inhibition of the sodium pump. This situation leads to accumulation of Na^+ and Ca++ in these cells, encouraging endosmosis thus leading to swelling/ bursting of cells and consequent narrowing of blood vessels creating hypertension. In plant cells, however, the rigid cell wall does not allow the cells to burst.

Ca^{++}-ATPase System: Ca^{++} is an important ion, taking part in signal transduction pathways in virtually all cells leading to control of many functions including muscle contraction. Free Ca^{++} has a low concentration in cytosol (~10^{-7}M) relative to that outside the cytosol or in ER (~10^{-3}M). Ca^{++} concentration is also low near the muscle fibres and all Ca^{++} is accumulated in a complex network of vesicles called sarcoplasmic reticulums or SRs (SR is a specialised type of endoplasmic reticulum) in the cytoplasm of muscle cells. Flow of Ca^{++} ions down its steep gradient, *i.e.* from SR to cytosol or from outside the cell to its interior, is one means of transmitting signals rapidly across the membrane. The maintenance of steep gradient of Ca^{++} across the membrane is, therefore, essential for cell function. Low Ca^{++} ion concentration in cytosol is maintained by Ca^{++} pumps actively transporting Ca^{++} ions out of the cytosol to SR or outside the cell. One of these pumps is an ATPase. Another Ca^{++} pump is an antiporter, driven by Na^+ electrochemical gradient.

Nerve impulses induce SR to release Ca^{++} leading to rise in cytoplasmic level of Ca^{++}, thus stimulating muscle contraction. Relaxation of muscles requires that cytosolic Ca^{++} levels are reduced to the resting level; this is achieved by Ca^{++}-ATPase, which is most abundant in SR membrane, and pumps Ca^{++} ions from cytosol into SR. The enzyme Ca^{++}ATPase is similar to Na^+, K^+-ATPase and the mechanism of its function is also similar in many ways (Fig.). Two Ca^{++} ions are transported into SR per ATP molecule hydrolysed.

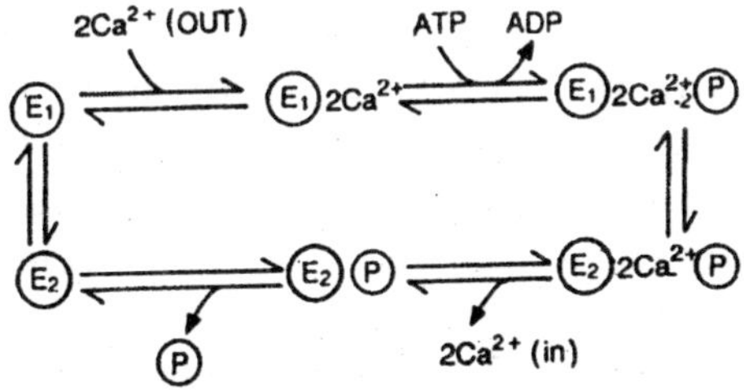

Mechanism for pumping cycle of Ca $^{2+}$***-ATPase from sarcoplasmic reticulum (redrawn from Garrett and Grisham, 1995).***

H^+,K^+-ATPase: In the stomach, a highly acidic environment (pH=0.8 to 1.0) is essential for digestion of food. The pH in the parietal cells of the gastric mucosa is 7.4, thus providing a pH gradient of 6.6, which is maintained by H^+, K^+-ATPase enzyme. This enzyme, through hydrolysis of ATP, pumps H^+ ions out of the mucosal cells into the stomach in exchange for equal number of K^+ ions, thus making the transport electrically neutral as against sodium pump or calcium pumps (described above), which are electrogenic. K^+ ions are pumped back out of the cells together with Cl^- ions, thus together making HCl inside the stomach (Fig.). H^+, K^+-ATPase bears similarities with Na^+, K^+-ATPase and Ca^{++}-ATPase in many ways.

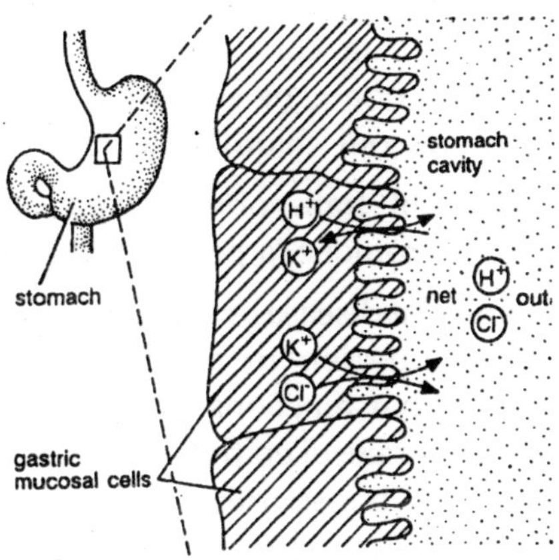

Proton (H^+) and (Cl^-) transport into the stomach mediated by H^+, K^+-ATPase and a K^+/CP co-transport system of gastric mucosal cells with co-transport of K^+ (redrawn from Garrett and Grisham, 1995).

ABC Transporter Superfamily (for Transport of Peptides and Drugs): The ABC transporters represent a class of ATPases (carrier proteins) that were characterised for the first time from bacteria. Atleast 50 such ABC transporters are now known, most of them from prokaryotes. However, an increasing number of ABC transporters are now being discovered from eukaryotes also. Each of these ABC transporter has an 'ATP binding cassette', hence the name ABC transporter (Fig.). These are considered to be of great clinical importance, one of them being responsible for the disease cystic fibrosis. These transporters help in transport of a great variety of substances including amino acids, sugars, inorganic ions, polysaccharides, peptides and even proteins. Following are some examples of ABC transporters:

(i) One of the first eukaryotic ABC transporters was discovered due to its ability to pump hydrophobic drugs out of the eukaryotic cells, and was described as 'multidrug resistance (MDR) protein', whose overexpression makes cancer cells resistant to a variety of drugs used in cancer chemotherapy.

(ii) Malaria parasite *(Plasmodium falciparum)* resistant to antimalaria drug chioroquine was shown to have amplification of a gene encoding an ABC transporter which pumps out chioroquine.

(iii) In yeast, an ABC transporter is responsible for exporting a mating pheromone (a peptide, 13 amino acids long).

(iv) In humans, the disease cystic fibrosis was shown to be due to a mutation in a gene encoding an ABC transporter, that functions as a Cl^- ion channel in the plasma membrane of epithelial cells. It has been shown that some ABC transporters can function both as carrier protein and as ion channel.

Osteoclast H^+ Pump and other H^+ ATPases: Osteoclasts are multinucleate cells that break down bones during normal bone remodelling. H^+ ion transporting ATPases are found in these osteoclasts and help in providing calcium for soft tissues like nerves and muscles. This calcium is released due to pumping of protons (H^+) in an extracellular space created between the bone and the osteoclast. The protons make an acidic solution, which dissolves the bone releasing Ca^{++} ions, CO_3^{2-} ions and calcium phosphate (Fig.).

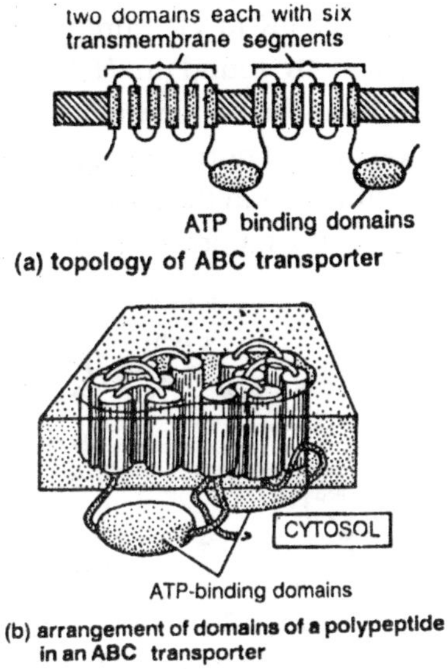

A typical ABC transporter, showing two domains of six transmembrane segments and two ATP-binding catalytic domains (redrawn from Alberts et. al., Molecular Biology of the. Cell, 1994).

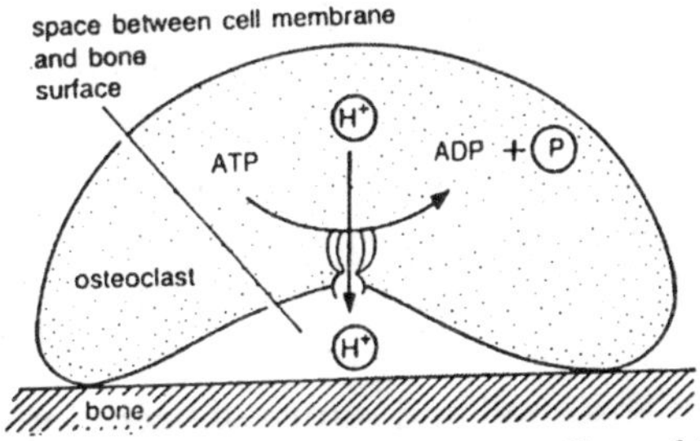

Proton pumps on the border of osteoclast cells used for pumping protons into the space between the cell membrane and the bone surface (redrawn from Garrett and Grisham, 1995).

Proton ATPases also exist in vacuoles, lysosomes, endosomes, Golgi apparatus, coated vesicles, etc., They also occur in yeast and bacteria and perform varied functions, which are beyond the scope of this book.

Light driven Active Transport Systems: Two light driven transport systems, which have been studied in detail include bacteriorhodopsin or bR (a H^+ pump) and halorhodopsin or hR (a Cl^-pump), both found in *Halobacterium halobium,* an archaebacterium that thrives on high-salt media (4.3M NaCl). This organism carries out normal respiration to provide energy, if oxygen is plentiful. But in the absence or shortage of oxygen, bacteriorhodopsin and halorhodopsin capture light

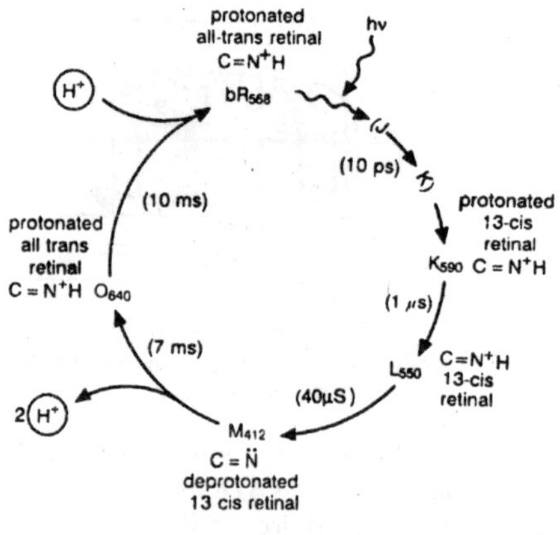

Reaction cycle of bacteriorhodopsin. Intermediate states are indicated by letters, where subscripts represent absorption maxima of the states. All-trans and 13 cis N̈ ***represent configurations of retinal chromophore and C=N or C=*** $\overset{+}{N}$ ***H represent protonation state.***

energy, through transport of protons. Absorption of a photon by bR_{568} form of bacteriorhodopsin converts all trans-configuration to the 13-*cis* isomer. Passage through several intermediate steps results in the outward export of $2H^+$ ions per photon absorbed and return of bacteriorhodopsin to its all trans-configuration. This establishes a proton gradient, later used to drive ATP synthesis and movement of molecules across the cell membrane (Fig.).

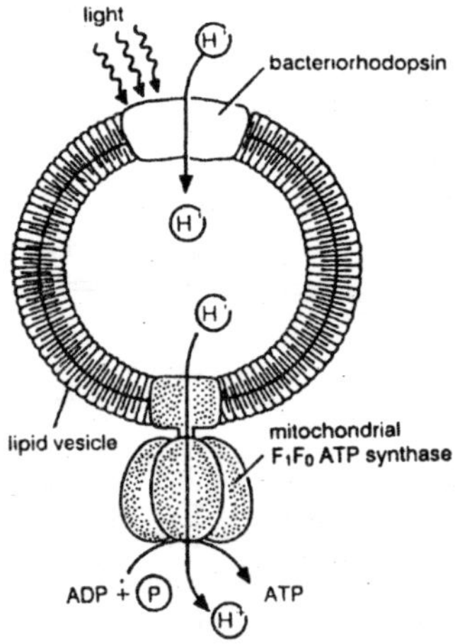

Light-driven proton transport drives the synthesis of ATP in H. lialobium; proton gradient established by bR can be utilised by ATP synthase for synthesis of ATP (redrawn from Garrett and Grisham, 1995).

In addition to outward transport of H^+ ions facilitated by bR_{568}, inward transport of Cl^- is mediated by hR (27kD), which also undergoes light driven conformational changes leading to outward transport of Cl^- (and not H^+ as in case of bR; see Fig.).

Ion-gradient Driven Active Transport Systems: Amino Acid and Sugar Transport (Coupled Transport-symport and Antiport): The gradients of ions (cations or anions) established by ATPase or by light driven transport may lead to 'secondary active transport' of substances like amino acids and sugars. These substances may move along with ions in the same direction (symport), or they may move in opposite directions (antiport). Anion transporter of erythrocytes is an example of antiport, while transports of sugars and amino acids with proton in *E. coli* are examples of proton symport. Na^+-symport for transport of melibiose, glutamate and other amino acids also exists in *E. coli.*

The best example of ion-substrate symport is the transport of lactose (lactose/ H^+ symport) using lactose permease system (LacY), where one molecule of lactose is transported with each

H^+ ion (Fig.). A proton gradient or electrical potential difference or both may be used for the transport of lactose. Lactose permease (47-kD; 417 residues) is an integral membrane protein (Fig.).

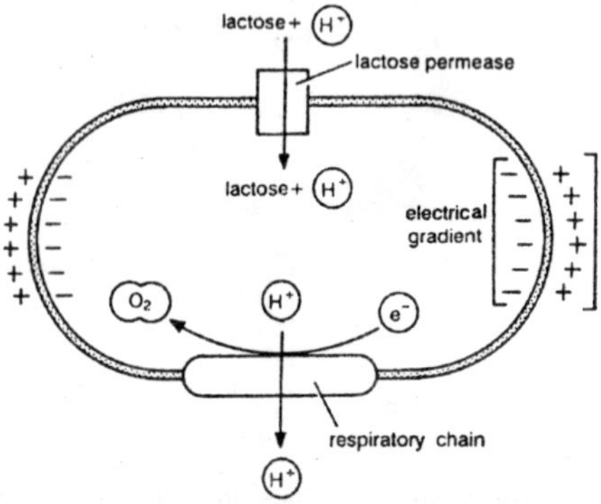

Lactose permease in the E. coli membrane, utilising a proton gradient for transport of lactose into the cell.

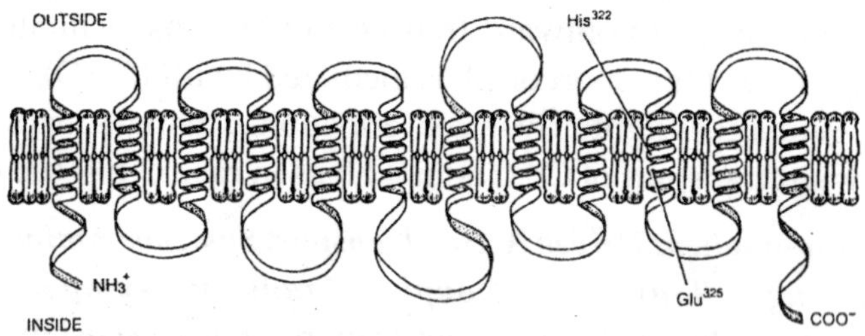

Arrangement of lactose permease in E. coli membrane showing 12 transmembrane segments.

Membrane Conveyance in Bacteria

E. coli, which is a Gram - negative bacterium, has an outer membrane outside the plasma membrane. Both these membranes (outer membrane and plasma membrane) contain transport proteins, which possess transmembrane domains. These domains are beta stands in outer membrane proteins and alpha helices in plasma membrane. The transmembrane α helices constitute membrane transporters, which are often found as a pair of domains, each containing six α helices (6 + 6).

Channels in Outer Membrane: The outer membrane of *E. coli* contains three types of channels (Fig.). (i) Porins (11-12Å in diameter) allow nonspecific passive transport of ions and hydrophobic nutrient molecules. Each *E. coli* cell has nearly 100,000 copies of these proteins which are usually trimeric but can also be monomeric. OmpF (outer membrane protein, F), OmpC, and PhoE of *E. coli* are some examples of porins, which range from 36,000 to 38,000 kD in molecular weight. They are the most abundant proteins in *E. coli* cells and are found as β strands in the outer membrane. (ii) Porin-like proteins contain specific binding sites and carry out facilitated diffusion of some nutrients, which are transported slowly through nonspecific porins. LamB (lambda receptor) of *E. coli* is the best example of porin like trimeric proteins replete with β structure, (iii) TonB-dependent receptors are found in outer membrane and are connected with TonB protein in the cytoplasmic membrane; these are used for transport of large nutrient molecules, which exist in low concentration outside (*e.g.*, vitamin B_{12}, Fe^{3+} chelator complex). FepA protein belongs to this receptor family.

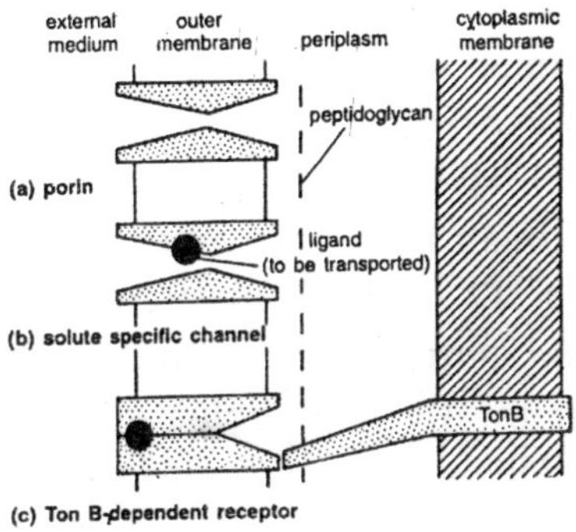

Three types of channels found in the outer membrane of E. coli.

Plasma Membrane Transporters: The transport systems in the plasma membrane are classified according to the nature of their energy source and include the following four types (Fig.). (1) Facilitated diffusion systems. These are represented

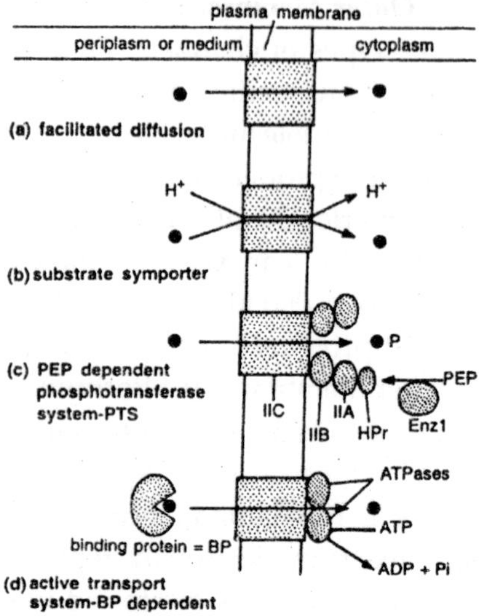

Four types of transport systems found in the plasma membrane of a bacterial cell.

by glycerol facilitator (GlpF), which has 281 residues with six transmembrane α-helices. GlpF has properties like those of channel type transporters and is likely to be gated, so that it opens only when the proper ligand binds at the binding site. (2) Secondary transporters with a 6+6 construction. These are represented by arabinose: H^+ symporter and xylose:H^+ symporter, both having strong sequence similarly to glucose facilitator of human hepatoma cells. The transporters of this class have each 12 hydrophobic transmembrane α-helices, 6 of them at NH_2-terminal end having similarity with another 6 α-helices at the COOH-terminal end (6+6 pattern). This pattern is found in more than 50 transporters in bacteria. There are following five clusters in this superfamily: (i) proteins catalyzing either H^+ symport or facilitated diffusion of sugars; (ii) oligosaccharide:H^+ symporters carrying out accumulation of lactose (LacY), sucrose (ScsB) and raffinose (RafB); (iii) phosphate ester (like hexose-p, glycerol-p and p-glycerate) including phosphate antiporters; (iv) drug resistance proteins which are perhaps drug: H^+ antiporters; (v) citrate: H^+ and α - ketoglutarate:H^+ symporters. LacY (lactose permease) described earlier belongs to this class. (3) PEP-dependent phospho-transferase systems (PTS). These have each a complex composition and involves phosphorylation of Enzyme I by PEP (phosphoenolpyrurate). The Enzyme I then transfers its phosphate to small protein HPr. The enzyme and HPr are then used for the translocation of many sugars. Further steps involve sugar specific Enzyme II with three domains (IIA, IIB, and IIC) of which IIA and IIB become phosphorylated, while IIC is a membrane spanning or channel domain, having 6-8 transmembrane helices as shown for Enzyme II for mannitol. (4) Periplasmic binding protein (BP) dependent systems. These involve transport of sugars, amino acids and ions by initial binding of these substances to periplasmic binding proteins, These transport systems have high affinity for their substrates and contain membrane associated transporter complexes composed of (i) two hydrophobic subunits, and (ii) two hydrophilic subunits which function as ATPases and belong to the class of ABC transporters.

Membrane Excitability in Animals (Neurotransmission and Ion Channels): One of the important characteristics of all living systems is their ability to respond rapidly to stimuli such as sights, sounds, smells, etc. In animals, this will certainly involve movement of muscles and intercellular communications.

These communications need to be very fast, certainly faster than the speed with which blood carrying hormones, or lymph flows in the circulatory system. Nerve impulses can move at a speed of 100m/sec or more and thus fulfil the requirement of quick response to stimuli. These nerve impulses are generated and transmitted through a complicated network connecting every part of the body to the brain, the latter itself having as many as 10^{12} cells.

The nervous system contains specialised receptor proteins in the membranes of excitable cells (cells which can be excited by stimuli). The stimulus causes a conformational change in these receptor proteins or causes a change in permeability of the excitable membranes. These changes in excitable membranes are propagated from one part of the cell to another and from one cell to another in a specific but reversible manner, carrying information from one part of the organism to another. These changes involve regular transport of ions and substances called neurotransmitters.

The progress in our knowledge in this area has been spectacular in recent years. However, since transmission of signals in the nervous system involving transport of ions and neurotransmitters takes place through nerve cells or neurons, a brief account of their structure will be presented here, before discussing the mechanism involved in the transmission of nerve impulses (neurotransmission).

Neurons and Neuroglia (or Glial Cells): Neurons and neuroglia are cell types unique to nervous system. While reception and transmission of nerve impulses are carried out by neurons, the protective and supportive functions are performed by glial cells (neuroglia = nerve glue). A neuron consists of three distinct regions - the cell body (soma), the axon and the dendrites. The cell body contains nucleus and the cell organelles (*e.g.* ER and mitochondria), but axon is simply an extension from the cell body, and so are the dendrites, except that the latter are much smaller in length and are branched, receiving nerve impulses and transmitting them to cell body.

The axon itself is a long (sometimes upto one meter in length) thin structure, whose primary function is to carry nerve impulses from the cell body to cell extremities or termini. Axons of neurons outside the brain, are covered by two layers (outer cellular sheath and the inner myelin sheath) derived from Schwann cells. Gaps between Schwann cells are called nodes of Ranvier, where no sheaths are found (Fig.). The axon terminates in structures called synaptic terminals, synaptic knobs and synaptic bulbs. The space between synaptic terminal of one neuron and a dendrite ending of an adjoining neuron is described as a synapse or synaptic cleft (Fig.).

Neurons can be of three types— (i) sensory neurons which acquire sensory signals, (ii) interneurons connecting one neuron to another neuron and having the function of receiving signals from one neuron and pass it on to another neuron, and (iii) motor neurons, which pass signals from neurons to muscle cells, thus causing muscle movement. In some cases (lower organisms), interneurons are missing, and sensory neurons are connected directly to motor neurons (Fig.).

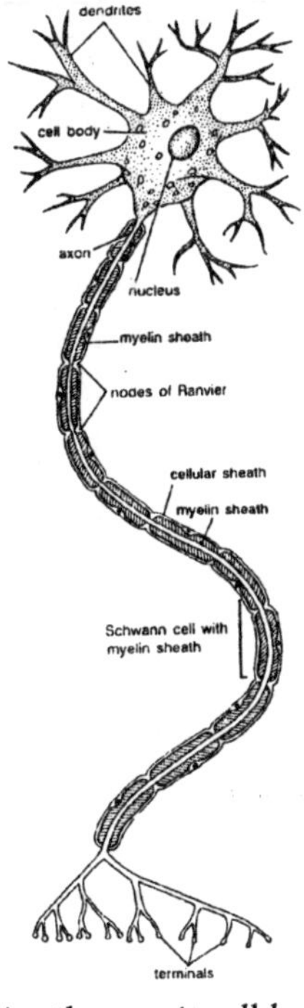

Structure of a neuron showing three parts-cell body, axon and dendrites.

In still other cases (*e.g.*, sea anemones), both interneurons and motor neurons are missing, so that sensory neurons are directly connected to muscle cells.

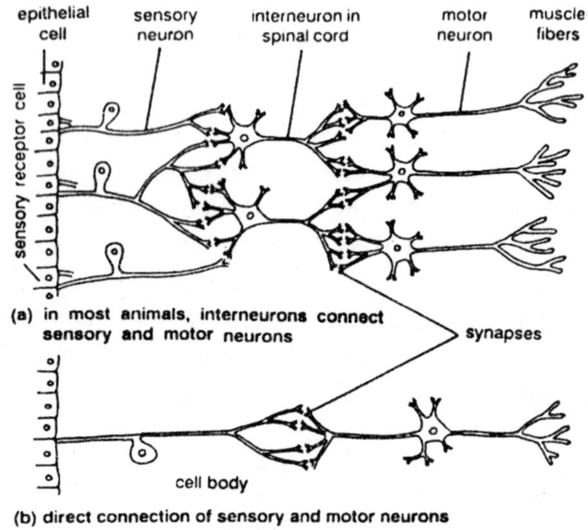

Connections ('synapses') between sensory neurons, interneurons and motor neurons.

Ion Gradients for Transmission of Nerve Impulse or Action Potential: The nerve impulses, also called 'action potentials', are transmitted from neuron to neuron in the form of transient changes in electrical potential differences (voltages) across the membranes of neurons (and other cells).

These potential differences are generated by ion gradients. At the resting stage, a neuron is rich in K^+ (20 times higher inside than outside; Fig.) and poor in Na^+ (9 times lower inside than outside) and Cl^- ions relative to extracellular fluid. This condition is maintained by Na^+, K^+-ATPase system, which sends out three Na^+ ions for every two K^+ ions imported. The potential difference at this resting stage is called 'resting potential' and is approximately -60mV (negative inside), at which no K^+ ions move across the membrane.

It actually ranges from 20mV to 200mV depending upon the organism and the cell type. This potential difference (V) at resting stage can be calculated, using Nernst's equation (expressing equilibrium condition) given below:

$$V = \frac{RT}{zF} l_n \left(\frac{C_2}{C_1}\right)$$

(V = the equilibrium potential in volts, *i.e.* internal potential minus external potential; C_2 and C, are concentrations of ions outside and inside respectively; R = the gas constant = 2 cal $mol^{-1} K^{-1}$; T = absolute temperature ; F = Faraday's constant = 2.3×10^4 cal $V^{-1}mol^{-1}$; z = the valence or charge of the ion; l_n = logarithm to the base e).

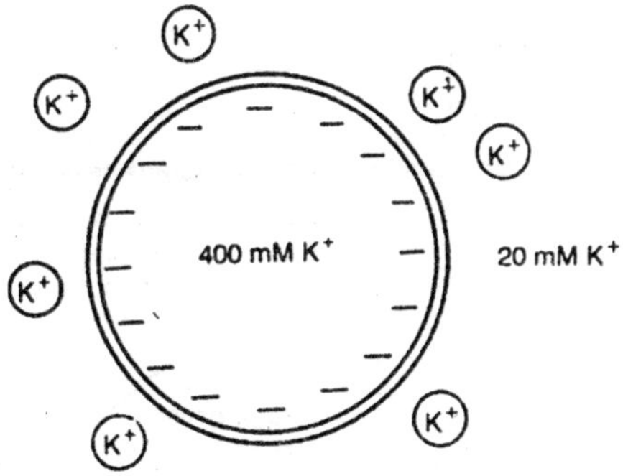

K^+ concentrations inside (400mN) and outside (20mM) a resting axon.

Action potentials are created, when the membrane is locally depolarised by approximately 20mV, changing it from -60mV (resting stage) to -40mV. (This is caused by the action of a neurotransmitter). These changes have a dramatic effect on voltage gated Na^+ and K^+ ion channels that are found on axon membrane throughout its length (Na^+ or K^+ ion channels are also found in other electrically excitable cells like, muscle, endocrine and egg cells), although their density and distribution along the length differ between unmyelinated axons (20 channels per μm^2, distributed uniformly; unmyelinated means myelin sheath absent) and myelinated axons (10,000 channels per μm^2, clustered at nodes of Ranvier). These ion channels remain closed at the resting potential, but the gates of Na^+ channels open at -40mV, so that Na^+ ions begin to flow into the cell along its electrochemical gradient. As Na^+ ions enter the cell, the Na^+ ions depolarise the membranes still further, leading to the opening of additional Na^+ channels, till finally (within a fraction of a second) the potential reaches a value of about +30mV to +50mV. At this stage Na^+ influx slows and stops, because the potential is approaching now the Na^+ equilibrium potential (K^+ equilibrium potential is -60mV; Na^+ equilibrium potential is +30mV). As the Na^+ channels close (Na^+ ion channels have an automatic

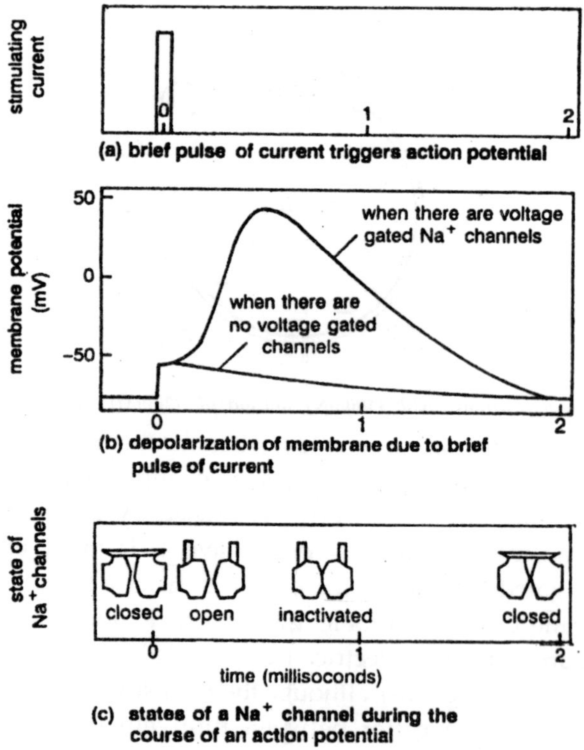

An action potential and its effect on the state of Na^+ channel (redrawn from Alberts et. al., Molecular Biology of the Cell. 1994).

inactivating mechanism), K^+ channels start opening. Now K^+ ions start moving out, ultimately changing the membrane potential to negative value, sometimes even overshooting the resting value of -60mV. At this point, K^+ channels close and resting potential is restored with the help of Na^+, K^+-ATPase (Fig.). These transient increase and decrease first in Na^+ and then in K^+ permeabilities, were first observed by Alan Hodgkin and Andrew Huxley, who shared 1963 Nobel Prize with J. C. Eccles.

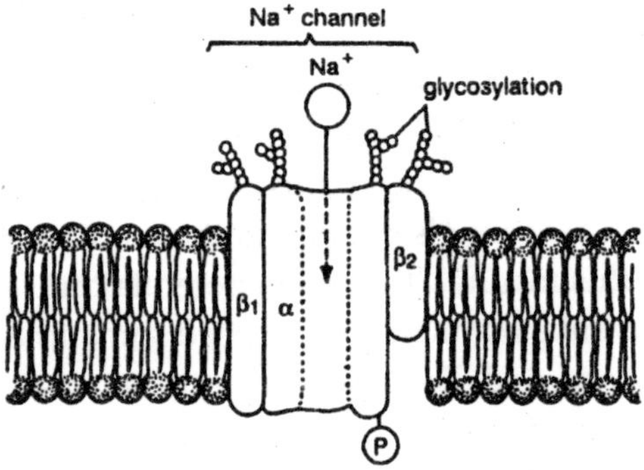

A Na^+ channel consisting of three subunits, α , β_1, β_2.

The changes in membrane potential are rapidly passed along the axonal membrane, so that Na^+ ions entering a

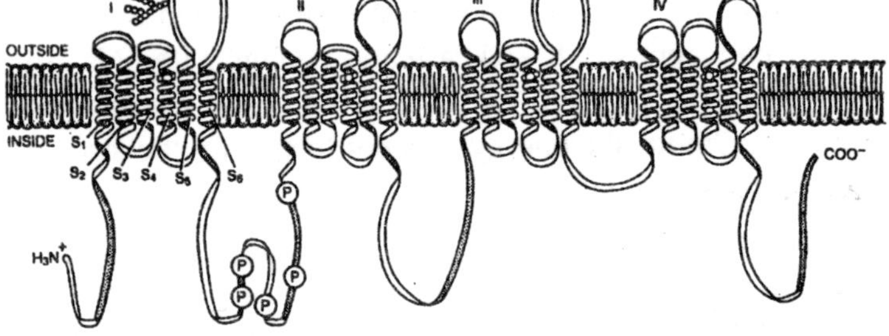

Arrangement of Na^+channel's alpha (α) subunit in the plasma membrane, showing four domains (1-1V), each consisting of six transmembrane alpha (α) helices (S1-S6) (redrawn from Garrett and Grisham, 1995).

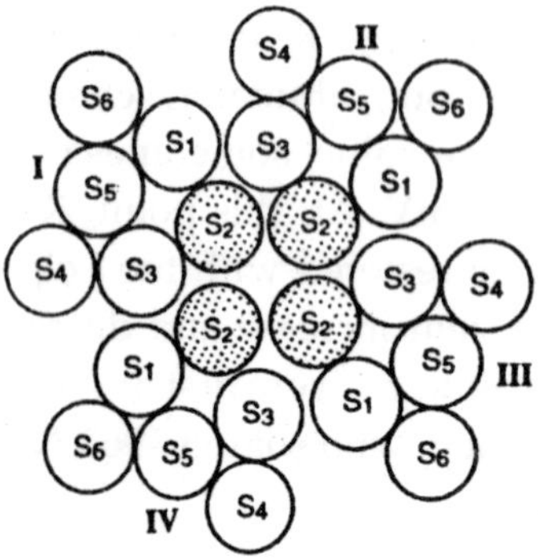

Four membrane spanning domains (I-IV) of Na^+ channel; four helical segments, one from each domain form the wall of the channel.

region in an axon diffuse farther along the axon length. This raises Na^+ concentration there, thus depolarising the membrane and causing Na^+ channels to open in these adjacent regions of the axon. In this manner, the action potential moves down the axon in a wavelike manner, with a speed sometimes exceeding 100 meters per second. The action potential moves only forward and can not move backward, due to inactivated Na^+ channels. The inactivated Na^+ channels are unable to reopen, until a few milliseconds after the membrane returns to its resting potential. Thus the recovery from this inactivated state needs about 10 milliseconds. Furthermore, the action potential is not diminished in intensity, despite travelling long distances (because ion gradient is maintained by Na^+, K^+-ATPase). It has been shown that the action potential is maintained due to an interplay between Na^+, K^+-ATPase and voltage gated Na^+ and K^+ ion channels, initiated by a stimulus at the postsynaptic membrane. Obviously, energy is spent to sustain the strength of the action potential.

A purified Na^+ channel from mammalian brain is a heterotrimer consisting of α-(260kD), β_{1-} (36kD) and β_2-(33kD) subunits, each exposed to extracellular surface and heavily glycosylated (Fig.). β_2 subunit is attached to α-subunit by disulphide bonds. The α–subunit contains four domains of 300-400 amino acids each, with approximately 50% identity (conserved sequences). Each domain has six regions (S1 to S6), each of helical structure spanning the membrane (Fig.). S4 has a sequence, which is highly conserved among Na^+, K^+ and Ca^{++} channels and has the voltage sensing mechanism in voltage gated Na^+ channels. Four S2 segments of an α -subunit form the walls of a Na^+ channel (Fig.).

Voltage gated potassium (K^+) channels have also been identified in many cases. The K^+ channels from rat synaptosomal membranes consist of a α -subunit of 76-80kD and a β -subunit of 38kD. Phosphorylation of the α -subunit leads to activation of K^+ channels. There are six transmembrane segments in α -subunit and the fourth of these six segments has homology with S4 segment (voltage sensor) of Na^+ channel. The arrangement of six transmembrane segments also resembles that of each of the four homologous domains (I to IV) described for Na^+ channel.

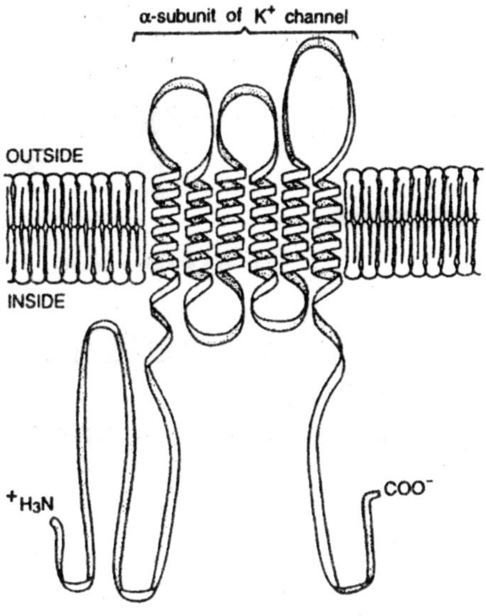

Arrangement of K^+-channel's alpha (α) subunit in the plasma membrane, showing six transmembrane segments.

Myelination and Propagation of Nerve Impulse: Earlier, we mentioned that Na^+ ion channels are more abundant and clustered at nodes of Ranvier in myelinated axons (10,000 channels per μm^2; Fig.). The myelin sheath greatly increases the rate at which, the action potential travels. In myelinated axon, depolarisation at one node of Ranvier is quickly transferred to the next node, so that the action potential really jumps from node to node, a process called saltatory conduction. In this process, action potential travels faster and the metabolic energy is conserved.

A disease 'multiple sclerosis' is actually caused due to demyelination, where myelin sheaths are destroyed in some regions of the central nervous system, due to unknown reasons. In this disease, the propagation of nerve impulse is greatly slowed leading to devastating neurological consequences.

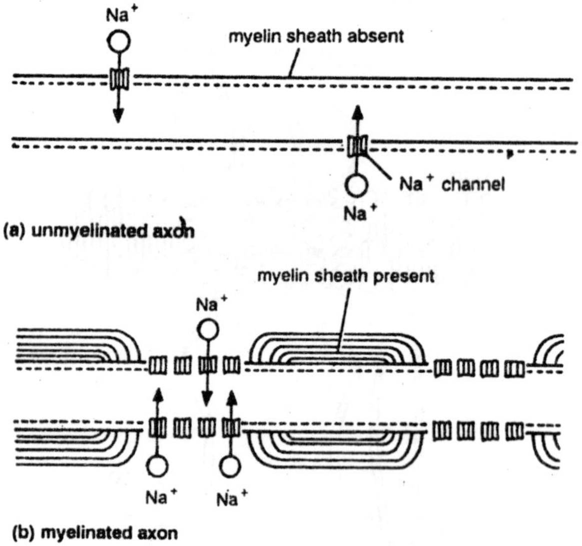

Na^+ channels in unmyelinated axon are infrequent and randomly distributed, but in myelinated axon, they are clustered in large numbers in the nodes of Ranvier between the regions surrounded by myelin sheath (redrawn from Garrett and Grisham. 1995).

Cell-Cell Communication at Synapse: A neuron transmits a signal to another neuron through a synapse and the same neuron may involve in several synapses (1 to 10,000). While in midbrain, there is only one synapse per post-synaptic cell, there may be 10,000 synaptic knobs impinging a single spinal motor neuron. In human forebrain also, the ratio of synapses to neurons is 40,000 : 1.

A List of Some Neurotransmitters.

Sl. no.	*Class of neurotransmitters*	*Neurotransmitters*
1.	Cholinergic agents	Acetylcholine
2.	Catecholamines	Norepinephrine (noradrenaline), epinephrine (adrenaline), L- dopa, dopamine, octopamine
3.	Amino acids and their derivatives	Gamma-aminobutyric acid (GABA), alanine, aspartate, cystathione, glycine, glutamate, histamine, proline, serotonin, taurine, tyrosine
4.	Peptides	Cholecystokinin, enkephalins and endorphins, gastrin, gonadotropin, neurotensin, oxytocin, secretin, somatostatin, substance P, thyrotropin releasing factor (TRF), vasopressin, vasoactive intestinal peptide (VIP)
5.	Gases	Carbon monoxide (CO), nitric oxide (NO)

The synapses may be electrical synapses or chemical synapses. In electrical synapses, the gap between presynaptic and postsynaptic cells is small, only 0.2nm, but in chemical synapse this gap is 20nm - 50nm wide. In electrical synapse, the arrival of action potential at presynaptic membrane leads directly to depolarisation of the postsynaptic membrane, and a new action potential is initiated in the postsynaptic cell. On the other hand, in a chemical synapse, the action potential causes the presynaptic cell to secrete a chemical substance called a neurotransmitter (Table).

This neurotransmitter has an affinity for the receptor located on postsynaptic membrane and therefore binds there, initiating a new action potential. The electrical synapse involves *fast synaptic transmission* that lasts for a short duration. The chemical synapse, on the other hand, involves *slow synoptic transmission,* which lasts for a longer duration and was the subject of Nobel Prize for Medicine for the year 2000 (also Curr. Sci, 10 November, 2000).

Acetylcholine as a Neurotransmitter: In cholinergic synapses, at the synaptic knobs, there are synaptic vesicles containing acetylcholine molecules (approx. 1000 molecules/ vesicle). When the action potential arrives at such a knob, special voltage-gated Ca^{++} channels open and Ca^{++} ions enter the synaptic knob, causing acetylcholine containing vesicles to attach and fuse with the knob membrane.

The vesicles then open and release acetylcholine into the synaptic cleft (space between presynaptic and postsynaptic membranes). Acetylcholine molecules then bind to acetylcholine receptor molecules located in the postsynaptic membrane and cause the opening of Na^+ and K^+ ion channels leading to the generation of action potential in the postsynaptic neuron (Fig.).

Acetylcholine receptor is itself (nicotinic receptor only) an ion channel, which was the first ion channel to be purified and sequenced; it was also the first to be reconstituted in synthetic lipid bilayer and was the first for which electrical signal of a single open channel was recorded.

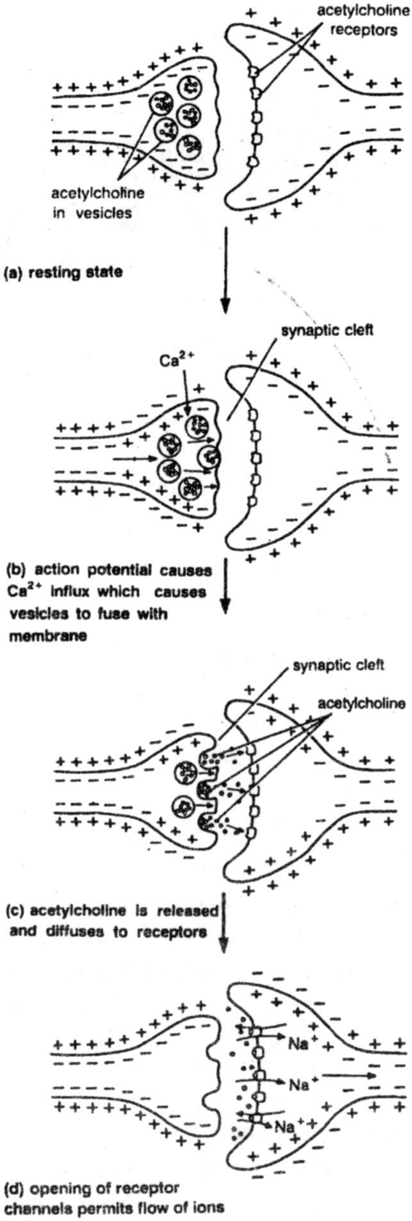

Cell-cell communication in the synapse involving four steps (a-d).

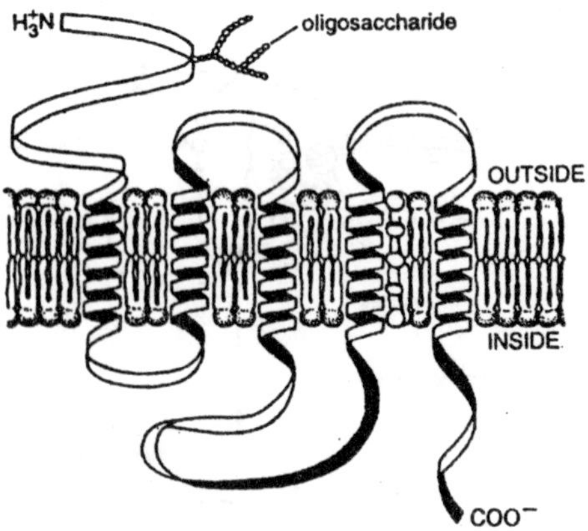

Arrangement of acetylcholine receptor alpha (α) subunit in the post-synaptic membrane.

The fusion of acetylcholine containing vesicles is facilitated by the presence of synapsin-1, a 75kD protein located in the vesicle membrane. This protein binds calmodulin due to influx of Ca^{++} (calmodulin is regulated by Ca^{++}) and gets phosphorylated due to a kinase enzyme leading to the fusion of vesicles with the knob membrane.

Acetylcholine receptors found in postsynaptic membranes can be muscarinic receptors (stimulated by muscarine) or nicotinic receptors (stimulated by nicotine). The former (found in smooth muscles and glands) are transmembrane proteins, that interact with G proteins and the latter (found in sympathetic ganglia and motor end plates of skeletal muscle) are ligand gated cation channels. Nicotinic acetylcholine receptor is a transmembrane glycoprotein of 270kD molecular mass and consisting of five subunits $\alpha_2\beta\gamma\delta$. Each subunit includes five hydrophobic regions, which span the membrane in helical form.

Each subunit has a binding site for acetylcholine (Figs.). Nicotine locks the ion channels of nicotinic receptors in their open configuration. When acetylcholine (the ligand) binds nicotinic acetylcholine receptor, a conformational change opens the channels (Fig.), which is equally permeable to Na^+ and K^+, the former rushing in and latter rushing out. Since the Na^+ gradient is steeper, Na^+ influx greatly exceeds K^+ efflux.

The Na^+ influx depolarises the membrane initiating an action potential. Muscarinic receptors are 70-kD glycoproteins and are members of the 7-transmembrane segment (7-TMS) family of receptors. Binding of acetylcholine to these receptors, through interaction with G proteins, leads to inhibition of adenyl cyclase, stimulation of phospholipase C and opening of K^+ channels (Fig.). Several toxins including insecticides/pesticides and nerve gases (used in chemical warfare) actually affect the above acetylcholine receptors and lead to block in nerve impulses, stop breathing and cause death by suffocation.

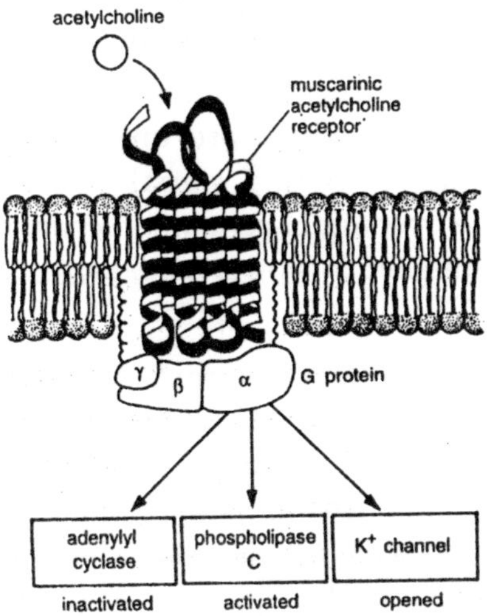

Muscarinic acetylcholine receptor consisting of seven transmembrane segments, and its binding to G-protein causing inactivation of adenyl cyclase, activation of phospholipase C and opening of K^+ channel (redrawn from Gerrett and Grisham, 1995).

After every cycle of synaptic signal transmission, acetylcholine is degraded with the help of acetylcholinesterase enzyme to resensitise the acetylcholine receptor. The synaptic vesicles are formed again by endocytosis and restocked with freshly formed acetylcholine (acetylcholine enters through H^+ pump with the help of acetylcholine transport protein; this H^+ pump is a V-type-ATPase) to start another cycle of nerve impulse transmission.

The Effect of Cl^- Channels: The concentration of Cl^- ions is much higher outside the cells than in the cytosol (Table). Therefore, when the channel opens, more Cl^- ions will move inside due to concentration gradient and hyperpolarise the membrane (interior being already negatively polarised at the resting stage), unless the membrane potential stops such a flow. This leads to excitation of the cell.

G-protein Linked Receptors and Enzyme-linked Receptors: Many of the signaling molecules that are secreted by axon terminals (*e.g.*, neuropeptides) regulate ion channels only indirectly. These neurotransmitters or signaling molecules bind to receptors, which are linked to G-protein or an enzyme inside, initiating signal transduction pathway leading to the opening of certain ion channels. This action or signal transmission is slower and more complex and lasts longer.

Psychoactive Drugs Attack Neurotransmitter-gated Channels: Although the different neurotransmitter-gated ion channels have structural and functional similarity, there is sufficient diversity among these channels to allow designing of drugs having specificity for individual channels. This basic principle has allowed in practice to design drugs targeted against narrowly defined group of neurons and their synapses, thus influencing specific brain functions. 'Curare' is a drug which blocks acetylcholine receptors on skeletal muscle, so that it can be used by a surgeon for keeping a muscle relaxed during operation.

Most other drugs used for treatment of diseases like insomnia, anxiety, depression and schizophrenia exert their influence at chemical synapses through binding transmitter gated ion channels. Two other drugs, 'valium' and 'librium' used as barbiturates and tranquilisers bind to GAB$\bar{A}$ receptors, potentiating the inhibitory effect of GABA, so that lower concentration of GABA is allowed to bind to receptors to open Cl^- channels. As more information about ion channels is becoming available, new generation of psychoactive drugs to alleviate the miseries of mental illness will become available.

Muscle Contraction Involves Sequential Activation of Five Different Ion Channels: When a nerve impulse stimulates a muscle cell to contract, the events take place in the following sequence involving five different ion channels:

(i) When the nerve impulse as an action potential, reaches axon terminals and depolarises the plasma membrane there, it transiently opens voltage-gated Ca^{++} channels, so that Ca^{++} ions flow inside due to a concentration gradient. Increase in Ca^{++} ions in the cytosol leads to release of acetylcholine from synaptic vesicles.

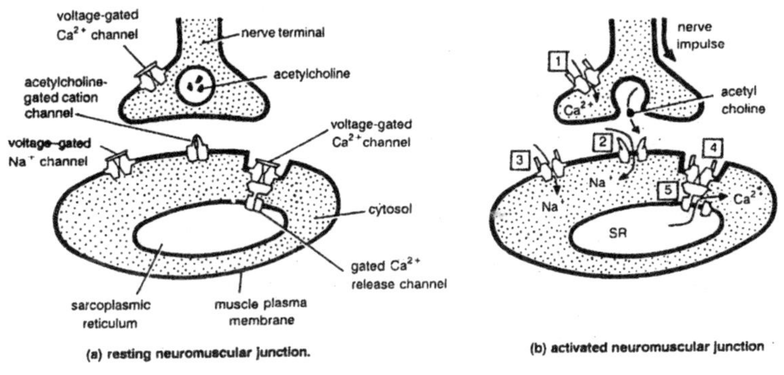

A system of ion-channels at neuromuscular junction involved in muscle contraction (redrawn from Alberts et. al., Molecular Biology of the Cell, 1994).

(ii) Acetylcholine binds to acetylcholine receptors in the muscle, opening the Na^+ channels associated with receptors, allowing more Na^+ to enter the cytosol of muscle cell, causing localised depolarisation.

(iii) Localised depolarisation opens voltage gated Na^+ channels permitting entry of more Na^+ ions into the cytosol of muscle cell causing further depolarisation; this leads to opening of more voltage-gated Na^+ channels and the action potential propagates involving the entire plasma membrane of muscle cell.

(iv) The depolarisation of entire plasma membrane of muscle cell activates voltage-gated Ca^{++} channels in specialised regions. This causes release of Ca^{++} within the cytosol; this then causes opening of gated Ca^{++} release channels of sarcoplasmic reticulum (SR) to release stored Ca^{++} ions, thus increasing Ca^{++} concentration in the cytosol. This causes myofibrils in the muscle to contract.

6

Significance of Membrane

Eukaryotic cells have developed an elaborate internal membrane system. This membrane system allows eukaryotic cells *firstly,* to take up macromolecules from cell surface by a process called endocytosis (sometimes involving 'coated pits' and 'caveolae'), forming structures called endosomes and *secondly,* to throw out substances by a process called exocytosis through structures called vesicles. The endosomes, in their turn, either deliver the macromolecules to lysosomes for digestion or throw them back to the cell surface for reuse (Fig.).

The pathway involving endosomes is described as endocytic pathway. Besides this endocytic pathway, eukaryotic cells also have means of delivering newly synthesised proteins and carbohydrates to the exterior (by the above mentioned process called exocytosis) or from one compartment to another through a pathway, which together with exocytosis is described as biosynthetic secretory pathway, involving multiple compartments of the cell (Fig.). Thus the biosynthetic secretory pathway includes not only exocytosis, but also the transport between ER and Golgi (both ways) and also the transport from Golgi to lysosomes.

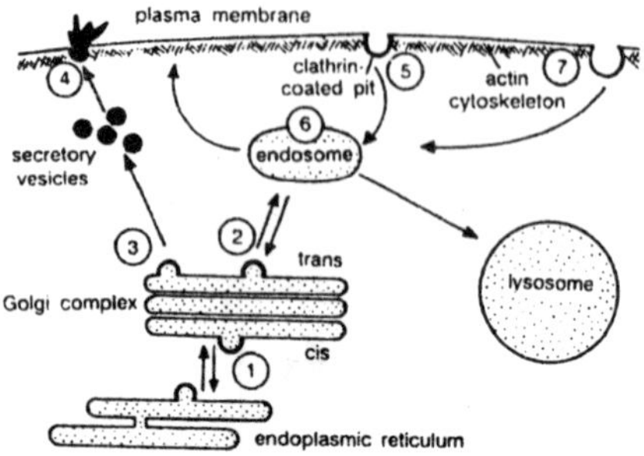

The role of endosomes and vesicles in endocytosis and exocytosis (redrawn from Science, 12 April, 1996).

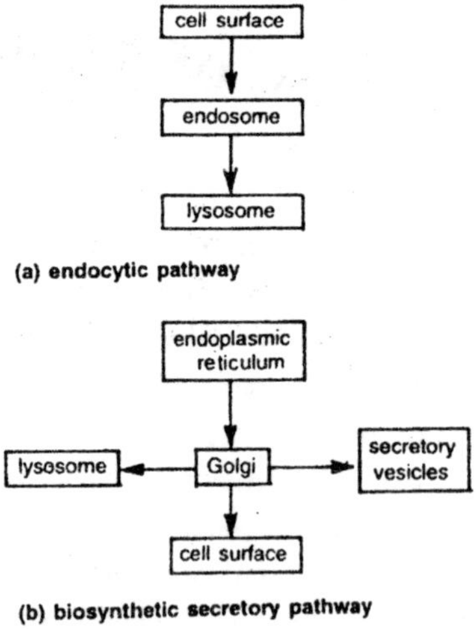

Outlines of endocytic and biosynthetic secretory pathways in a eukaryotic cell.

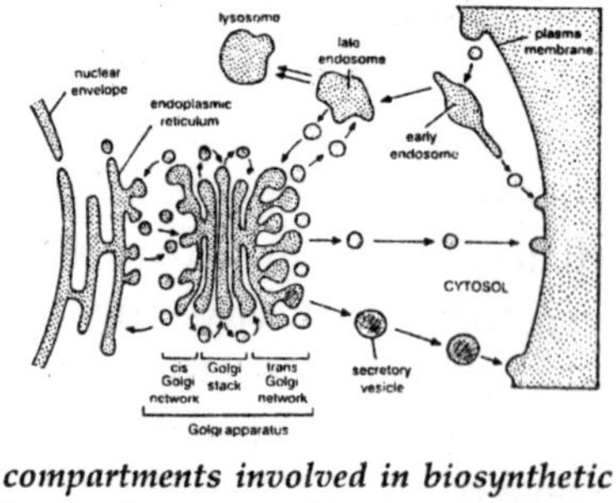

Intracellular compartments involved in biosynthetic secretory and endocytic pathways, by means of transport vesicles (redrawn from Alberts et. al., Molecular Biology of the Cell, 1994).

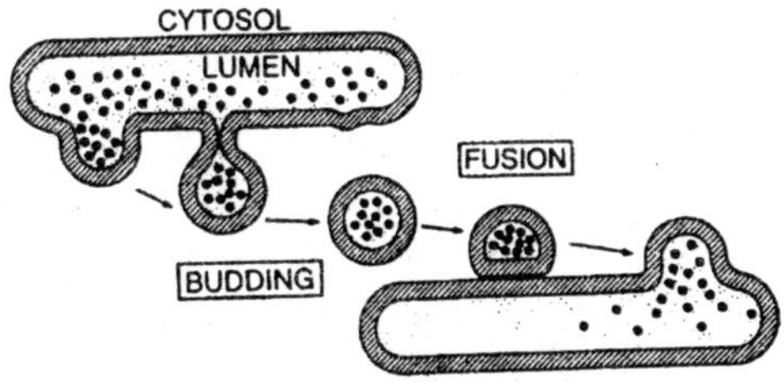

Vesicle transport involving budding off from one compartment and fusion with another compartment.

In endocytic as well as in biosynthetic secretory pathways, different compartments send material to one another, by means of numerous transport vesicles, which continuously bud off from membrane of one compartment and fuse with that of another (Figs.). This transport with the help of vesicles differs from transmembrane transport from cytosol to various organelles (involving a variety of channels), and also from two way gated transport between cytosol and the nucleus (involving nuclear pore). This chapter is devoted to this vesicular traffic involved in endocytosis and secretory pathways.

Protein Sorting and Vesicular Conveyance

Earlier it was believed that cargo from ER to Golgi was transported through vesicles using a default pathway, requiring no transport signals. However recently (after 1995), it was shown that transport signals are needed for this traffic at least in some cases. This cargo carried by vesicles first appears as pre-Golgi intermediates (PGI), which move on microtubule tracks to the *cis*-Golgi region. As the cargo moves through the stack of Golgi cisternae, it is modified by Golgi associated processing enzymes and reach the *trans*-Golgi surface, where sorting of cargo for various extracellular destinations takes place.

Recent work suggested that cargo-containing ER-derived vesicles, which first appear as PGI, actually form the early Golgi compartments or *cis*-Golgi, which mature gradually

Examples of Some known Transport Signals
(K, Lys; D, Asp; E, Glu; L, Leu; R, Arg; Y, Tyr; Q, Gln; N, Asn; P, Pro; X, any amino acid; from Rothman and Weiland, 1966)

Signal	*Location in protein and with respect to membrane*	*Fate specified*
KDEL	COOH-terminus, luminal	Retrieval of proteins from Golgi to ER
KKXX	COOH-terminus, in cytoplasm	Retrieval of membrane proteins from Golgi to ER
XXRR	NH_2-terminus, in cytoplasm	Retrieval of membrane proteins from Golgi to ER
Propeptide	NH_2-terminus, luminal	Transport from Golgi to endosomes or lysosomes
Mannose 6-phosphate	Asn-linked oligosaccharides, luminal	Transport from Golgi to endosomes or lysosomes
Tyrosine-rich dileucine	Cytoplasmic domain	Transport from Golgi to endosomes or lysosomes
YQRL	Cytoplasmic domain	Transport from cell surface to Golgi
tfPXY (and similar)	Cytoplasmic domain	Transport from cell surface to endosomes

into late compartments by retrieval of the processing enzymes and the post-Golgi sorting determinants. This has been described as directed maturation of Golgi compartments, or "cisternal progression" model, which received support from the demonstration that retrograde transport from Golgi to ER does take place. The transport of large cargo complexes (too big to be carried by the vesicles, *e.g.*, procollagen precursors) from ER to Golgi and from *cis* Golgi to *trans*-Golgi without the aid of vesicles gave further support to this hypothesis.

A protein actually may or may not enter a vesicle budding from the ER. This choice is exercised with the help of a sorting signal which may consist of a discrete peptide domain (4-25 residues) or may be a conformationally determined epitope. A protein can also have multiple signals, each specifying the fate of the protein at one of the different successive steps during the journey of protein transport. Depending upon these sorting signals, there can be as many as three potential fates for a given protein using the vesicular traffic for its transport (Fig.).

(i) The membrane bound cargo protein may have a transport signal which may reside either on the cytoplasmic side or on the luminal side of the ER membrane taking part in vesicle formation. In the former case the signal binds directly to a coat protein and in the latter it binds to a receptor, whose cytoplasmic domain contains a transport signal which in its turn binds to coat protein (Fig.). A classical example of such a receptor is low density lipoprotein (LDL) receptor which is packaged into clathrin-coated vesicle and helps in the transport of LDL particles from plasma membrane into the cell. In this mode of vesicular transport, the concentration of the cargo protein in the vesicle will be higher than in the donor compartment (*e.g.*, ER).

(ii) The protein may have a retention signal that specifies lack of movement as shown above; such proteins may sometimes escape into the vesicle (Fig.) and are then transported to Golgi, but are retrieved back due to retention signal with the help of a receptor in the Golgi. In this mode of transport, the concentration of cargo is low in the vesicle.

(iii) The protein may lack both transport and retention signals and enter a vesicle at its prevailing concentration thus following default pathway (Fig.). Transport of cargo across Golgi stack appears to occur by such a bulk flow. It is thus obvious that the transport from ER to Golgi like other transport pathways may involve a transport signal or a retention signal or a default pathway. It has also been shown that the export from ER is generally mediated by a multiple of low efficiency signals that must bind simultaneously to multiple low affinity receptors. Thus the transport from ER to Golgi differs from other transport pathways which require each a single transport signal.

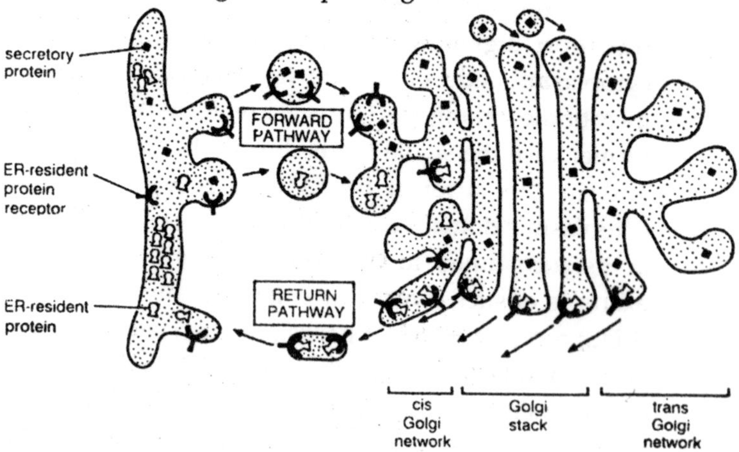

Mechanism to retain resident proteins in ER, using a retention signal (KDEL).

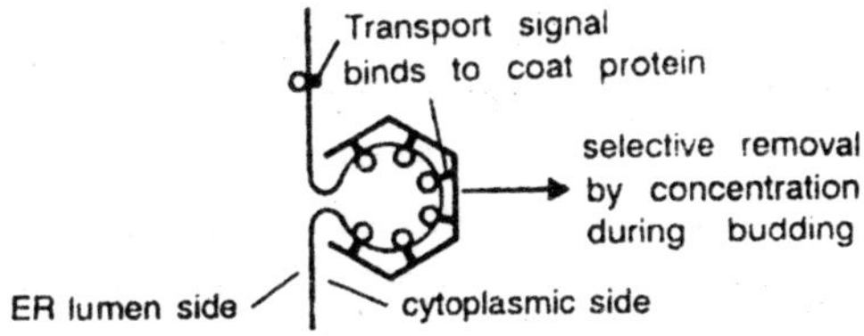

(a) transport signal binds to coat protein directly

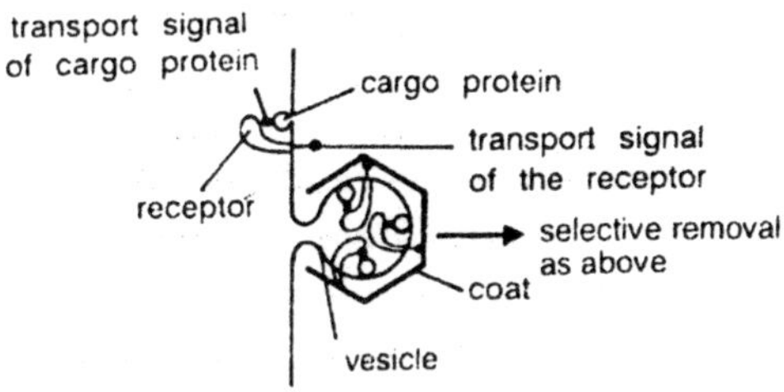

(b) transport signal binds to coat protein indirectly through a receptor

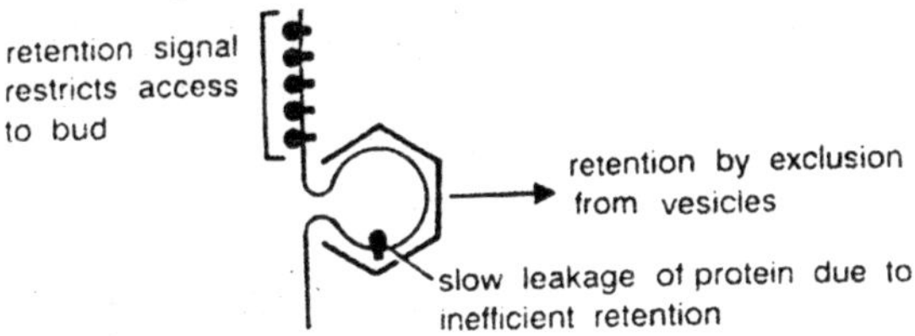

(c) retention signal restricts access to bud

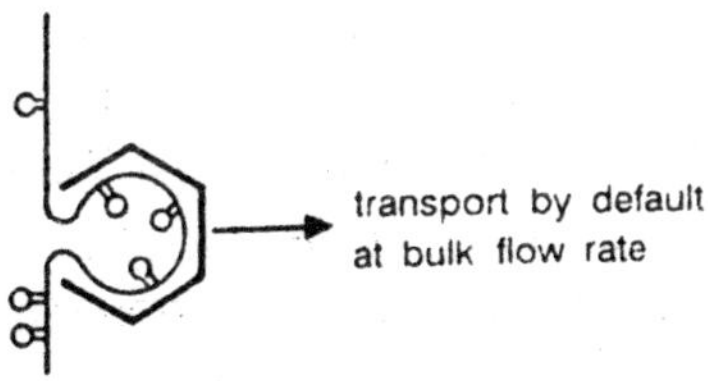

(d) no signal in protein (bulk flow by default)

Three possible fates of a given protein using vesicular traffic for its transport, depending upon the signal the protein possesses.

Retrograde Conveyance

The ER and Golgi retain their own distinct sets of proteins. However, the integral membrane proteins of ER and Golgi as well as the soluble proteins in the lumen of ER may escape in departing vesicles but are then returned to the donor compartment by retrograde transport. As mentioned above, presence of the sequence KDEL at the -COOH terminus helps retrieval of a protein from Golgi to ER with the help of a KDEL receptor. Similarly KKXX at the COOH terminus or XXRR at the amino-terminus also helps the retrograde movement of the membrane protein of ER (K=lysine; R=arginine; D=aspartic acid; L=glutamic acid; X=any amino acid).

Transport from Cis-Golgi to Trans Golgi:Flow Pattern in Golgi Stack, as a Distillation Tower (Anterograde and Retrograde Transport): After transport from ER to the cis face of the Golgi, the cargo is transported from cis face to the trans face of the Golgi. During this process, the cargo may also be retrieved back either from the first Golgi cisterna or from any of the successive cisternae through which the cargo transported from ER to Golgi passes from cis face to the trans face of the Golgi. This is possible because KDEL receptor is present in all cisternae as a gradient with highest concentration at the cis face.

This retrograde transport from Golgi to ER may follow one of the following two patterns (Fig.): (i) cross current flow, which assumes direct traffic from each cisterna of Golgi to ER, and (ii) counter current flow, which assumes percolation of cargo backwards layer to layer, so that any resident proteins of Golgi may get a chance to be retained in these cisternae (this will not be possible in cross current flow). It is possible that the cross current flow and counter current flow coexist in the Golgi, thus serving different purposes.

It has also been shown that the cells have the capacity to retrieve back the escaped ER proteins at every level of Golgi stack. In other words, if a protein escapes retrieval in the first cisterna, it can be captured in the next one and so on. An analogy, therefore, has been drawn between Golgi stack and distillation tower used by chemists to separate the components of liquid mixture. The Golgi stack can function as a distillation tower both in cross current flow and counter current flow. In any case, the proteins meant for retrieval should be concentrated at cis face and its concentration should gradually decrease towards trans face, which is consistent with the known gradient of KDEL receptor having its highest concentration at the cis face and lowest concentration at the trans face. Such a distribution is expected if distillation tower hypothesis is accepted for Golgi stack. In this distillation tower hypothesis, ER may also be regarded as the first plate of the distillation tower, greatly expanded in surface area as compared to other plates *i.e.* cisternae of Golgi.

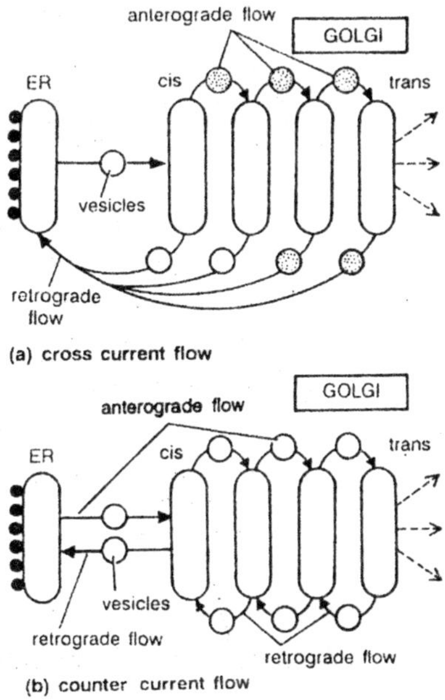

Two likely membrane flow patterns in the Golgi stack, which functions like a distillation tower.

Transport from the Trans-Golgi Network (TGN) to Lysosomes: The proteins, which are received in the Golgi apparatus from ER may be resident proteins or secretory proteins. The resident proteins are retained in Golgi as permanent residents, but the secretory proteins are sorted out in the trans-Golgi network (TGN) according to their final destination. The most important of these proteins (digestive enzymes) are those which are destined to be transported to the lysosomes.

Lysosomal hydrolases (containing N-linked oligosaccharides; N=Asn=asparagine) and membrane proteins for lysosomes are synthesised on the rough ER and transported to lysosomes through Golgi by means of transport vesicles which bud out from trans-Golgi network. There are mechanisms available which selectively sort out lysosomal proteins for transport to lysosomes. Mannose 6- phosphate (M6P) groups (as markers) are added to the N-linked oligosaccharides (N=Asn or asparagine) of the enzymes destined for lysosomes, when they are still in the cis-Golgi network. M6P is recognised by M6 receptors present as transmembrane proteins, in trans-Golgi network.

These receptors later help packaging enzymes in transport vesicles destined to be fused with 'late endosomes' or lysosomes'. The M6P receptor proteins, after delivery of enzymes to lysosomes, dissociate from enzymes (due to low pH) and return to trans-Golgi network via transport vesicles and used again there. The pH of lysosomes is maintained at 5.0 through an ATP-driven H^+ pump in the lysosomal membrane.

Transport from the Trans-Golgi Network to the Cell Surface (Exocytosis): Secretory Vesicles for Transport of Secretory Proteins: In the secretory pathways, a number of molecules are also directly secreted out of the cell. The process is called exocytosis and starts at the Golgi apparatus. The transport vesicles or secretory vesicles carrying the cargo to be exported leave the trans-Golgi network (TGN) in a steady stream. However, instead of merging with lysosomes, these vesicles arrive at the cell surface and fuse with the plasma membrane there. These transport vesicles carry lipids and hydrophobic membrane proteins for assembly of plasma membrane. They also carry secretory soluble proteins for regulated secretion of substances like hormones or neurotransmitters, etc. Most of the proteoglycans and glycoproteins of the extracellular matrix (ECM) are also secreted by this process (Fig.).

The secretory pathways comprising the above vesicular traffic may either involve constitutive secretion occurring in all cells or may involve regulated secretion occurring in cells specialised for secreting specific products. Examples of housekeeping exocytosis (which occurs continuously in all cells) include export of materials like hormones (insulin, epinephrine), enzymes (invertase, trypsin) or building blocks like collagen and proteoglycan. The examples of regulated exocytosis (which occurs in specialised cells, whenever required), on the other hand, include sperm acrosome, oocyte cortical granules, secretions of endocrine/exocrine cells, and neurotransmitters.

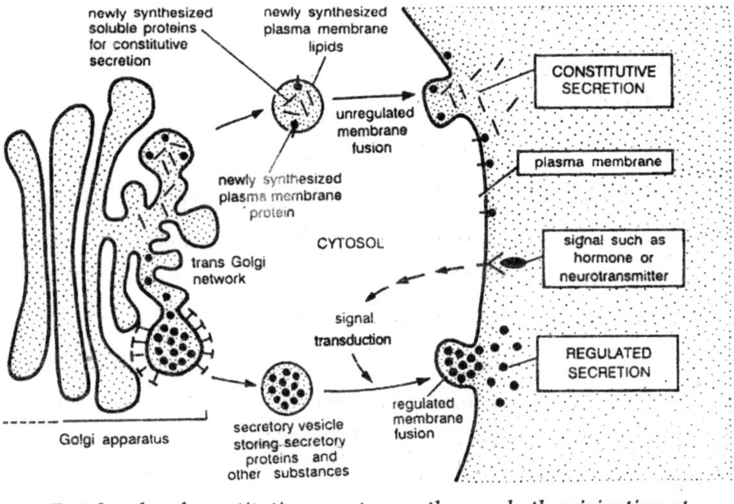

Regulated and constitutive secretory pathways, both originating at trans-Golgy network (redrawn from Alberts et. al., Molecular biology of the Cell, 1994).

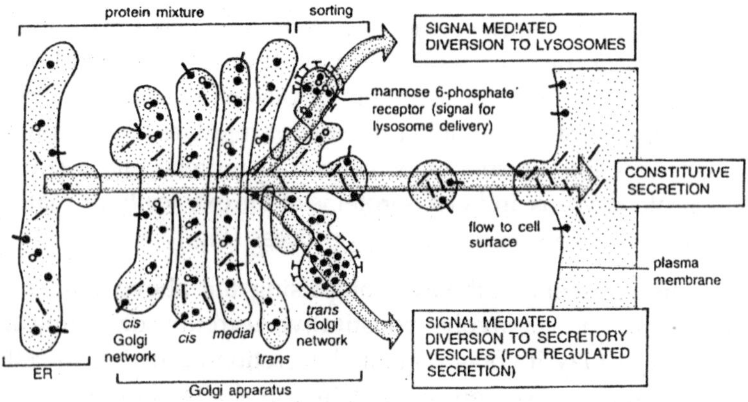

Three pathways of protein sorting in trans-Golgi network (i) including two signal mediated pathways and a constitutive pathway, (redrawn from Alberts et. al., Molecular Biology of the Cell, 1994).

Exocytosis of most cell granules has recently been studied in some detail and led to the development of the concept of 'fusion pore'. The regulated secretion takes place rapidly, but only on demand, so that the products are stored in the secretory vesicles (often called secretory granules or dense core vesicles), till there is a demand. Another characteristic of secretory vesicles is, that once loaded, it reaches the site of secretion (often plasma membrane), where it waits, until the cell receives signal to secrete. Products like hydrolases destined for lysosomes are tagged by M6P and then packaged into another class of specialised vesicles. Secretory vesicles are formed due to clathrin coated budding from trans-Golgi network. After the immature secretory vesicles bud off from Golgi, their clathrin coat is removed and contents become greatly condensed (upto 200 fold) as a result of acidification due to ATP-driven H^+ pump.

In summary, there are three types of secretory vesicles budding off from *trans* golgi network; *first,* for constitutive secretion on cell surface, *second,* for regulated secretion on cell surface and the *third,* form transport of products to lysosomes (Fig.). In addition to these pathways, there may be additional pathways in polarised cells, where different products need to be delivered to different domains on the cell surface. These pathways are slightly more complex.

Several secretory proteins are actually synthesised as inactive protein precursor molecules, from which active molecules are produced by proteolysis. These inactive precursors may be synthesised as pre-pro-proteins. "Pre-piece", consisting of ER signal peptide, is cleaved off earlier in rough ER and "pro-piece" is cleaved off shortly before secretion to yield mature active protein. Some polyproteins, carrying multiple copies of same amino acid sequence, are also synthesised for signals. This process also prevents a secretory protein from acting prematurely before it is secreted to perform its function.

As indicated above, a secretory vesicle, once loaded with a secretory protein reaches the cell surface and waits there till a signal is received. Sometime, this site of secretion is far away from Golgi as in case of nerve cells. In these nerve cells, vesicles, carrying secretory proteins such as peptide neurdtransmitters, are made in Golgi of cell body. These secretory vesicles secrete the contents (peptide neurotransmitters) at the tip of axon after travelling a distance of upto one metre. This journey is facilitated by motor proteins on the surface of the secretory vesicles, which propel themselves along axonal microtubules. Similar situation exists in polarised epithelial cells.

At the nerve axon termini, the secretory vesicles receive a signal initiated in the form of a chemical messenger such as hormone, which binds to the receptor on cell surface. Activation of receptor generates intracellular signals, often involving increase in Ca++ ion concentration. In case of nerve cell, the signal is an action potential triggered by a chemical transmitter binding to receptors elsewhere on the cell surface. Action potential causes an influx of Ca^{++} ions through 'voltage gated Ca^{++} channels'. This then triggers exocytosis, causing secretory vesicles to fuse with plasma membrane and release their contents to the extracellular space.

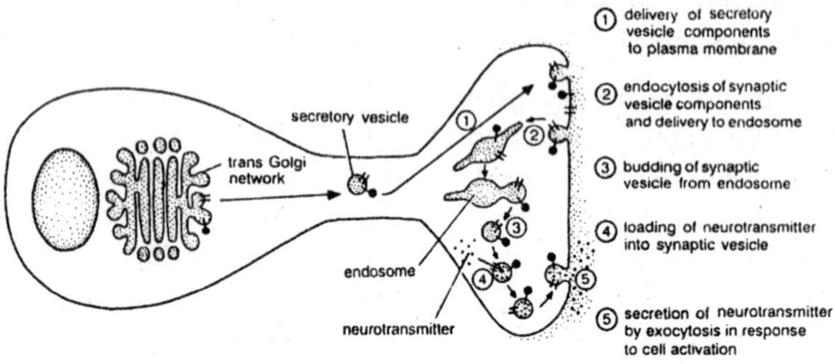

The formation of synaptic vesicle for secretion of neurotransmitters (redrawn from Alberts et. al., Molecular Biology of the Cell, 1994).

Synaptic Vesicles for Transport of Neurotransmitters: In the nerve cells, there is another class of specialised tiny synaptic vesicles (50nm in diameter), which originate from endosomes near the axon termini and carry neurotransmitter molecules (*e.g.* acetylcholine, glutamate, and gamma aminobutyric acid or GABA) to the synaptic cleft.

These neurotransmitters allow rapid signaling from cell to cell through chemical synapses. When an action potential arrives, these tiny synaptic vesicles release their contents within fraction of a millisecond.

Synaptic vesicles are retrieved back again by endocytosis to form endosomes. From these endosomes, vesicles bud off again to form synaptic vesicles, which may have carrier proteins in their membrane to assist in collecting neurotransmitter from the cytosol, where it is synthesised. This cycle continues between plasma membrane at axon termini and the endosomes found at the axon end, through the traffic of these synaptic vesicles involved in neurotransmission (Fig.).

Defects in synaptic transmission lead to several neurological disorders like Parkinsonism. In view, of this, it was the subject of the 2000 Nobel Prize in Physiology or Medicine awarded to Arvid Carlsson, Paul Greengard and Eric Kandel (for details, see Curr. Sci. 10 November, 2000).

Import of 'Annexins' in Exocytosis

During 1970s, a protein 'synexin' was identified, which helped in vesicle-plasma membrane contact, followed by fusion of vesicle membrane with plasma membrane. Later it was found that 'synexin' (now called annexin VII) is only one of the several proteins that bind to lipid membranes in a calcium dependent manner.

These proteins were called annexins. Although annexins are involved in a variety of intracellular trafficking events, they play an important role in membrane fusion and in pore formation during exocytosis. Annexin molecules of one membrane interact with annexin molecules of the second membrane, causing fusion of membranes. The channel forming property, of annexins also causes the formation of an exocytotic pore. This will lead to the expansion of the area of plasma membrane due to incorporation of membrane of the secretory vesicle.

Transport from Plasma Membrane via Endosomes: Endocytosis: Material to be transported from outside to the interior of the cell is progressively enclosed in a small portion of plasma membrane by formation of an invagination, which later pinches off as an intracellular vesicle. When the ingested material consists of macromolecules, the vesicles are described as endosomes but when this material consists of large particles or microorganisms, the vesicles are described as phagosomes. The phenomenon in both cases is described as endocytosis.

Endocytosis is also classified in (i) pinocytosis ('cellular drinking'), which involves ingestion of fluid and solutes, making vesicles 150nm in diameter and (ii) phagocytosis ('cellular eating'), which involves ingestion of large particles making vesicles measuring 250nm in diameter. While pinocytosis is a continuous process, phagocytosis is a triggered process. The best example of triggers in phagocytosis is antibodies which bind antigens and are then recognised by some receptors found on the surface of macrophages and neutrophils, the professional phagocytes in mammalian blood.

Pinocytic vesicles are often returned to the cell surface after delivering its contents to the interior of the cell, thus making a part of plasma membrane. In this sense, endocytosis and exocytosis often constitute an 'endocytic-exocytic cycle'. The endocytic part of this cycle often begins at regions called clathrin coated pits, which are formed to take up specific macromolecules, and within a minute are pinched off as clathrin coated vesicles.

These vesicles are formed at the rate of 2500/minute, which shed their coats within seconds and fuse with early endosomes. This phenomenon of endocytosis mediated by clathrin is described as 'receptor mediated endocytosis'. Clathrin coated secretory vesicles are also, formed from trans-Golgi network and are then involved in exocytosis.

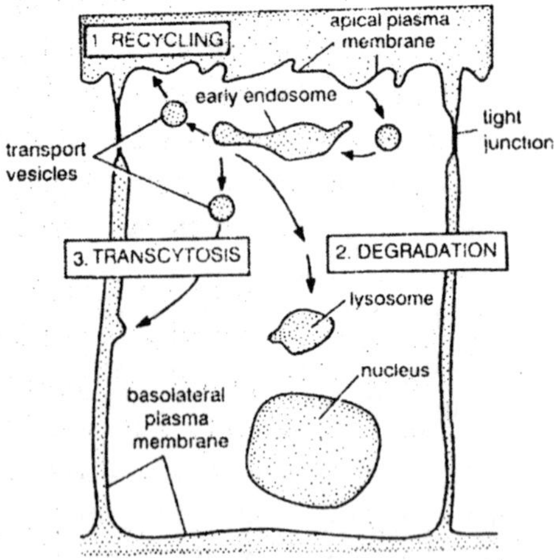

Three possible fates (1,2,3) of transmembrane receptor proteins, which are endocytosed and transported via endosomes (redrawn from Alberts et. al., Molecular Biology of the Cell, 1994).

The receptor proteins mediating this transport thus reach the endosomes and may follow anyone of the following three pathways: (i) recycling, when the endosome or a part of it returns back to the plasma membrane, depositing its contents on cell surface; (ii) degradation, when the endosome merges into or becomes a lysosome, where the contents undergo hydrolysis with the help of enzymes received from Golgi, and (iii) transcytosis, where some receptors on the cell surface transfer specific macromolecules from one domain of plasma membrane to another through endosomes (Fig.).

Caveolae and their Role in Potocytosis, Transcytosis and Signal Transduction: The cell membrane has many cellular indentations on its outer surface. These include a variety of pits and caves for different functions. For instance, as discussed above, 'coated pits' (so called, because their inner surfaces are covered by a dense layer of protein 'clathrin') play an essential role in receptor mediated 'endocytosis', a process in which cell carries proteins and other macromolecules into the cytoplasm. 'Caveolae' (tiny caves, discovered in 1950s and so named by E. Yamada) are another class of cellular indentations formed due to fusion of small vesicles to the cell membrane, and coated with protein 'caveolin'.

They are meant *firstly,* for drawing into the cells interior, small molecules like vitamins by a process called 'potocytosis', *secondly,* for transfer of molecules from the blood through the endothelial cells to the other side of these cells by a process called transcytosis and *thirdly,* for signal transduction, where the stimuli like growth signals are transmitted from outside into the cell.

In the phenomenon of potocytosis, the caveolae remain tethered to the membrane, the extracellular opening is closed and the concentration of substance inside the caveolae becomes high so that the substance crosses the caveolae's membrane into the cytoplasm. In contrast to this, in 'endocytosis', coated vesicles break free from the membrane and move into the cytoplasm.

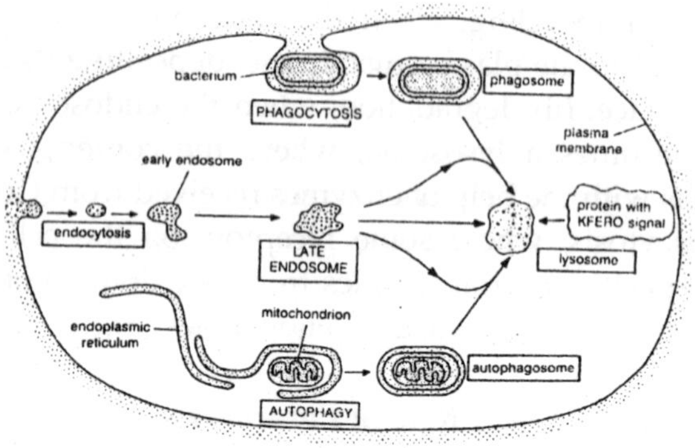

Four pathways for delivery of molecules to lysosomes for degradation (modified from Alberts et. al., Molecular Biology of the Cell, 1994).

Delivery of Molecules to Lysososmes for Digestion: The materials for degradation or digestion are delivered to lysosomes by following four different pathways (Fig.): (i) endosomes, (ii) auto-phagosomes, (iii) phagosomes, (iv) proteins with KFERO signal sequence.

(i) In the first pathway involving endosomes, macromolecules are taken up from outside and delivered into small, irregularly shaped intracellular vesicles called early endosomes. From these early endosomes the molecules may be recycled to plasma membrane or may pass to late endosomes, which simultaneously also receive from Golgi, the vesicles containing lysosomal hydrolases. These late endosomes have mild acidic medium (pH 6.0) inside, where hydrolytic digestion of macromolecules begins. These late endosomes then become lysosomes, due to loss of some membrane proteins, accompanied with further decrease in internal pH (pH 5.0).

(ii) Autophagy involves disposal of obsolete parts of the cell (like old mitochondria, which have lost their utility; in liver, a mitochondrion has a life of only about 10 days). The obsolete parts like organelles are enclosed in a membrane derived from ER and thus give rise to an autophagosome, which then fuses with a lysosome or with a late endosome.

(iii) Phagocytosis involves degradation of large particles and microorganisms (*e.g.* macrophages and neutrophils). These particles are engulfed in plasma membrane to form phagosomes, which later form lysosomes.

(iv) Signal peptides, like KFERO (K = lysine, F= phenylalanine, E = glutamatic acid, R = arginine and O = glutamine) whenever associated with a protein, may also help the protein to reach the lysosomes for degradation.

Polarised Cells and Vesicular Conveyance

Most epithelial and nerve cells are polarised with following two distinct domains of plasma membrane; apical domain facing the lumen (*e.g.* gut) and basolateral domain covering the rest of the cell *i.e.*, the base and the sides of the cell. The apical domain generally has specialised features, such as cilia or microvilli.

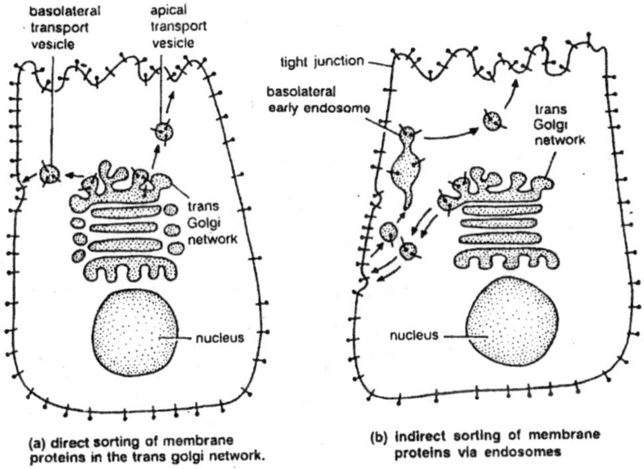

Sorting of plasma membrane proteins in a polarised epithelial cell, using direct pathway in trans Golgi or an indirect pathway via endosome.

The two domains are demarcated by a ring of tight junctions preventing diffusion of lipids and proteins from one domain to the other (Fig.). Consequently, the lipid composition of two domains also differs, apical domain being greatly enriched in glycolipids, which protect this exposed surface from damage by a variety of enzymes in the lumen.

The distribution of different proteins in different domains is though achieved sometimes by random delivery of proteins followed by selective retention and elimination, but in many cases the delivery of proteins is specifically directed. For instance, digestive enzymes are secreted at the apical domain of the cells lining the gut, and products like laminin or other components of basal lamina are secreted on the basolateral surface of these cells. A nerve cell is an extreme example of a polarised cell, with axon terminals on one end, and cell body and dendrites on the other end. While axon terminals are specialised to send signals, dendrites are specialised to receive signals. The axon termini are actually equated with the apical domain and the cell body/dendrites equated with basolateral domain of a polarised epithelial cell.

It has been shown that in the polarised cells (including nerve cells), proteins meant for different domains travel together from ER to trans-Golgi network (TGN). It is in the TGN, that these proteins are sorted out and dispatched in secretory or transport vesicles to appropriate domains of the plasma membrane in the polarised cell. In some cases, the proteins for apical and basolateral domains have distinct sorting signals, which direct them to their corresponding domains either directly or through an endosome (Fig.). In other cases, proteins for only one of the two domains has a sorting signal, while the proteins for the other domain, reach the target by a default pathway.

Molecular Mechanism of Vesicular Transport: The cell contains a variety of membrane bound compartments, which not only maintain their identity but also receive from or send specific products to other specific compartments. If these products, mainly proteins/lipids, are to be transported in the direction of concentration gradient (as in passive transport across a membrane), the problem will be simple, but the transport has to be selective, quite often unidirectional, which may be directed against the concentration gradient (as in active transport across a membrane). These processes require free energy and make use of vesicles, which behave in a very disciplined manner (as discussed above). How is it achieved at the molecular level?

The vesicle budding may involve anyone of the following three mechanisms:

(i) In the first model, an enveloped virus or a nucleoprotein particle adheres to cell surface or to the surface of an intracellular compartment and bud off in the form of a vesicle. A reverse situation could involve budding out of a vesicle from an organelle into the cytoplasm.

(ii) In the second model, a local change in the surface area of the two monolayers of a membrane may lead to membrane curvature inducing the formation of a bud.

(iii) In the third and most popular model, it is assumed that due to action of some coat proteins (at sites where cargo needs to be exported), the membrane is deformed and the cargo is packaged to form the vesicle.

A coat is thus used as a mechanical device to bud off vesicles, atleast in some cases. It is thus obvious that the formation of some vesicles involves coat proteins, while that of others does not. Most vesicular transport in eukaryotic cells, however, does involve vesicles coated with distinctive proteins on the cytosolic face and the coat is discarded before the vesicle fuses with target membrane. The discarded coat is often retrieved back to the donor compartment to be used again in vesicular traffic.

Coat Proteins and Coated Globule

Coats are spherical protein shells, 50-100nm in diameter (analogous to virus capsids), having a fixed composition and consisting of many copies of the same subunits. Subunits, belonging to these coat proteins, are recruited from the cytosol to the donor membrane, deforming the attached segment of this donor membrane, thus leading to the formation of a vesicle encased in the coat. The coat is later discarded to allow the vesicle to fuse with the acceptor membrane. There are four types of coats that have already been characterised- two clathrin coats and two COP coats (Table). Other coats include the following: (i) striated coat on caveolae involved in internalisation of folate and other receptor molecules; (ii) a lace like coat surrounding buds and vesicles at the trans-Golgi network (TGN); (iii) a neuronal specific coat molecule with sequence homology to a subunit of COPI and (iv) an immunological valiant of COPI associated with vesicle traffic between endosomal membranes. These coats are responsible for the formation of three types of coated vesicles shown in Figure. More such coats for vesicular traffic will certainly be discovered in future.

A transport vesicle should have a distinct pilot protein to recognise its target or acceptor compartment. This will facilitate docking of the vesicle at its destination followed by fusion with the target membrane. The accepting or target compartment, similarly should have a responding receptor which will enable the pilot protein of the-vesicle to recognise the target. These requirements of the pilot and receptor proteins in the vesicle and the target compartment are fulfilled by the presence of proteins called SNAREs.

Clathrin Coated Vesicles (CCV): During receptor mediated endocytosis, clathrin coated vesicles capture receptor proteins. Some receptors (*e.g.* insulin and epidermal growth factor or EGF) may be bound with a ligand, while others (*e.g.* LDL receptor) may remain without a ligand. The binding of a ligand to receptor may be facilitated by an interaction with the plasma membrane adaptor protein complex (α-adaptin, β-adaptin, AP50 and AP17). The receptor has -COOH terminal chain hanging in the cytoplasm and can recruit the adaptor protein (adaptin) to a coated pit, where clathrin assembles and forms hexagonal facets of a polygonal lattice (Fig.). The receptors destined to be internalised, are included and enriched in these pits, while others remain at the cell surface. Clathrin involved in this bud formation has three heavy and three light chains. They together form a structure called triskelion (Fig.). Using ATP and Hsc70 (heat shock cognate protein), the polygonal lattice acquires pentagonal facets, giving curvature to form a coated bud. Another protein 'dynamin'(a GTPase) helps in the closure of the vesicle.

Four types of coated vesicles (SAR is closely related to ARF; TGN = trans-Golgi network (from Science, April 12, 1996).

Type of coated vesicle	*Subunit of coat*	*GTPase*	*Origin*	*Destination*	*Inhibited by brefeldin A*
AP-1 clathrin	Clathrin, AP-1 adapter	ARF	TGN	Preiysosomes	Yes
AP-2 clathrin	Clathrin, AP-2 adapter	ARF	Plasma membrane	Endosome	Yes
COP I	Coatomer	ARF	ER-Golgi	Golgi-ER	Yes
COP II	COP II proteins	SAR	ER-Golgi	Golgi	No

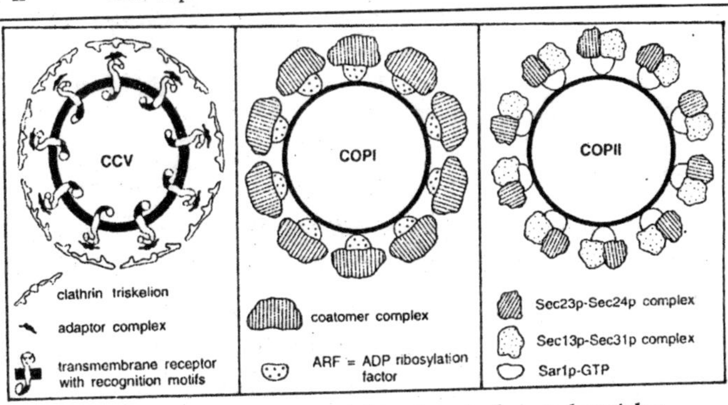

Structural organisation of three types of coated vesicles.

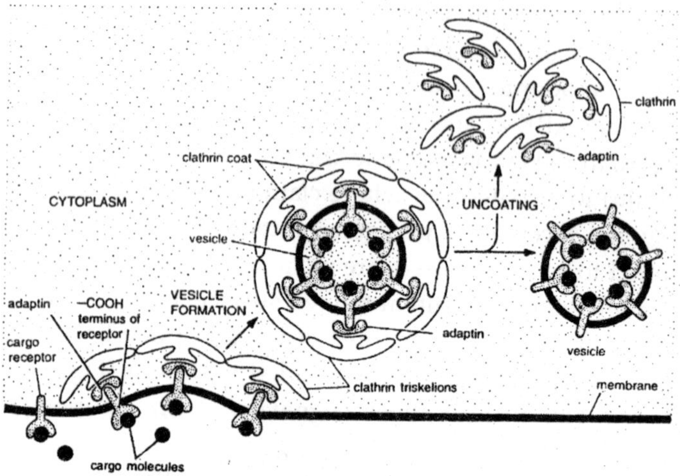

Selective transport, mediated by clathrin-coated vesicles; note the binding of adaptin to clathrin triskelions and cargo receptors, (redrawn from Alberts et. al., Molecular Biology of the Cell, 1994).

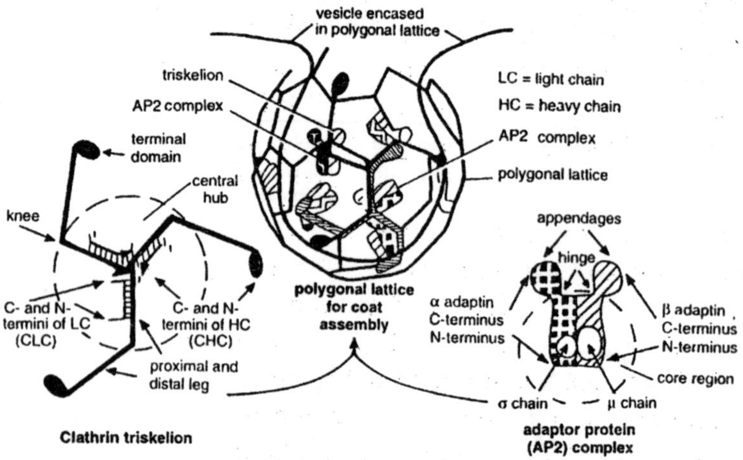

Structure of clathrin triskelions and AP2 (adaptor protein) complex and a model for coat assembly (redrawn from Ann. Rev. Biochem, 1997).

The activity of dynamin is regulated by a kinase-phosphatase (phospho-rylation-dephosphorylation) cycle, leading to membrane fission that will separate the vesicle from the membrane.

The protein complex called adaptin also plays a significant role both in binding of the clathrin coat and in trapping various transmembrane receptor proteins, which in turn capture specific cargo molecules inside the vesicle. In this manner, a set of specific cargo molecules, bound to their corresponding receptors gets enclosed in clathrin coated vesicles. Although the clathrin cage of different clathrin coated vesicles, carrying different cargos to different targets, is the same, the adaptins differ and mediate the capture of different types of cargo receptors. Once the clathrin coated vesicle pinches off, the coat is lost very rapidly. Hsc70 acts as an uncoating ATPase and provides energy to remove the coat.

Clathrin coated vesicles are also involved in traffic from trans-Golgi network (TGN) to lysosome. The clathrin coated vesicles in trans-Golgi network capture receptors involved in traffic of lysosomal or vacuolar proteins. This is mediated by a distinct adaptor complex (β' adaptin, γ adaptin, AP47 and AP19), which functions like the adaptor complex described above for interaction of receptor with a ligand.

In other cases, some membrane proteins (like mannose-6-phosphate receptor) are involved not only in the traffic of endogenous lysosomal precursor proteins but also in capturing of the ligands for receptor mediated endocytosis. Thus, the protein sorting and cargo packaging during budding will be governed by a series of protein interactions. Cell free budding reactions have also been used for understanding the clathrin mediated transport processes.

Coatomer Coated Vesicles (COPI vesicles): Till about 1985, clathrin was viewed as the only essential coat protein for all vesicular traffic. Later, it was found that mutants lacking clathrin were capable of affecting vesicular traffic. Similarly, it was also shown that not all Golgi-associated vesicles were coated by clathrin. Consequently, another soluble complex comprising the coat assembly protomer called coatomer was isolated. It was also shown using cell-free systems that coatomer and ARF {adenesine diphosphate (ADP) ribosylation factor} are required to form vesicles (ARF is a GTPase, used for GTP hydrolysis).

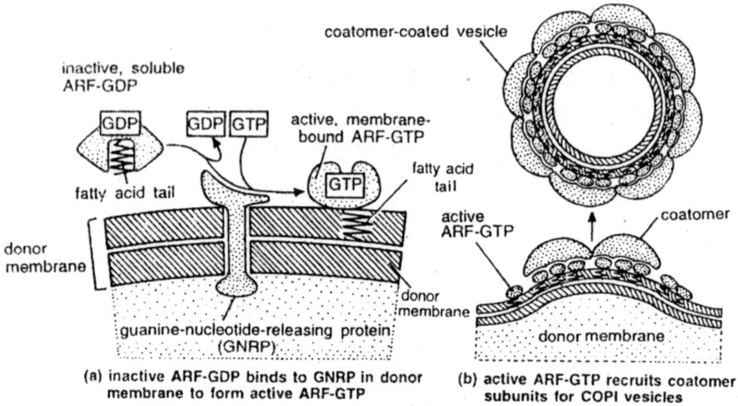

A model for the formation of coatomer coated (COPI) vesicle, showing the role of ARF (redrawn from Alberts et. al., Molecular Biology of the Cell, 1994).

Coatomer-coated vesicles mediate non-selective vesicular transport of the default pathways, which includes transport from ER to Golgi, from one Golgi cisterna to another and from trans Golgi network (TGN) to plasma membrane. Coatomer consists of seven individual coat protein subunits called COPs. These include $\alpha,\beta,\beta',\gamma,\delta,\varepsilon,$ and ξ.

Atleast, one of them shows homology to adaptin of clathrin coated vesicles. However, coatomer coats require ATP for their formation, while clathrin coat does not need ATP. Further, the coat of the clathrin coated vesicles is lost rapidly, after these vesicles are pinched off, but the coatomer coat is retained until the vesicle docks with its target membrane.

Both the assembly and disassembly of coatomer depends on ARF, which is a GTP binding protein. The GTP binding proteins can be either the monomeric GTPases (ARF is a GTPase) or the trimeric G-protein. Both of them are important for vesicular traffic. For the discovery of G-protein, the 1994 Nobel Prize in Medicine was awarded to Drs.

Martin Rodbell and Arthur Gilman. The ARF, when bound to GTP, recruits coatomer subunits (Fig.). When the coatomer coated vesicle docks with its target membrane, a specific GTPase-activating protein in the target membrane assists ARF to hydrolyze its GTP to GDP. This allows the vesicle coat to undergo disassembly, permitting membrane fusion to take place.

ER-derived Transport Vesicles (COPII vesicles): In addition to the coatomer coated vesicles, which play a role in membrane traffic between ER and Golgi, there is yet another group of vesicles, which bud off from ER. These are called ER derived transport vesicles , (also called COPII to emphasise their similarities with COPI vesicles, which are the coatomer coated vesicles).

The COPII vesicles are coated with COPII proteins, which in yeast consist of five subunits: (i) a monomeric small GTP binding protein; (ii) Sar1p; (iii) heteromer Sec23-Sec24p; (iv) heteromer Sec13p-Sec31p and (v) Sec12p. The Secl2p remains in the ER as a landmark, guiding the budding machinery to appropriate site (Fig.). This is regulated by GTP binding and hydrolysis. Sarlp is recruited due to interaction with Secl2p and promotes exchange of GDP for GTP. Sarlp then recruits the Sec23p and Sec13p complexes to produce functional vesicles. Sec23p serves as a Sarlp-specific GTPase activating protein (GAP).

This ER budding reaction is neither stimulated by coatomer and/or ARF, nor are the subunits of clathrin coated or COPI vesicles found in these ER derived COPII vesicles. However, Sarlp is similar to ARF, and the GTP binding proteins are involved both in COPI and COPII vesicles. Mammalian equivalents of the COPII subunits have also been detected by molecular cloning and immunological cross-reactions.

In summary, COPII handles anterograde budding and COPI mediate both anterograde and retrograde budding (Fig.). Both vesicles are free of ER resident proteins, but contain the same set of target molecules (Sec22p, Boslp, Betlp) and several other polypeptides to be sorted out and transported to Golgi complex.

However, budding of COPI (but not COPII) vesicles is inhibited by brefeldin A, an attribute of ARF. However, as pointed out earlier, several polypeptide constituents of COPI and COPII are distinct. This suggests that each may be responsible for the transit of some common and some distinct cargo proteins.

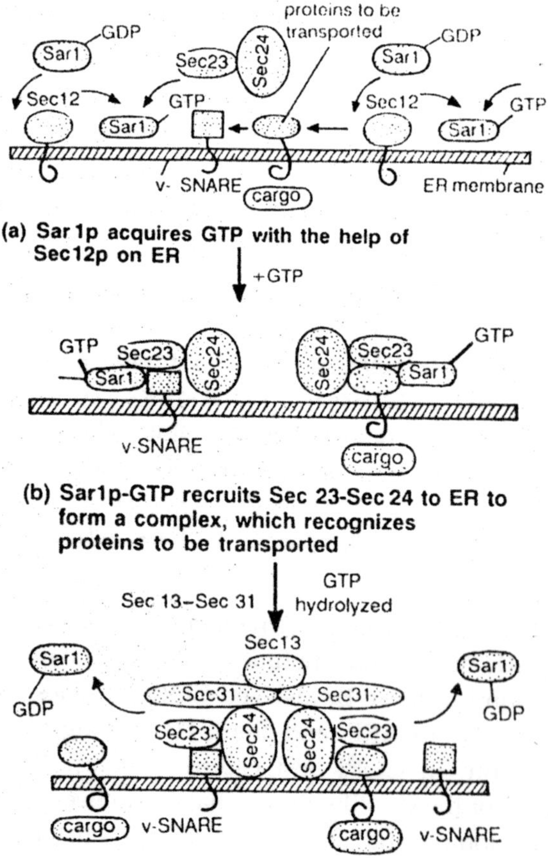

(a) Sar1p acquires GTP with the help of Sec12p on ER

(b) Sar1p-GTP recruits Sec 23-Sec 24 to ER to form a complex, which recognizes proteins to be transported

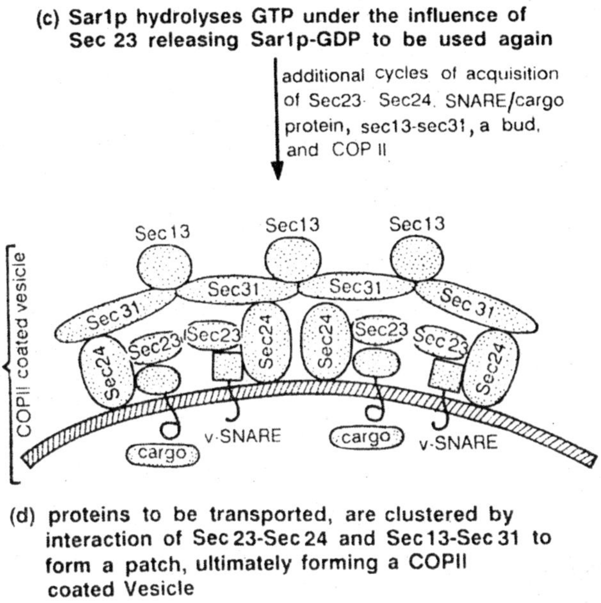

A model showing different steps in the formation of COPII (ER-derived) transport vesicles, showing the role of Sarlp (redrawn from Science, 15 March, 1996).

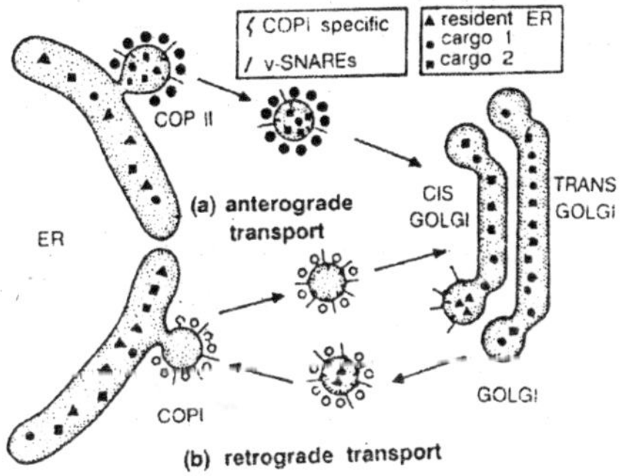

Role of COPI vesicles in anterograde and retrograde transport and that of COPII vesicles in only anterograde transport (redrawn from Science, 15 March, 1996).

COPI and COPII vesicles are also generated from the nuclear envelope. They contain each a large number of proteins, although major cargo is transported by COPII. Several proteins are exclusively transported by COPII. These include Gaslp, Hiplp, and Gaplp in yeast and VSV G protein in mammalian cells.

SNARE Hypothesis and Fusion Machine (V-SNAREs, t-SNAREs and Rab Proteins): The vesicles, after collecting the cargo from a donor compartment, have to travel and recognise their target membranes. It is believed that proteins called SNAREs play an important role in this recognition process (SNARE is SNAP receptor/element; SNAP = soluble NSF attachment protein; NSF = N-ethylmaleimide-sensitive fusion protein). A vesicle with its own SNAREs (v-SNAREs) finds the desired target membrane with a compatible set of SNAREs (t-SNAREs) and bring about membrane fusion. This phenomenon is described as SNARE hypothesis, proposed and supported during 1980s and 1990s (Fig.).

SNAREs consist of structural features called α -helices or coils. During fusion, four α -helices, generally consisting of one syntaxin and three non-syntaxin proteins, form a stable four-helix complex, also called the fusion machine, which mediates the fusion event.

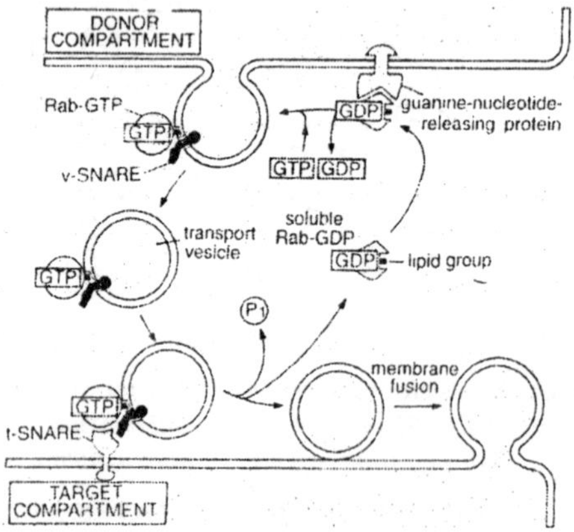

Roles of Rah protein, v-SNARE and t-SNARE in the formation of fusion machine and in ensuring specificity in the docking of transport vesicle (redrawn from Alberts et. al., Molecular Biology of the Cell, 1994).

Syntaxins, first discovered in 1992 as proteins involved in docking of synaptic vesicles, were later found to be conserved proteins that reside on the organelles, and with other non-syntaxin SNARE proteins take part in the fusion of transport vesicles. The genome of budding yeast has 8 syntaxins including the plasma membrane syntaxins Ssolp and Sso2p. Similarly, the genome of *Arobidopsis* has 24 syntaxins arranged in 8 main groups (SYP1 to SYP8), most of them orthologous (homologous by ancestry) to syntaxins of yeast and mammals. At the target membrane, the constitution of t-SNARE may differ, depending upon whether it is a plasma membrane or an intracellular membrane (*e.g.* Golgi or endosome/lysosome).

For t-SNAREs of the plasma membrane, one helix is supplied by a syntaxin and the other two (fused) α -helices are supplied by a single protein, SNAP-25 (SNAP-25 was first discovered as a synaptosomal-associated protein, differentially expressed in some neurons). In the intracellular membranes, on the other hand, the corresponding α -helices of t-SNAREs are derived from a heavy chain, that is homologous to syntaxin and two separate (not fused, as in plasma membrane) non-syntaxin light chains (Fig.).

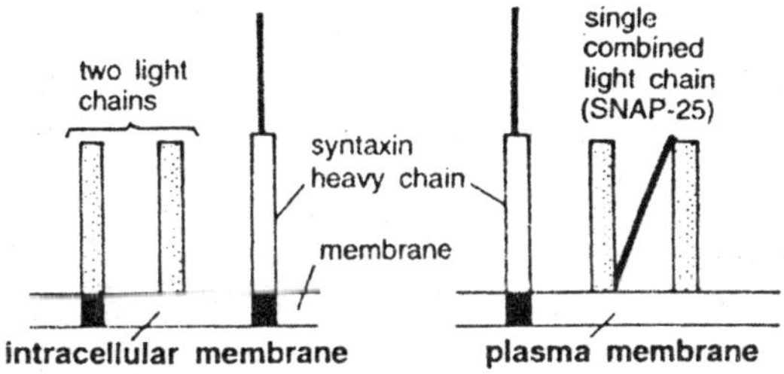

Constitution of t-SNARE at intracellular and plasma membranes.

Enough variation occurs among SNAREs to confer specificity to the vesicles and the target membranes found in the cell. As an example, the SNAREs involved in the fusion of yeast vacuoles include three t-SNAREs including Vam3 (a syntaxin). Vam7 and Vtil, and a v-SNARE including Nyvl.

Similarly, ER derived COPII vesicles contain v-SNAREs including syntaxin5, membrane, which help in targeting and fusion with Golgi having protein complexes like TRAPP and Sec34/35p.

It is believed that v-SNAREs on a transport vesicle reach the target membrane and grab t-SNAREs. The SNAREs then intertwine in a tight four-helix *'trans'* complex (also called SNARE *pins)*, which causes fusion and results in the formation of *'cis'* complex (Figs.). When the SNARE hypothesis was first proposed, the proteins NSF (an ATPase) and its cofactor SNAP were also believed to be involved in the formation of fusion machine and in the actual fusion event, but later (1998-2000) it was shown that the fusion event is much simpler, involving only SNARE proteins. Now it is known that NSF (Sec 18 in yeast) and SNAP (Sec 17 in yeast) perhaps play a role in dissociation of stable *cis*-SNARE complex into its constituent SNAREs to be used again. The energy for this dissociation comes from hydrolysis of ATP due to NSF.

The crucial recognition step involving SNAREs is controlled by a class of monomeric GTPases, called Rab -proteins, which help in the correct fit between a t-SNARE with its corresponding v-SNARE.

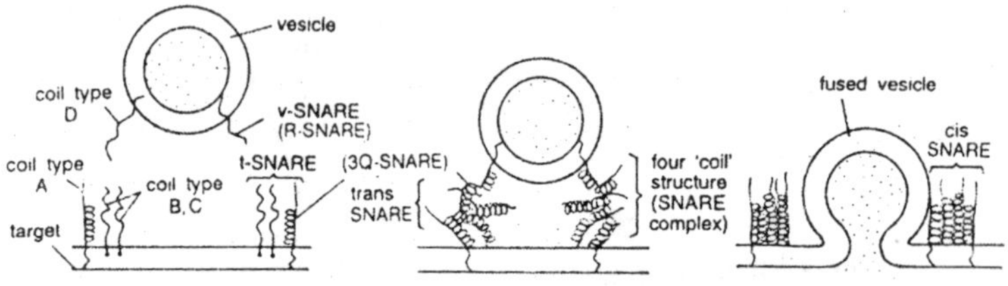

Three steps involving participation of v-SNARE and f-SNARE in the formation of trams-SNARE, which leads to membrane fusion and formation of m-SNARE.

When a vesicle finds the correct target membrane, the binding of v-SNARE to t-SNARE causes the vesicle to remain bound for long enough, so that Rab protein may hydrolyze GTP bound to it (Fig.). This locks the vesicle on the target membrane for fusion. Many types of these Rab-proteins are found. The first of these Rab-proteins, called Sec4 was discovered in yeast. This was responsible for docking of secretory vesicles.

Summarising the above, the vesicular transport involves the following steps; (i) vesicles with v-SNARE bud from the donor membrane, under the direction of a coat, (ii) vesicles travel to the target and lose their protein coats, (iii) vesicles attach to the target having cognate t-SNAREs, through coordinated action of Rab (bound to GTP) and a tethering protein (*e.g.*, pl 15), (iv) *SNAREpins* or *trans-SNARE* complexes assemble together forming a four α -helical bundle, which facilitates membrane fusion and results in the formation of *cis*-SNARE complex, (v) After membrane fusion, NSF and its cofactor SNAP bring about disruption of *cis*-SNARE into its components to be used again.

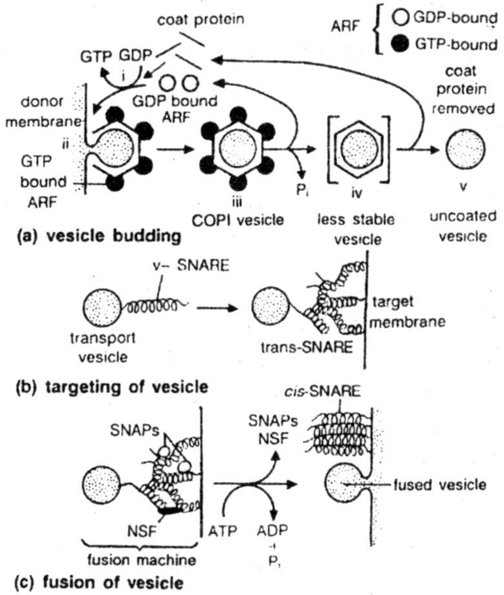

Different steps in the formation of fusion machine, involving budding, targeting and fusion of a transport vesicle.

Vacuolar fusion in yeast is, however, different from the above vesicular fusion as shown in a report published in 2001, suggesting that SNAREs may cause fusion indirectly. Although *trans-SNARE* complexes are formed in vacuoles destined to fuse, these *trans-SNARE* complexes may disassemble before fusion and a macromolecule (V0 part of vacuolar proton pump), which is a dimer of proteolipid rings, helps in fusion of vacuoles (for more details, consult Nature Feb. 1, 2001).

Regulation of Membrane Traffic by Phosphoinositides: For a proper understanding of the mechanism of vesicular traffic, there are a variety of questions that need to be answered. These questions pertain to problems of regulation and include questions like the following: What regulates vesicle formation?. What regulates coat assembly and disassembly? What distinguishes the forward vesicles from the recycling vesicles that carry the same proteins, but move in opposite directions? These questions demand that the vesicular traffic must have temporal and spatial specificity.

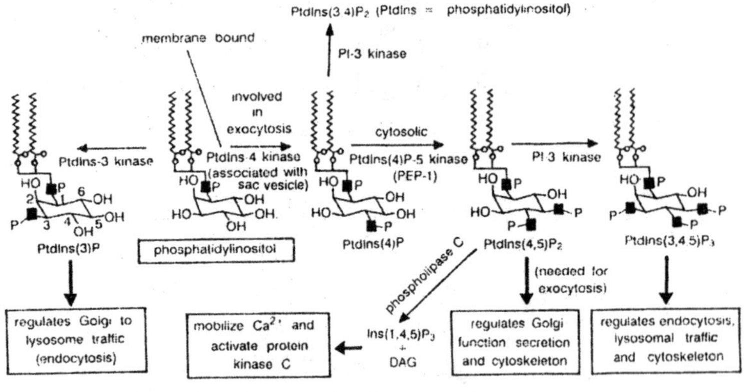

(a) sequence of phosphorylation reaction involving PtdIns and PIs

Sequence of phosphorylation reactions involving Ptdins and PIs and structures of InsPPs (redrawn from Science, 15 March, 1996).

Both proteins and lipids participate in this regulation. The proteins playing a major role in the regulation of membrane traffic include GTPase, while the lipids playing a similar role include phosphatidylinositol (abbreviated as Ptdins; may also be called inositol phospholipids) and phosphoinositides (PIs). The PIs are the phosphorylated derivatives of Ptdins and include Ptdins (4, 5) P2 and Ptdins (3,4,5) P3. Phospholipids, as we know, generally have a head group consisting of glycerol. Unlike these phospholipids, Ptdins and PIs have a head group consisting of inositol ring, which is versatile and can be modified at several positions.

Consequently, due to phosphorylation using a set of kinases, phosphoinositides or PIs are formed (Fig.), which regulate vesicular traffic, the cytoskeleton and the cell growth. Even the metabolites of PIs such as inositol tri-phosphate or Ins (1,4,5)P3 and DAG formed due to action of phospholipase C on Ptdins (4,5)P2, can function as regulators. Three cytosolic proteins, PEPl, PEP2, PEP3 (PEP = priming of exocytosis proteins) have also been identified to be involved in the priming of the exocytosis of secretory granules through formation of secretory vesicles.

Of these three enzymes, PEP1 is a Ptdins (4) P-5 kinase and PEP3 is Ptdins transfer protein (PITP). Ptdins-4 kinase, involved in the synthesis of Ptdins (4) P (the substrate for PEP1) and associated with secretory vesicles, also plays an important role in exocytosis. Therefore, cytosolic PEP1 and PEP3 in concert with Ptdins-4 kinase take part in the synthesis of Ptdins (4,5) P2, which is needed for a critical step in exocytosis.

Phosphoinositides in Yeast and Mammals: In yeast, a gene *SEC14* has been cloned and was shown to encode $Sec14_p$, which is a PITP. A mutation in this gene blocks post-Golgi secretory traffic, but the precise site of action of $Secl4_p$ is not known. The activity of Secl4p, however, involves binding and exchange of phospholipids.

It senses composition of phospholipids in the Golgi membrane and helps in maintaining the appropriate lipid composition in the membranes of Golgi complex. It is believed that the yeast Secl4p is required for vesicle budding. A mammalian gene for PITP protein has also been isolated and was shown to be necessary for vesicle formation. This protein PITP thus has been shown to have a general role in cytoplasmic transport and in phosphorylation of Ptdins and its metabolism.

Another gene *VPS34* from yeast was found to encode Ptdins-3 kinase. It was shown to be essential for the sorting and delivery of soluble vacuolar hydrolases from the late Golgi to the vacuole (equivalent to lysosome of higher eukaryotes), so that in mutants for this gene there is a defect in a specific vesicle-mediated transport process.

Another protein Vpsl5p which is also a kinase, is needed for activation of Vps34p, so that any defect in Vps15p blocks this activation, leading to defects in the transport process. A complex that resembles Vps34p-Vps15p was also identified in mammalian cells and was assumed to play a similar role in transport from trans-Golgi-network (TGN) to lysosome. It is believed to generate a patch in the TGN, that is rich in Ptdins (3) P.

In mammals, a PI-3 kinase (PI-3 kinase is different from Ptdins-3 kinase), called p85-pl10 has been shown to have a function involving endocytic pathway membrane traffic. This protein transduces signals of tyrosine-phosphorylated receptors into a variety of intracellular responses.

There is evidence that this PI-3 is not involved in the actual formation of clathrin coated vesicles or their internalisation, but through its association with PDGF receptor, it helps in post-endosomal sorting (PDGF=platelet derived growth factor). Phosphatases including inositol-5-phosphatases which remove phosphate from 5' position of inositol ring (5-phosphatases), also play a role in vesicular transport. Synaptojanin (a protein rich at the nerve terminal), which colocalises with dynamin (a GTPase, involved in the fission of clathrin coated vesicle) at the nerve ending, is involved in endocytic pathway.

A List of Proteins, Directly or Indirectly Implicated in Vesicular Traffic, and Participate in PI Metabolism or Bind PI Metabolites.

Protein or protein complex	*Function Link to Ptdins (phosphatidylinositol)*	*Putative function in traffic*
Coatomer (COPI)	Binds InsPPs	Generation of vesicle buds at the endoplasmic reticulum-Golgi complex boundary
ARF1 (GTPase)	Activates phospholipase D (44); activity regulated by Ptdins (4, 5) P_2	Promotes recruitment of coatomer and TGN clathrin coat
Vps34p (Ptdins-3 kinase)	Synthesis of Ptdins (3) P	Serine-theonine kinase; essential for Golgi → vacuole transport in yeast
Vps 15p (protein kinase)	Recruits Vps34p to membrane and activates it	Essential for Golgi → vacuole transport in yeast
Secl4p (PITP)	Senses Ptdins-phosphatidylcholine content of membranes	Required for TNG → plasmalemma transport in yeast
Mammalian PITP (PEP3)	Mediates Ptdins exchange and phosphorylation	Role in budding from the TGN and in exocytosis of secretory granules
PtdIns(4)P-5 kinase (PEP1)	Synthesis of PtdIns(4, 5) P_2	Role in exocytosis of secretory granules
Synaptotagmin	C2b domain binds InsPPs	Putative role in exocytosis and endocytosis
AP2	Binds InsPPs and PIs	Recruits clathrin coats at the plasmalemma

Contd....

Protein or protein complex	***Function Link to Ptdins (phosphatidylinositol)***	***Putative function in traffic***
AP 180 (AP3)	Binds InsPPs	Neuron-specific clathrin adaptor
Dynamin	PH domain binds Ins (1, 4, 5) P_3 and Ptdins (4, 5)P_2	Fission reaction of plasmalemma-derived clathrin-coated vesicles
Synaptojanin (5-phosphatase)	Substrates include Ptdins (4,5)P_2, Ins (1,4,5) P_3, Ins (1,3,4,5)P_4	Neuron-specific protein with putative role in synaptic vesicle recycling
p85-pl 10 (PI-3 kinase)	Synthesis of Ptdins (3,4,5) P3 and other Pis	Implicated in recycling through early endosomes
Rab5 (GTPase)	Regulated by PI-3 kinase	Role in endosome fusion
Actin-binding proteins (Proflin, gelsolin, α –actinin, cofilin, β -spectrin, and others)	Bind Ptdins (4,5)P_2	Regulate function of actin-based cytoskeleton
Rho family (GTPases)		
Rho	Binds and activates PtdIns(4)P-5 kinase	Regulates function of actin-based cytoskeleton, implicated in clathrin-independent endocytosis
Rac	Activated by p85-pl 10 (PI-3 kinase)	
Rac, Cdc-42	GTP-bound forms bind and activate p85-p110 PI-3 kinase	

Both synaptojanin and dynamin are rapidly dephosphorylated after neurotransmitter release. Amphiphysin is another neuronal protein (colocalised with synaptojanin and dynamin), which interacts with clathrin adaptor AP2 and is thus implicated in synaptic vesicle endocytosis. Synaptojanin is believed to be a phosphatase and regulates the amounts of specific Ptdins metabolites. Another phosphatase concentrated at Golgi complex is OCRL protein, which is believed to be involved in vesicular traffic at the Golgi complex.

Several GTPases (*e.g.* ARF1, Rab protein) assist PIs in their role in vesicular traffic. For instance, ARF1 helps in the assembly of the COP1 coat and clathrin coat at the TGN by generation of high concentration of Ptdins(4,5)P2. Rab proteins similarly play a role in exocytic and/or endocytic pathways.

For instance Rab5 is known to activate membrane fusion in endosomes and stimulates transferrin endocytosis. Rho family is another class of GTPases involved in vesicular traffic. The variety of proteins or protein complexes that are directly or indirectly implicated in vesicular traffic and participate in PI metabolism or bind to PI metabolites are listed in Table.

7

Role of Cell Nucleus

Robert Brown for the first time in 1833 discovered a prominent body within the cell and termed it nucleus. A synonymous term for this organelle is the Greek word karyon. A German biologist, J. Hammerling, demonstrated in 1934 that the nucleus determines the characters of the cell and ultimately the characters of the individual. He conducted certain experiments using two species of a green alga, *Acetabularia*. The two species, namely *A. crenulata* and *A. mediterranea* used in this experiment differ in the shape of their caps. While in *A. crenulata* the cap has loose rays, in *A. mediterranea* an umbrella-like cap is found.

The nucleus in both the species is situated in rhizoid at the bottom of stalk. If cap is cut off, it will develop again and its shape will be that of the original type. However, if after removing the caps, stalk of one species, is grafted on rhizoid (containing the nucleus) of the other species, shape of cap will be determined by nucleus and not by stalk (Fig.). If the nucleus belongs to *A. crenulata*, shape of cap will be of the *crenulata* type and if the nucleus comes from *A. mediterranea*, cap will be of *mediterranea* type. When both nuclei are present, shape of cap will be intermediate. This experiment demonstrated clearly for the first time that characters of an individual are controlled by nucleus of the cell or cells. This controlling attribute of the nucleus is now well established and is known to be due to the presence of chromosomes in this organelle.

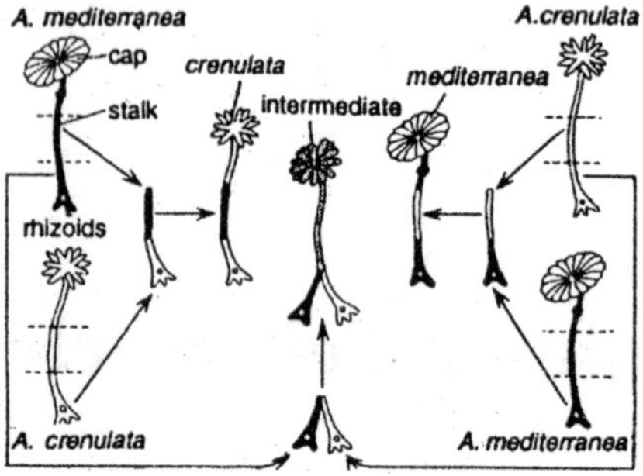

Hammerling's experiment in Acetabularia showing relative roles of nucleus and cytoplasm (redrawn from Swanson: The Cell, 1971).

On the basis of presence or absence of well-defined nucleus, living organisms were earlier classified into two groups by molecular biologists. These groups are (i) prokaryotes, the individuals which do not have a well-organised nucleus and will therefore include viruses, bacteria and blue-green algae; and (ii) eukaryotes, which would include the remaining types, which have a well-organised nucleus. However, according to a phylogenetic classification proposed in 1996, living organisms are classified into the following three groups (i) bacteria; (ii) archaea and (iii) eucarkya.

The nuclear equivalent of a prokaryotic organism is known as prokaryon or more commonly as nucleoid rather than a nucleus. The 'prokaryon' or 'nucleoid' does not have a true chromosome; it is not enclosed in a nuclear envelope and does not divide by regular mitosis.

The nuclei may even be absent in some specialised cells of eukaryotes. For instance mature mammalian red blood cells are also without any nuclei. This is why they are often called as red blood corpuscles rather than cells. A nucleus may be described as having three important parts, namely, nuclear membrane or nuclear envelope, nucleolus and chromosomes. The fluid, in which nucleolus and chromosomes are present and which is enclosed in nuclear membrane, is called nucleoplasm.

NUCLEAR COVER

Nuclear boundary of interphase and prophase nuclei is called nuclear membrane or nuclear envelope. It breaks down at the end of prophase and is reformed at the end of the nuclear division. It consists of a double membrane having two unit membranes (Fig.). The space between two unit membranes varies in width and is known as perinuclear space. Outer membrane is continuous with the endoplasmic reticulum.

Each unit membrane is 7.5 nm (1 nm = 10 Å) in diameter and perinuclear space may vary from regular 15 nm wide spaces to irregular cavities several hundred times wide. Outline of nuclear envelope is smooth and interrupted by pores which appear circular in surface view. Diameter of these pores varies from 30 nm to 100 nm.

It is obvious that at the boundary of these pores, outer and inner unit membranes are joined. These pores provide direct contact between nucleus and cytoplasm and allow import and export of protein and RNA (particularly export of messenger RNA, which is synthesised in the nucleus and then reaches cytoplasm for protein synthesis).

The inner nuclear membrane is lined by the nuclear lamina, which is composed of A and B type lamins (specialised type of intermediate filament proteins). Similarly, the outer membrane is surrounded by a network of intermediate filaments, which are not as well organised as the nuclear lamina (Fig.).

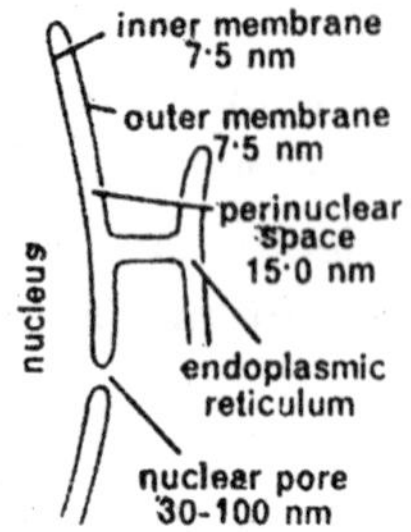

Nuclear membrane showing double structure.

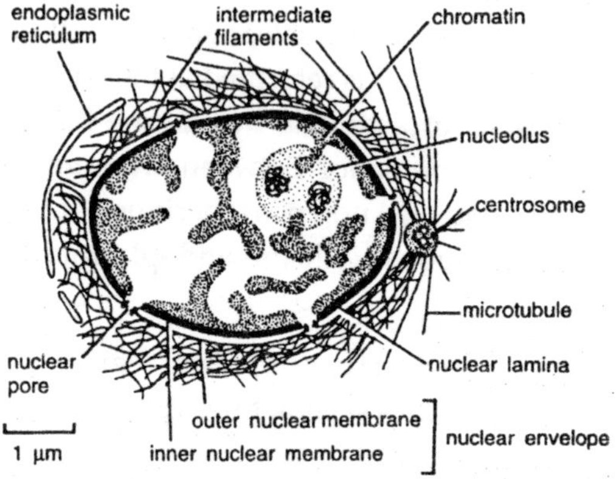

Structure of nuclear envelope.

Disassembly and Reassembly of Nuclear Envelope

As mentioned above, the nuclear envelope disassembles at the onset of mitosis and is reassembled at the end of mitosis. The mechanism of assembly involves (i) the attachment of vesicles to the chromatin, followed by (ii) the fusion of vesicles to form a double membrane system. The binding of vesicles to the chromatin requires both chromatin and membrane bound proteins, but does not require ATP. On the other hand, the fusion of membrane bound vesicles to form the nuclear membrane does require ATP and GTP hydrolysis, that is also required in membrane fusion events during exocytosis and endocytosis. The vesicles used for assembly of nuclear envelope form a subset of ER-derived vesicles, and are distinct from the majority of other ER-derived vesicles (COPII). Lamin-depolymerisation and polymerisation during disassembly and reassembly of the nuclear envelope also involves reversible phosphorylation.

Nuclear Pore Complex (NPC)

Nuclear pore occupies a central position among the major cellular structures, but still remains one of the least understood structures. However, during the late 1980's and early 1990's, significant progress was made towards a better understanding of the structure and function of the nuclear pore. During this period, new pore proteins were identified (particularly in yeast), the genes for several of these proteins were cloned, a number of mutants in these pore proteins were isolated and detailed mechanism of nucleocytoplasmic traffic was proposed. Further, the pore was reconstituted *in vitro*, a number of 'signal sequences' and one or more 'signal sequence receptors' were identified, and a new 'basket-like structure' was found attached to the inner side of the nuclear pore. (Consult review by Douglass J. Forbes in *Ann. Rev. Cell Biol.*, 1992 for detailed account).

The nuclear pore is a large complex structure of 125 million daltons or 30 times the size of a eukaryotic ribosome. The pore is 120nm in diameter and 50nm in thickness. It consists of four separate elements: (i) the scaffold, which includes majority of the pore, (ii) the central hub or transporter, which carries out active transport (both import and export) of proteins and RNAs, (iii) short thick filaments attached to the cytoplasmic side of the pore and (iv) a newly discovered basket attached to the nucleoplasmic side of the pore.

The scaffold is a stack of three closely apposed rings, namely the cytoplasmic ring, the nucleoplasmic ring and a central ring of thick spokes. Each ring has a eight-fold symmetry. The spokes of central ring are attached to the transporter on the inner side, and to the nucleoplasmic and cytoplasmic rings on the outer side. Interspersed between the spokes are aqueous channels, 9nm wide, which allow diffusion of proteins and metabolites between the nucleus and the cytoplasm.

The transporter is a proteinaceous ring, 36-38nm in diameter and consists of two irises of eight arms each. The two irises are assumed to be stacked atop one another and open sequentially, each like the diaphragm of a camera, to let a nuclear protein or RNA pass through from the nucleus to the cytoplasm. On the cytoplasmic side of the pore, thick fibres (3.3nm in diameter) extend into the cytoplasm. On the nuclear side, a large basket like structure is found, which consists of eight filaments (each 100nm long), extending from nucleoplasmic ring of the pore and meeting a smaller ring (60nm in diameter) within the nucleus. This basket may play an important role in RNA export. The detailed structure of nuclear pore complex is shown in Figure.

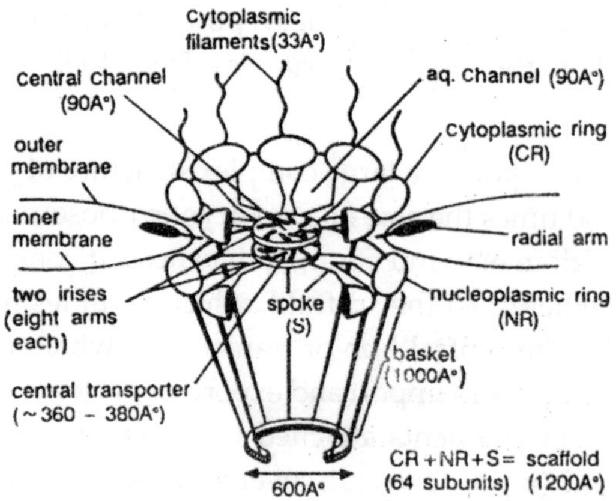

Detailed structure of the nuclear pore, showing iris and transporter.

Nucleocytoplasmic Transport

Nuclear pore complexes (NPCs) are the sites of exchange of macromolecules between the cytoplasm and the nucleus. Each NPC has a mass of 125 megadaltons in higher eukaryotes and contains about 100 different polypeptides called Nup (nuclear pore proteins or nucleoporins). Following are some of the characteristic features of many of these nucleoporins: (i) modification of O-linked N-acetyl glucosamine; (ii) presence of short degenerate repeats (*e.g.*, FXFG repeats in Nupl53p and p62, and GLFG repeats in Nup98p; in FXFG and GLFG repeats, each letter stands for an amino acid; X means any amino acid. The nuclear pore complex has a passive diffusion channel, 9nm in diameter, permitting diffusion of many but not all small proteins including cytochrome c. Several small proteins like histones (<9nm) and other larger proteins (>9nm and upto 25nm) pass through NPC by an active transport process. The active process is facilitated by (i) energy, (ii) signal sequence and (iii) saturability, so that the process is mediated by carrier molecules.

The transport through NPCs involves both import to and export from the nucleus. All nuclear proteins are imported from the cytoplasm where they are synthesised and all tRNAs/ mRNAs are exported to the cytoplasm, where they are used for protein synthesis. There are also molecules that are first exported to the cytoplasm and then reimported. For instance, some of the small nuclear RNAs (snRNAs) involved in RNA splicing include Ul, U2, U4, and U5. They are exported out of the nucleus after transcription.

In the cytoplasm, they assemble with Sm core proteins and undergo a number of modifications such as cap hyper-methylation involving conversion of the cap m^7GpppN5′ to $m^{2,2,7}$GpppN. These partly mature U snRNPs re-enter the nucleus and associate with proteins specific for U snRNPs. In case of U4, the U4 snRNP re-enters the nucleus and associates with U6 RNA.

Thus the snRNPs complete their assembly by export followed by reimport in the nucleus. The situation is reverse in case of ribosomal proteins. They enter the nucleus, get incorporated into ribosomal subunits and are then reexported as parts of ribosome subunits. It has been estimated in HeLa cells, that 100 ribosomal proteins and 3 ribosomal subunits travel through each pore each minute. This demonstrates that transport through NPC is a major activity. For a detailed account, the readers may consult two recent reviews (Science, 15 March, 1990, pages 1513-1518; 24 April, 1997, pages 779-787).

Signals for transport across the pore. The import and export of proteins and RNPs across the NPCs are facilitated by the presence of signal sequences. A number of these signal sequences that have been studied and characterised are listed in Table. Some of these sequences, described as 'classical' nuclear localisation sequences (NLSs), are characterised by one or more clusters of basic amino acids. The two examples of NLSs include signal sequences in large antigen of SV40 and the bipartite NLS of nucleoplasmin.

It has been shown that both these NLSs use the same receptor. While NLSs are used for import, similar export signal sequences are also known, which are described as nuclear export signal (NES). These NES sequences have already been found in atleast following three cases: (i) human immunodeficiency virus (HIV) Rev protein, (ii) PKI, an inhibitor of protein kinase A and (iii) transcription factor IIIA (TFIIIA) used for transcribing 5SRNA genes, tRNA genes, etc. The only solitary example of a signal sequence that directs both import and export by shuttling between the nucleus and the cytoplasm is the M9 domain of hnRNP protein, such as RNP protein Al, also called-hnRNPAl (a human protein involved in mRNA export).

The export of RNA from the nucleus is actually characterised by the following three features— (i) the mRNA needs to be released from the retention process which allows the precursor mRNA to stay in the nucleus for post-transcriptional processing events; (ii) RNAs are exported in

Signal Sequences Involved in Protein Transport Across the Nuclear Pore Complex (NPC)

Function	*Signal (length)**	*Amino acid sequence**
1. Import	SV40 large T antigen NLS (7)*	PKKKRKV
	Nucleoplasmin bipartite NLS (16)*	KRPAAIKKAGQAKKKK
2. Export	HIV-l0Rev NES (9)*	LPPLERLTL
	TF III A NES (19)*	QPPDASKADPALPVLENLTLK L
	PKI NES(IO)*	ALKLAGLDI
3. Targets import receptor to nucleus	IBB domain of import in (41)*	RMRKFKNKGKDTAEL RRRRVEVSVELR KAKK DEQILKRRNV
4. Confers rapid shuttling	hRNPAI M9 (38)*	NQSSNFGP MKGGNFGG RSSGPYGGGG QYFA KP RNQGGY

* length represents number of amino acid residues; figures in parentheses represent numbers of amino acid residues.

the form of RNPs (ribonucleoproteins), where associated proteins (*e.g.*, Rev with NES domain or TFIIIA) actually carry the signals; (iii) many signals may be involved in the export of large RNPs making the study of the mechanism difficult. The only well defined example of RNA export thus is U snRNAs with hypermethylated cap ($m^{2,2,7}$ GpppN), which binds to the proteins (cap binding proteins complex or CBC) involved in export, thus forming RNPs.

Import of Nuclear Proteins: The following four factors are known to be required in nuclear protein import: (i) importin-α (also called NLS receptor; called SRPlp in yeast) (ii) importin-β (also called p97 or PTC97), (iii) the small GTPase Ran, and (iv) ppl5 (also called p10 or NTF2). Importin is also called karyophorin. The import actually involves several stages including the following—the protein to be imported has an NLS which helps in binding of protein to importin $\alpha-\beta$ heterodimer, the latter thus acting as a receptor, the receptor site being present in subunit importin α. An importin-β binding (IBB) domain in importin-α subunit helps not only in interaction with importin-β, but also facilitates translocation through NPC to the nucleus. The NLS-protein-receptor complex docks to the nuclear pore complex via importin–β and is subsequently translocated through the pore by an energy-dependent mechanism. It also requires Ran and ppl5. The energy required for translocation across the NPC comes atleast partly from GTP hydrolysis, which is facilitated by Ran (a GTPase). The Ran GTPase needs the nuclear protein, RCC1 (a Ran activating protein).

The function of ppl5 will be known in future only. Since the distance to be travelled by NLS-protein-receptor complex is atleast 100nm and one GTP can help movement (through motor protein kinesin or the myosin power stroke) to only 8-10nm, it is estimated that the movement of a NLS-protein receptor complex would need 10 GTP molecules. After the translocation, the constituents of NLS-protein-receptor complex become separated, of which the protein remains in the nucleus and importin-β and importin-α are recycled to the cytoplasm, the former rather rapidly and the latter rather slowly due to the requirement of dissociation from NLS (Fig.).

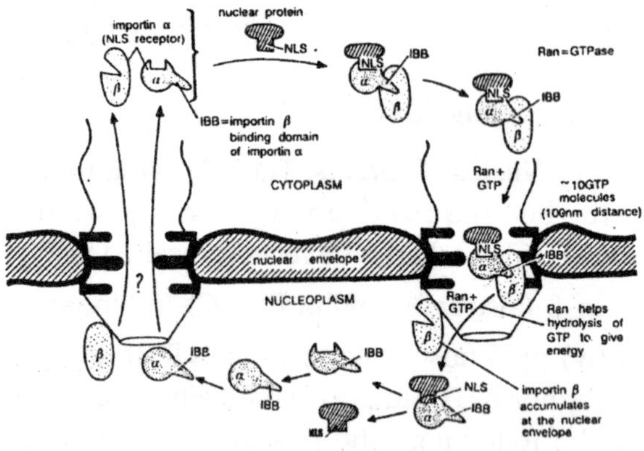

Steps involved in the import of nuclear proteins (redrawn from science, 15 March 1996).

Export of RNA from the Nucleus: RNA export from the nucleus across NPC is also mediated by some signal sequences in the proteins that associate with RNA to form RNPs. The

RNA to be exported may contain response elements. The best studied such protein is HIV-1 Rev protein. An intron in unspliced HIV-1 RNAs contains RRE (Rev response element), where several Rev molecules can bind and allow export of unspliced RNA.

Rev protein has a RNA binding domain and an 'activation domain' the latter being a nuclear export sequence (NES). When coupled with a heterologous protein, the NES of Rev protein directs the rapid export of the fusion product. When NES directs export of a protein the bound protein is also exported automatically. A search for a receptor for NES suggested that human proteins hRip or Rab and yeast protein Riplp are the possible candidates for such a receptor (Rip = Rev-interacting protein; Rab = Rev activation domain binding protein).

These proteins seem to be related to nucleoporins, but their role in export is not yet fully understood, although atleast two models are available. In one model sequential interaction of Rev-NES first with Rip and then with nucleoporins takes place, while in the second model Rev-Rip complex is translocated across NPC through interactions between Rip and other nucleoporins (Fig.).

Export and Reimport of RNAs: Two examples of export followed by reimport of RNA are 5S rRNA and U SnRNAs. Two proteins (TFIIIA and ribosomal protein L5) seem to be involved as mediators in export of 5S RNA. TFIIIA seems to contain a sequence similar to Rev NES. Similarly for export of U SnRNAs, a nuclear monomethyl cap binding protein complex (CBC) seems to be involved. CBC contains two proteins (CBP80 containing NES like sequence and another nucleoplasmic protein CBP20).

Another human protein hnRNPAl and several other hnRNP proteins are also involved in export. They shuttle rapidly between the nucleus and the cytoplasm. The protein hnRNPAl remains bound to polyA-RNA. A short domain M9 of hnRNPAl confers the shuttling behaviour. More information about these shuttling proteins will become available in future.

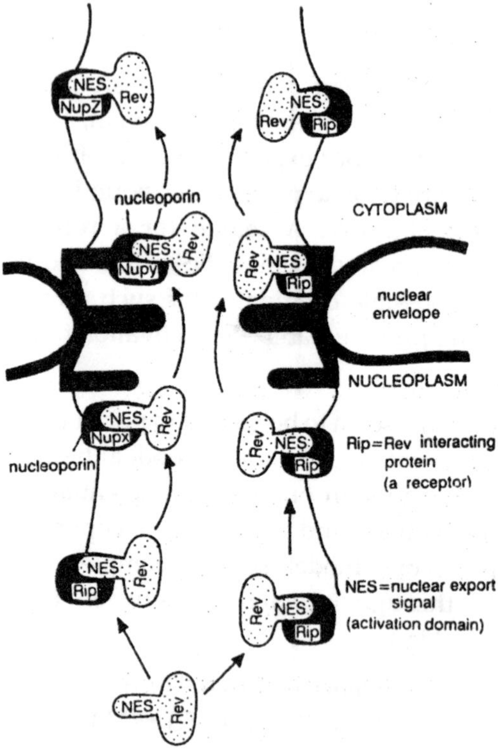

Two models for Rev-mediated export of RNA from the nucleus (redrawn from Science, 15 March 1996).

Origin of Nucleus

There are atleast two contrasting theories available for evolutionary origin of the nucleus: (i) Karyo genic hypothesis. According to this hypothesis the nucleus and its surrounding membranes were gradually acquired through some unspecified segregating process. (ii) Endokaryotic hypothesis. According to this hypothesis, the nucleus, like other eukaryotic organelles (*e.g.*, mitochondria and chloroplasts) enclosed in double membrane, has been derived through capture by an engulfing species. In this case, the guest (the nucleus), rather than being under the control of the host, has taken over control of the host. This hypothesis is simple and explains the origin of nucleus, chloroplasts and mitochondria by the same mechanism, rather than two separate mechanisms needed, one for the origin of the nucleus and the other for the origin of chloroplasts and mitochondria.

The Nucleus

In higher organisms, every cell nucleus has a spherical, colloidal body called nucleolus, which is associated with a particular nucleolar organising chromosome (Fig.). A special region in this chromosome is known as the nucleolar organising region (NOR) to which usually the nucleolus remains associated (Fig.). Quite often, more than one nucleoli in the same nucleus may also be observed. These several nucleoli may subsequently coalesce and give rise to a larger single nucleolus.

While chromatin mainly consists of DNA, nucleolus mainly consists of RNA, acidic dyes and basic dyes; phospholipids and alkaline phosphatase are also found. Nucleolar DNA had also been reported in a number of cases. This DNA is believed to represent the nuclear organiser.

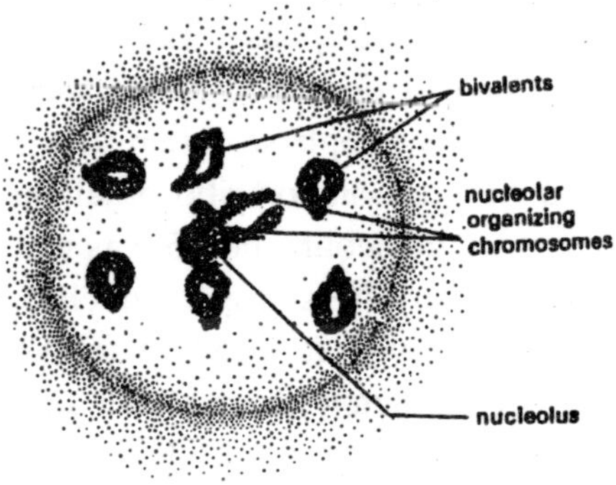

Diakinesis cell showing attachment of a bivalent with nucleolus.

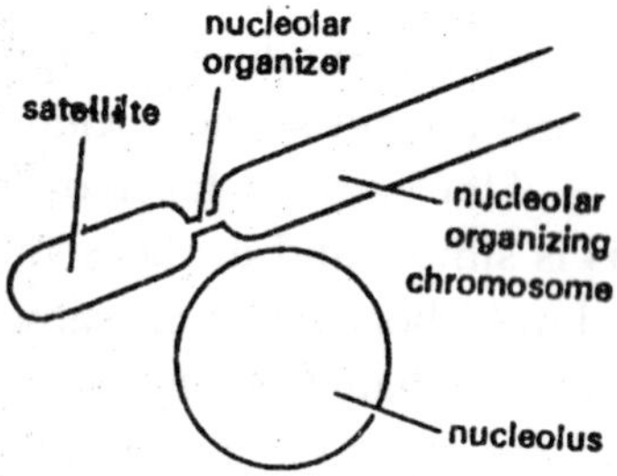

A satellited chromosome ad an attached nucleolus.

The nucleolus was first described in 1781 by Fontana. Ever since then, vast literature has been published on the nucleolus which has been adequately covered in a monograph entitled *"The Nucleolus and Ribosome Biogenesis"* published in 1985. This monograph was written by the distinguished French molecular biologist, Asen Hadjiolov, who suddenly passed away in April 1996. Since the publication of the above monograph, considerable work has been done, which was adequately covered in a special issue of the journal *Chromosoma* brought out in the year 1997 in the memory of Dr. Hadjiolov. The present status of he biology of nucleolus is briefly summarised here.

Nucleologenesis

Nucleolus can be seen as a very conspicuous structure in the interphase nucleus. It disappears during mitosis and reappears at the next interphase. The process by which the nucleolus is formed, is described as nucleologenesis. During prometaphase to early telophase, when the nucleolus remains disappeared, a number of non-ribosomal nucleolar proteins (*e.g.*, B23, fibrillarin, nucleolin and p52) as well as U3 snoRNA are found in (i) the peripheral regions of chromosomes and in the (ii) nucleolus derived foci (NDF) found as cytoplasmic particles 1-2 μ in diameter; the number of these NDFs can reach as many as 100 per cell at mid- to late-anaphase, but later their number declines to few or none at telophase.

The decline in the number of NDF approximately coincides with the appearance of prenucleolar bodies (PNBs) and reforming of the nucleoli. The nucleolar shuttling phosphoprotein, Nopp 140, however, did not follow the above pattern of localisation. It remains dispersed throughout the cytoplasm during pro-metaphase to early telophase, and is not found in NDF. These observations suggest that the NDF and prenucleolar bodies are the precursors of the newly formed nucleoli, but the forces that bind them together to form nucleoli are still unknown.

Nucleologenesis can also be induced in cultured cells by experimental treatment. It has been shown that the nucleolus disappears upon hypotonic shock of the interphase cells and reappears when these cells are returned to isotonic medium,

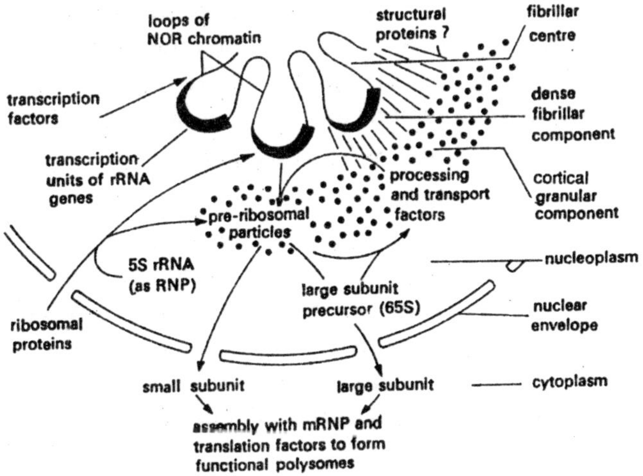

Three regions of the nucleolus showing their roles in ribosomal RNA (rRNA) synthesis.

although the cells continue to remain at interphase. Axtinomycin D also blocks the formation of nucleoli from prenucleolar bodies (PNBs), suggesting that the nucleolus formation requires active transcription of ribosomal RNA (rRNA) genes by RNA polymerase I.

Nucleolus and the Ribosome Biogenesis

The nucleolus is the site of ribosome biosynthesis, where the synthesis of ribosomal RNA (rRNA) and the assembly of ribosome takes place. It has been shown that the genes for ribosomal RNA are clustered at the nucleolar organiser region in the form of tandemly repeated ribosomal DNA (rDNA) units. The initiation, production and maturation of ribosomes in the nucleolus seem to proceed from centre to the periphery in the following three distinct regions: (i) Fibrillar centre (FC), where rRNA genes of NOR (nucleolar organising region) are located; the transcription of rRNA genes (RNA synthesis on DNA template) also takes place in this region. (ii) Dense fibrillar component (DFC), which surrounds the fibrillar centre and where RNA synthesis progresses. The 80S ribosomal proteins (rps) also bind to the transcripts in this region. (iii) Cortical granular component (GC), which is the outermost region and where processing and maturation of pre-ribosomal particles occurs. These three regions of the nucleolus and their roles in ribosome formation are shown in Figure.

The transcription for the synthesis of pre-rRNA actually occurs in FC and particularly at its edge in a region described as transcription zone (txn). In this region are observed the structures described as `christmas trees' by O. Miller. The ribosomal precursors (pre-rRNAs) move from one compartment to the next for different stages of processing and are subsequently transported to the cytoplasm to make mature ribosomes.

Small Nucleolar RNAs (snoRNAs) and rRNA Processing

Like small nuclear RNAs (U snRNAs; *e.g.*, Ul, U2, U4, U5, U6, etc.) found in the nucleus, small nucleolar RNAs (U snoRNAs; *e.g.*, U3, U7, U8, U14, etc.) are found in the nucleolus. During the last more than a decade, the list of snoRNAs has grown to over 50, which can be grouped into two major categories (excluding 7-2/MRP); (i) those derived from evolutionarily conserved DNA sequences called boxes C and D (box C = 5'-RUGAUGA-3, box D = 5'-CUGA-3') present at the 5' and 3' ends respectively, and (ii) those with an AC A motif at the 3' end. Most of the snoRNAs of box C/D class are encoded within introns of other genes and are important

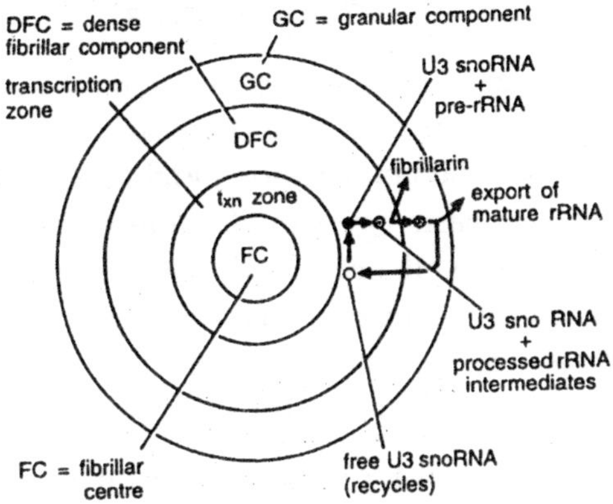

A cycle involving association and dissociation of U3 snoRNA with pre-rRNA in the nucleolar regions.

for rRNA methylation and rRNA processing. It is believed that U3 snoRNA associates with the nascent pre-rRNA and accompanies it, when it passes through the different domains of the nucleolus during its processing. This U3 snoRNA recycles from the granular component (GC) to the dense fibrillar component (DFC) for association with another nascent pre-rRNA (Fig.).

While some of the snoRNAs are ubiquitous (*e.g.*, U3 and U14), there are others, which are described either only in vertebrates or only in yeast. Seven snoRNAs (U3, U8, U14, U22, SnR10, SnR30, RNA component of RNAase MRP) are now known to be required in the processing of pre-rRNA. Of these U3 and U14 are bound to ETS and/or ITS1, which are removed by early processing (the precursor rRNA consists of 5'-ETSl-18S-ITSl-5.8S -ITS2-28S-ETS2-3'; ETS = external transcribed spacer; ITS = internal transcribed spacer). It is not known, however, whether, these snoRNAs act as chaperones to help in correct folding of the pre-rRNA, so that the correct sites are exposed for cleavage or whether the snoRNAs themselves are involved directly in cleavage reactions.

Chromosomes: the Genetic Factor

E. Strasburger in 1875 discovered thread-like structures which appeared during cell division. These thread-like structures were called chromosomes (chroma = colour) due to their affinity for basic dyes. In all types of higher organisms (eukaryote), the well organised nucleus contains definite number of chromosomes of definite size and shape. These chromosomes are invisible in the nucleus but can be easily seen during cell division, whether mitosis or meiosis.

At leptotene stage of meiotic prophase, chromosomes appear as beaded structures, bead-like nodules being known as chromomeres. Size of chromomeres and interchromomeric regions are not constant, so that every leptotene has its own particular pattern. The DNA is though known to concentrate in the chromomeres, but is believed to be present in the interchromomeric regions also. A diploid nucleus has two chromosomes of each type. Two similar chromosomes, are known as homologous chromosomes, which come in contact at zygotene and pair lengthwise throughout their length.

Number, Size and Shape of Chromosomes

Chromosome number varies from $2n = 4$ $(n = 2)$ in *Haplopappus gracilis* (Composite) to $2n = > 1200$ in some pteridophytes. In *Aulacantha* a radiolarian, a diploid number of approximately 1600 chromosomes is found (consult Swanson, *Cytology and Cytogenetics)*. While '*n*' normally signifies the gametic or haploid chromosome number, '2n' is the somatic or diploid chromosome number in an individual. In polyploid individuals, however, it becomes necessary to establish an ancestral primitive number, which is represented as '*x*' and is called the base number. For instance, in common wheat (*Triticum aestivum*), $2n = 42$; $n = 21$ and $x = 7$, showing that common wheat is a hexaploid ($2n = 6x$).

A chromosome is normally measured at mitotic metaphase and may be as short as 0.25 μ (μ = .001 mm) in fungi and birds, or as long as 30 μ in some plants like *Trillium*. As a rule, most metaphase chromosomes fall within a range of μ in fruitfly (*Drosophila*), 5 μ in man and 8-12 μ in maize.

Chromosome shape is usually observed at anaphase, when the position of primary constriction or what is also called centromere determines chromosome shape. This constriction or centromere can be terminal, sub-terminal or median in position. The terminal centromere will give rod shaped chromosome, a sub-terminal one would give J-shaped and a median centromere would give a V-shaped chromosome (Fig.).

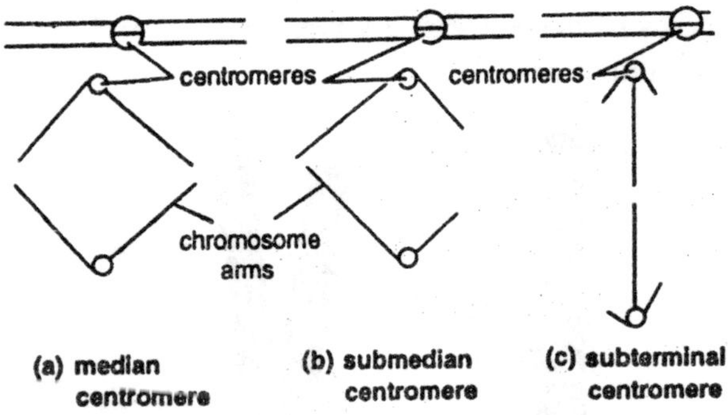

Different positions of centromeres controlling shapes of chromosomes at anaphase (redrawn from De Robertis et. al., Cell Biology, 6th Edn).

Morphology of Chromosomes

Corresponding to different positions of centromere, chromosomes would be called (i) acrocentric or telocentric, having terminal centromere, (ii) submetacentric having sub-terminal centromere and (iii) metacentric having median centromere.

Besides centromere, which produces a primary constriction in chromosomes, secondary constrictions can also be observed in some chromosomes. Such a secondary constriction if present in the distal region of an arm would pinch off a small fragment called trabant or satellite. The satellite remains attached to rest of the body of the chromosome by a thread of chromatin. Secondary constrictions may be found in other regions also and are constant in their position, so that these constrictions can be used as useful markers. Secondary constrictions can be distinguished from primary constriction or centromere, because chromosome bends or shows angular deviation only at the position of centromere. Chromosomes having a satellite are marker chromosomes and are called SAT- chromosomes. The chromosome extremities or terminal regions on either side are called telomeres. If a chromosome breaks, the broken ends can fuse due to lack of telomeres. A chromosome, however, can not fuse at the telomeric ends, suggesting that a telomere has a polarity which prevents other segments from joining with it. Telomeres have been studied in great detail at the molecular level in recent years).

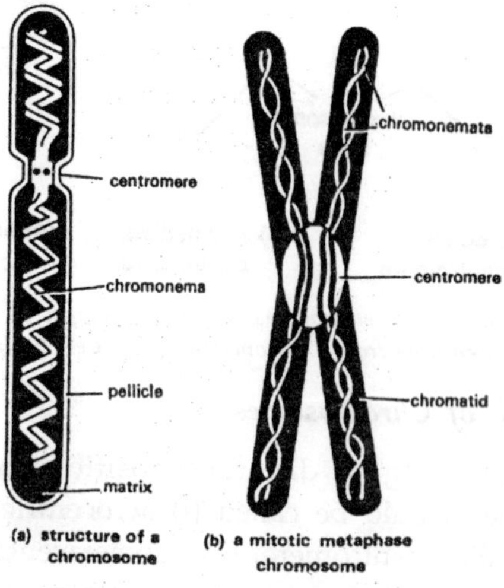

Structure of a chromosome and chromatids.

Detailed study of chromosome morphology reveals a coiled filament throughout the length of a chromosome. This filament is called chromonema (Vejdovsky, 1912). The chromonemata form the gene-bearing portions of the chromosomes. The chromonemata are embedded in the achromatic substance known as matrix (Fig.). Matrix is enclosed in a sheath or pellicle. Both matrix and sheath are non-genetic materials and appear only at metaphase when the nucleolus disappears. It is believed that nucleolar material and matrix are interchangeable *i.e.*, when matrix disappears, nucleolus appears and *vice-versa*. It would be necessary here to make a distinction between chromonema and chromatid. While a chromatid is a half chromosome, two chromatids being connected at the centromere, the chromonema is a structure which is of a sub-chromatid nature and there can be more than one chromonemata in a chromatid (Fig.).

Karyotypes

A group of plants or animals comprising a species is characterised by a set of chromosomes, which have certain constant features. These features include chromosome number, size and shape of individual chromosomes and other attributes listed above. The term karyotype is given to the group of characteristics that identifies a particular chromosome set

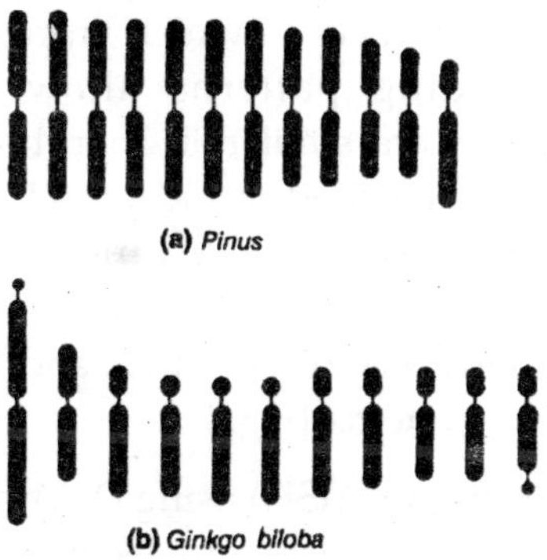

(A) A symmetric and (B) an asymmetric karyotype (redrawn from Stebbins. Chromosomal Evolution in Higher Plants, 1971).

and is usually represented by a diagram called idiogram, where chromosomes of haploid set of an organism are ordered in a series of decreasing size. The karyotypes of different groups are sometimes compared and similarities in karyotypes are presumed to represent evolutionary relationships.

Karyotype also suggests primitive or advanced feature of an organism. A karyotype showing large differences between smallest and largest chromosome of the set and having fewer metacentric chromosomes, is called asymmetric karyotype, which is considered to be a relatively advanced feature when compared with symmetric karyotypes. A symmetric and an asymmetric karyotype are shown in Fig. In 1931 G.A. Levitzky, a Russian scientist suggested that in flowering plants there is a predominant trend towards karyotype asymmetry. This trend has been carefully studied in the genus *Crepis* of the family composite. In several cases it was shown that increased karyotype asymmetry was associated with specialised zygomorphic flowers.

The technique of karyotype preparation does not allow identification of chromosomes with similar morphological attributes (*e.g.*, size of chromosome, position of centromere, etc.). The development of chromosome banding techniques during late 1960's and early 1960's proved very useful for the preparation of karyotypes in which linear differentiation due to distinct banding patterns allow identification of chromosomes that are similar in morphology. The banding technique allows detection of GC or AT rich regions or the regions with repetitive DNA. A variety of different kinds of bands (*e.g.*, Q, C, G or R bands) have been used in animal materials. Similarly, Giemsa C bands and N bands have been utilised in plant systems (Fig.).

In situ hybridisation (ISH) using DNA probes, labeled with radioactive or non-radioactive molecules, can also be used to locate the position of specific DNA sequences on chromosomes (Fig.). DNA may also be labeled with fluorochromes to allow the use of one or more colours to locate the positions of one or more DNA sequences simultaneously on the same chromosome. These techniques are described as fluorescence in situ hybridisation (FISH) and multicolour fluorescence in situ hybridisation (McFISH). They have been extensively utilised in animals (including humans) and plants in recent years.

Karyotypes can also be prepared by a relatively recent technique called flow cytometry. In this technique a suspension of many thousands of chromosomes is made and the suspended chromosomes are stained with a DNA binding fluorochrome. As these chromosomes pass through the cytometer, the fluorescence is measured for individual chromosomes giving a histogram, each peak in this histogram representing one chromosome or a group of chromosomes of same size. The technique allows detection of difference as small as 1.5 to 4.0 Mb (megabase = 10^6 bases), so that aneuploidy or duplications/ deletions can be easily detected. Karyotypes of many plant species like tomato, faba been and wheat have actually been prepared using the technique of flow cytometry.

Euchromatin and Heterochromatin: When chromosomes are stained with stains like acetocarmine or feulgen (basic fuchsin) at prophase, a linear differentiation into regions having dark stain and those having light stain becomes conspicuous. In 1930's and 1940's Emil Heitz and other cytologists studied this aspect. The darkly stained regions were called heterochromatic and light regions were called euchromatic (Fig.).

Heterochromatic regions are constituted into three structures namely chromomeres, chromocenters and knobs. Chromomeres are regular features of all prophase chromosomes, large enough to reveal them, but their number, size, distribution and arrangement are specific for a particular species at a particular stage of development.

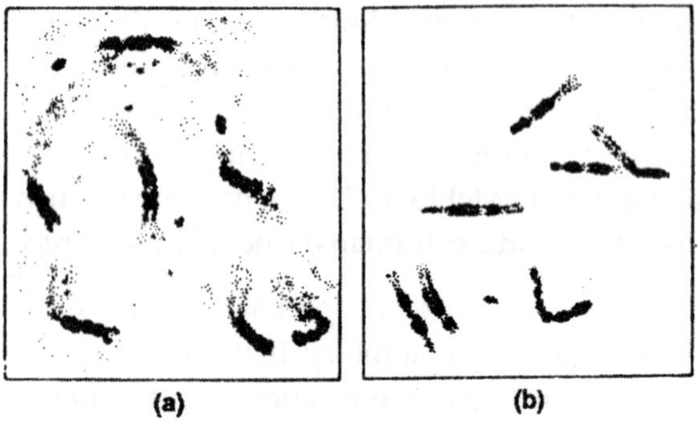

Chromosomes showing euchromatin and heterochromatin. (A) early prophase (B) late prophase (redrawn from Stebbins: Chromosomal Evolution in Higher Plants, 1971).

Chromocenters are heterochromatic regions of varying size which occur near the centromeres in proximal regions of chromosome arms. At mid-prophase, many chromocenters can be resolved into strings of chromomeres, which are larger than chromomeres found in distal regions. In some dipteran salivary glands, the chromocenters of different chromosomes fuse to form a large chromocentre (Fig.). The relative distribution of chromocenters are sometimes considered to be of considerable evolutionary value.

Knobs are spherical heterochromatin bodies which may have a diameter equal to the chromosome width but may reach a size having a diameter which is several times the width of the chromosome. Very distinct chromosome knobs can be observed in maize at pachytene stage. Knobs are valuable chromosome markers for distinguishing chromosomes of related species and races.

Constitutive and Facultative Heterochromatin

Certain heterochromatic regions of chromosomes, particularly those proximal to centromeres are constant, and are called constitutive heterochromatic regions serving as chromosome markers. There are other heterochromatic regions called facultative heterochromatic and represented by whole sex chromosomes which become heterochromatic only at certain stages. For instance in female humans, one X-chromosome is inactivated or becomes heterochromatic only facultatively. Similarly in plants accessory chromosomes in general, and among dioecious genera like *Melandrium* and *Rumex*, one or both sex chromosomes may undergo partial or complete heterochromatinisation.

It is established that DNA replicates in heterochromatic region at a time different than that in euchromatic regions. It is also established that genes in heterochromatic region are inactive, but the earlier belief that no genes are found in heterochromatic regions is not correct because, genes could be located in heterochromatic regions in several cases like *Drosophila* and tomato. The genes in heterochromatic region perhaps become active for a short period. Y chromosome is another example of heterochromatic chromosomes having inactive genes in several dioecious plants and animals.

Single-stranded and Multi-stranded Hypotheses for Chromosomes: When chromosomes are compared in related species which differ widely in DNA content, such differences may be attributed to one of the two causes: (i) lateral multiplication of chromonemata leading to multiple strandedness or (ii) tandem duplication, where length-wise duplication instead of lateral multiplication is responsible for difference in DNA content. This later condition will retain the single stranded feature of chromosomes.

Although multiple strandedness has been demonstrated in several cases of plants like *Vicia faba* and animals like dipteran salivary gland chromosomes, there are evidences against such a hypothesis to become a generalisation. In *Vicia faba* chromosomes, sub-chromonemata were actually observed, while in related *V. sativa* they could not be observed. In other genera like *Allium* and *Lolium* also, it has been shown that increase in DNA content is mainly brought about by tandem duplication rather than by lateral multiplication leading to multiple stranded feature. Therefore, the two hypotheses assuming single stranded and multiple stranded nature of chromosomes are complementary and not exclusive to each other.

Chemical Composition of Chromosomes: The major chemical components of chromosomes are DNA, RNA, histone proteins and nonhistone proteins. Calcium is also present in

Chemical Composition of Chromatin (per cent) from Various Sources

Source	*DNA*	*Histone*	*Nonhistone*	*RNA*
Pea embryonic axis	39.0	40.0	11.0	10.0
Pea vegetative bud	40.0	52.0	4.0	4.0
Pea growing cotyledon	43.5	34.5	16.0	6.0
Rat liver	37.0	37.0	25.0	1.0
Cow thymus	40.2	46.0	13.5	0.3
Sea urchin blastula	39.2	41.0	19.0	1.0
Sea urchin larva	33.4	29.0	35.0	2.6

addition to these constituents. The relative proportions of different components are given in Table for a variety of organisms, which suggest that there is more protein than DNA in chromatin in all cases DNA.

As we know, DNA is the most important chemical component of chromatin, since it plays the central role of controlling heredity. Quantitative measurements of DNA have been made in a large number of cases which were reviewed by M.D. Bennett and I.J. Leitch in 1995 (*Annals of Botany* 76: 113-176). The most convenient measurement of DNA is picogram (10^{-12} g) which is equivalent to 31cm of double helical DNA.

It has been found that quantity of DNA varies greatly in cells from different kinds of organisms. The haploid genome of mammals usually contains 1000 times DNA content of bacteria. Other eukaryotes may similarly have 10 to 100 times the bacterial DNA content.

It is interesting to note that a human diploid cell has 174cm (5-6 picograms) of DNA, so that all cells in a human being may have DNA equal to 2.5 x 10^{10} km (100 g), a length which is equal to 100 times the distance from earth to sun. Similarly a diploid cell of *Trillium* has 37 meters (120 picograms) and that of *Drosophila* salivary glands has 91 meters (293 picograms) of DNA. In comparison of these enormous lengths, the DNA of bacteria measures only 1.1mm-1.4mm.

Histones: There are five fractions of histones, which have been differently designated by different workers (Table; current designations in the last column). H1 histone is most easily removed and so is least tightly bound. This may thus be concerned with holding together a chromosome fibre. H3 and H4 are extremely conserved, having same structure in different species and should thus have a common structural role.

Old and New Standard Designations for Different Kinds of Histones Isolated from Eukaryotic Chromosomes.

Types of histone	*Designations*		
	Old		*New*
	Bonner et. al., 1968	*Johns, 1971*	*Lewin, 1975*
1. Lysine rich	I b	f 1	H1
2. Slightly lysine rich	II bl	f 2a2	H2A
	II b2	f 2b2	H2B
3. Arginine rich	III	f 3	H3
	IV	f 2al	H4

Histones, isolated from diverse materials showed considerable similarity. It is also assumed that general similarities in histones have been conserved during evolution. This feature alone suggested that these proteins should play a structural role rather than a regulatory role.

However, some important chromatin reconstitution and other experiments conducted in recent years have established that histones do play a regulatory role. This regulatory role of histones is more of general nature rather than specific and is exercised by repressing the activity of genes.

Non-histones: In comparison to histones, the non-histone proteins display higher but still limited diversity. In a variety of organisms, number of non-histones can vary from 12 to more than 20. Heterogeneity of these proteins suggested that these proteins are not as conserved in evolution as histones. The non-histone proteins differ even between different tissues of the same organism suggesting that they regulate the activity of specific genes.

Chromatin reconstitution experiments described in 1973 by R.S. Gilmour and J. Paul of Institute for Cancer Research at Glasgow (U.K.), established conclusively for the first time that specific non-histone proteins switch on specific genes. The results of these experiments were later confirmed in a number of cases (Barrett *et. al.*, 1974; Groner *et. al.*, 1975). During 1960's and 1990s, many transcription factors have been shown to be non-histone proteins, providing further evidence that non-histone proteins exercise positive control on the activity of specific genes.

Ultrastructure of Chromosomes

In the past, study of chromosome ultrastructure was an important area, where electron microscope had failed to give us a clear picture of organisation of DNA. For the study of chromosomes with the help of electron microscope, whole

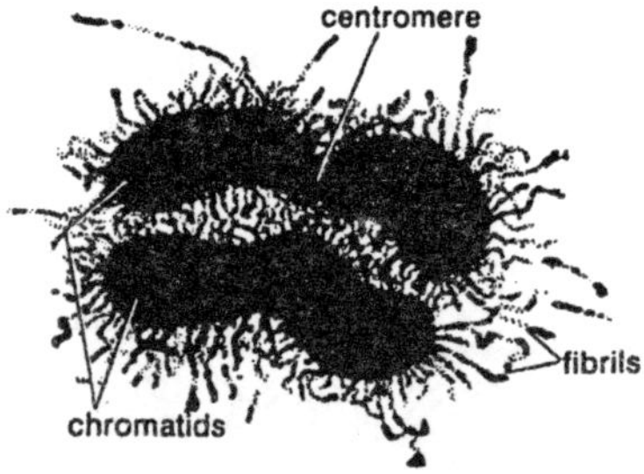

Ultrastructure of chromosome (drawn from an electron micrograph. Du Praw: Cell and Molecular Biology, 1969).

chromosome mounts as well as sections of chromosomes were studied. Such studies demonstrated that chromosomes have very fine fibrils having a thickness of 2nm–4nm (Fig.). Since DNA is 2nm wide, there is possibility that a single fibril corresponds to a single DNA molecule. However, whether these fine fibrils represent the natural state of DNA or is an artifact was not known. Moreover, in these fibrils the structure corresponding to protein component of the chromosomes was also not known, and different positions of proteins were shown in different chromosome models.

A meaningful picture of the structure of chromosome could be earlier drawn from available data on ultrastructure of eukaryotic chromosomes. If a single chromatid has a single long DNA molecule, as has been proved, we have no choice but to believe that DNA should be present in a coiled or folded manner. This can also be inferred from the fact that the thickness of a chromosome is usually hundred times that of DNA and the length of DNA found in a chromosome is several thousand times the length of the chromosome.

The manner of coiling and folding of DNA was a matter of debate and dozens of important models for this purpose were available during 1960's and early 1970's A popular model was the folded fibre model (Fig.) given by E.J. Du Praw in 1965. However, the most important and universally accepted model is nucleosome model proposed in 1974. It is not desired here to present these different models, or else to discuss their merits or demerits. Nucleosome concept will be described briefly here.

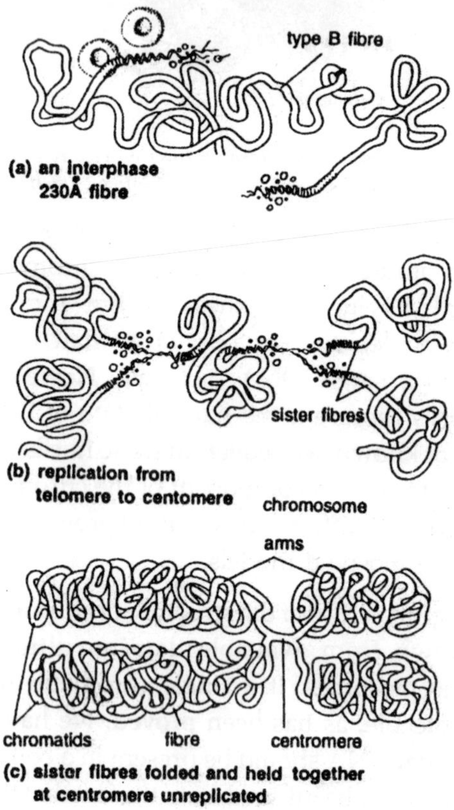

Structural organisation in a chromosome according to folded fibre model (redrawn from Du Praw: Cell and Molecular Biology).

Structure of Chromosomes at Molecular Level

Nucleosome-subunit of Chromatin: In 1974, R.D. Kornberg and J.O. Thomas proposed an attractive model for basic chromatin structure involving DNA and histones. They suggested that DNA interacts with a tetramer ($H3_2$-$H4_2$) and two molecules of an oligomer (H2A-H2B), so that a tetramer involving two molecules each of the histones H3 and H4, is associated with two molecules each of the histones H2A and H2B and with 200 base pairs of DNA. This makes a repeating unit (Fig.). One molecule of H1 is also associated with each repeating unit. They also proposed that the tetramer makes the core of the unit and oligomers determine the spacing thus giving a flexible structure. This model is supported from biochemical and electron microscopy results. P. Oudet *et. al.*

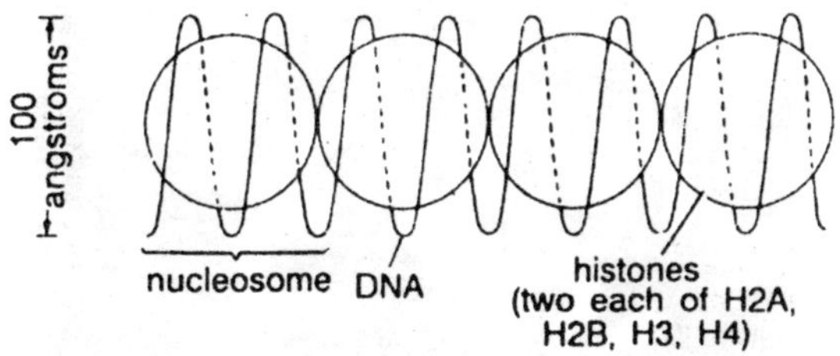

Original proposal for nucleosome repeating units, with DNA wound on a series of beads; actual shape of histone complex or the path of DNA was not known (redrawn from Sci. Amer. Vol. 244, 1981).

(1975) proposed the term nucleosome for repeating units which were observed as beads on strings (or string on beads) under electron microscope.

Nucleosome (12.5nm in diameter) = 200 base pairs + 2 molecules each of H2A, H2B, H3, H4.

Telomere: In recent years the structure of telomeres in a wide variety of organisms has been studied to demonstrate that telomeres are highly conserved elements throughout the eukaryotes, both in structure and function. Telomeric DNA has been shown to consist of simple randomly repeated sequences, characterised by clusters of G residues in one strand and C residues in the other. Another feature is a 3' overhang (12-16 nucleotides in length) of the G-rich strand. Some of the telomeric DNA sequences found in eukaryotes are given in Table.

The same repeated sequence is found at the ends of all chromosomes in a species and the same telomere sequence may occur in widely divergent species, such as humans, some

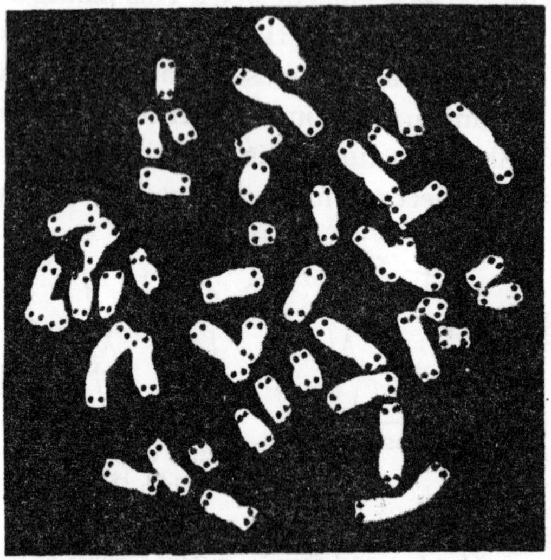

A metaphase plate of mitotic chromosomes, hybridised in situ with a probe having telomeric DNA repeat sequences; the telomeric sequence can be seen at the ends of all chromosomes.

Repeated Telomeric DNA Sequences in Some Organisms

	Telomeric DNA repeat	*Organisms*
1.	AGGTT	*Homo sapiens, Physarum, Neurospora, Trypanosoma*
2.	GGGGTT	*Tetrahymena, Glaucoma*
3.	GGG(G/T)TT	*Paramecium*
4.	GGGGTTTT	*Oxytricha, Stylomychia, Euplotes*
5.	AGGG(T/C)TT	*Plasmodium*
6.	AGGGTTT	*Arabidopsis* (a higher plant)
7.	AGGGTTTT	*Chlamydomonas*

Contd...

	Telomeric DNA repeat	*Organisms*
8.	(A)$G_{(2-5)}$TTAC	*Schizosaccharomyces pombe* (fission yeast)
9.	$G_{(1-3)}T$	*Saccharomyces cerevisiae* (budding yeast)
10.	$G_{(1-8)}A$	*Dictyostelium* (a mold)

a cellular slime molds (trypanosomes) and fungi like *Neurospora.* At every telomere, as much as 10 kilobases of this repeat sequence may occur. The telomeric DNA is also complexed with non-histone proteins, the complex structure being associated with nuclear lamina, as shown in *Oxytricha,* a ciliated protozoan. The telomeric DNA is synthesised under the influence of telomerase, an enzyme which has been shown to be a ribonucleoprotein, whose RNA component works as a template for synthesis of telomeric DNA repeats and protein component has reverse transcriptase (RT) activity.

Recently (in 1997), proteins have been isolated from telomerase in yeast and a ciliated protozoan *(Euplotes)* which could be the RT component of telomerase. These were pl23 in *Euplotes* and Est2 in yeast. In recent years, efforts have also been made to understand, how the telomere length is monitored in chromosomes, because uncontrolled activity of telomerase will lead to indefinite elongation of telomeres. Proteins binding to telomere repeats have been identified, which block the elongation of telomeres. These include Raplp in budding yeast, Tazlp in fission yeast and TRF in humans. The significance of these proteins lies in the following two observations made in recent years: (i) Shortening of telomere tract (repeat sequence) is associated with senescence and aging; (ii) Controlled elongation of telomere is an essential step in tumour formation and oncogenesis. However, even in tumour cells, this telomere length does not increase in an uncontrolled manner, and the elongation is regulated. However, we still do not know, 'how does the cell measure the telomere length, and how is this information used to regulate the length of telomeres' ?

Kinetochore and Centromeric DNA Sequences: As earlier described, centromere is a unique region of a chromosome characterised by a *constriction,* where the two chromatids remain joined together after chromosome replication. On each of these centromeres, specialised DNA-protein complexes known as kinetochores assemble. Each chromosome has two kinetochores, one on each sister chromatid, facing in opposite directions. These kinetochores are the sites for binding of kinetochore microtubules (spindle), which assist in the movement of chromosomes during anaphase.

The DNA sequences representing the centromere contain the information specifying the assembly of kinetochore. These centromeric DNA sequences have been isolated and characterised in a number of organisms but, unlike the telomeric sequences, have not been found to be conserved. For instance, each of the 17 chromosomes of budding yeast *(S. cerevisiae)* contains a different centromere sequence about 125 base pairs long, although there are substantial regions of homology between centromeres of different chromosomes. These centromeres in budding yeast, each bind to a single microtubule and can move chromosomes of 0.26-3 megabases in size.

Further the centromere in budding yeast contains three DNA sequence elements (CDEI, CDEII, CDEIII). In the centromere of the budding yeast, there are also found centromeric proteins, called centromere DNA-binding factors (CBF), which include (i) CBF1 binding to CDEI and (ii) CBF3 binding to CDEIII. It is believed that binding of CBF3 to CDEIII is more important and is involved in kinetochore assembly.

The centromeric region of fission yeast chromosomes, on the other hand, is more like that of higher animals and plants. It is much larger (50-150kb long) and contains atleast four classes of repetitive DNA elements (L, K and B sequences flanking a core sequence, cc2), which seem to be responsible for full centromere function. Centromeric DNA sequences have also been examined in some mammals, and in a number of plant materials (maize, barley, rice, *Sorghum bicolor* and *Brachypodium sylvaticum*, etc.). These centromeres of fission yeast, mammals and higher plants are much more complex than those from budding yeast, and are called regional centromeres. They include both unique and repetitive DNA sequences, several kilobases or megabases in length (as shown above for fission yeast).

For instance, in mammals, centromeres consist of many different and much longer DNA sequences, that are both unique and repetitive in nature. Several of these sequences form much larger kinetochores, each of them binding 30 or 40 microtubules instead of one in budding yeast. It is believed that much of the repetitive DNA sequence (called satellite DNA) in mammalian centromeres is required for the special chromatin organisation at the centromere. However, it is shown that these tandemly repeated centromeric DNA families are poorly conserved between species.

The best studied centromeric satellite sequence is alpha-satellite DNA or alphoid DNA, that is found in all human and primate centromeres. The basic units of alpha-satellite are diverged, and consist of 171bp long monomers (arranged in a tandem manner), that are organised into higher order repeat units (making upto millions of base pairs). A small sequence, called CENP-B box (see below) is found only in a subset of these monomers. Alpha-satellite DNA is also believed to play an important role in centromere function. Similarly, minor satellite (monomer sequence of 300bp) in mouse also represents repetitive DNA elements related to centromeric function.

Centromeric sequences have also been isolated in a number of cereals and other members of grass family but none of them could be shown to perform centromere function. These include (i) CCS1 from Triticeae (CCS=cereal centromere sequence); (ii) BCS1 and BCS2 from barley (BCS=barley centromeric sequence); (iii) RCS1 from rice (RCS=rice centromeric sequence); (iv) MCS1 from maize (MCS=maize centromeric sequence); (v) pSau3A9 (745bp) from sorghum (this sequence has also been shown to be conserved in distantly related monocot plant species but not in dicotyledons).

A number of centromeric proteins have also been identified in mammalian cells. These include the following: (i) centromere proteins (CENP-A, B, C, D and E); (ii) inner centromere proteins INCENPs) and (iii) chromatid linking proteins (CLiPs). One of these proteins, called centromere protein B (CENP-B), is found associated with most human and mouse centromeres and its amino acid sequence is highly conserved among mammals. The protein CENP-B has also been shown to be related to a family of transposes found in a family of transposons.

The binding site for 'CENP-B' is the 'CENP-B box', 17bp long, which is a degenerate motif (5'N......... TTCGNNNNA NNCGGGN3') found in diverse animal systems. This suggests that other than the 'CENP-B box', there is little sequence similarity between centromeric DNA sequences of different mammalian centromeres. This 'CENP-B box' is, however, absent in human and mouse Y chromosomes.

Similarly, centromeres of the chromosomes of African green monkey (AGM) also have few, if any 'CENP-B boxes'. Further, the absence of CENP-B protein and CENP-B boxes (DNA sequence) from some active centromeres, and the presence of CENP-B at some non-centromeric locations strongly argue that binding of CENP-B protein is neither necessary, nor sufficient for centromere function.

The isolation and cloning of functional centromeric DNA sequences as above, is a prerequisite for construction of artificial chromosomes. The two other sequences, necessary for this purpose are telomeres and replication origins. Such artificial chromosomes have already been constructed in yeast and are called yeast artificial chromosomes or YACs. Mammalian (or human) artificial chromosomes (MACs or HACs) have also been reported in 1997. In future, construction of plant artificial chromosomes (PACs) may also become possible.

Function of Chromosomes

The function of chromosomes is to carry the genetic information from one cell generation to another. That DNA, which is the only permanent component of chromosome structure, is the sole genetic material has been shown by a variety of experiments. Also, the manner in which DNA stores the genetic information will be dealt elsewhere. The replication of chromosome depends on a very precise replication of DNA.

Special Types of Chromosomes

Chromosomes dealing eukaryotes was devoted to structure and function of chromosomes as observed in mitotic or meiotic cells in plants and animals. In certain organisms there are special tissues where these chromosomes take up a special structure. Lampbrush chromosomes of the vertebrate oocyte and giant chromosomes of salivary gland cells of dipterans are such special types of chromosomes. Due to special significance of these chromosomes, a relatively detailed account of these two types of chromosomes will be presented.

Lampbrush Chromosomes: As indicated earlier, chromosome structure at the same stage of cell division remains constant in the different kinds of cells in the same organism. Chromosomes of a special kind are, however, found in a variety of primary oocyte nuclei in vertebrates (mainly amphibians) as well as in some invertebrates. These chromosomes, known as lampbrush chromosomes, are found during the prolonged diplotene stage of first meiotic division in primary oocytes of amphibians, and in spermatocyte nuclei of *Drosophila*.

The lampbrush chromosomes are characterised by a remarkable change in structure. The change in structure includes an enormous increase in length. These chromosomes may sometimes become even larger than polynemic giant salivary gland chromosomes.

The largest chromosome having a length upto 1mm has been observed in urodele amphibian. The chromosomes seem to have a chromomeric pattern with loops projecting in pairs from majority of chromomeres. One to nine loops may arise from a single chromomere. The size of loops varies with an average of 9.5 μ in interchromomeric fibres.

The pairs of loops in these chromosomes give them the characteristic lampbrush appearance (Fig.). Frequently these loops exhibit a thin axis (which probably consists of one DNA double helix) from which fibres project which are covered with a loop matrix consisting of RNA and protein. The number of pairs of loops gradually increases in meiosis till it reaches maximum in diplotene.

As meiosis proceeds further, number of loops gradually decreases and the loops ultimately disappear due to disintegration rather than reabsorption back into the chromomere. H. Ris, however, had thought that the loops were integral parts of chromonemata which are extended in the form of major coils.

It is also believed that the loops represent the modified chromosome structures at the loci of active genes. It has been observed that, if the activity of these genes is stopped by actinomycin D (actinomycin D stops synthesis of RNA on DNA template), the loops will collapse, suggesting that the loops mainly consist of RNA.

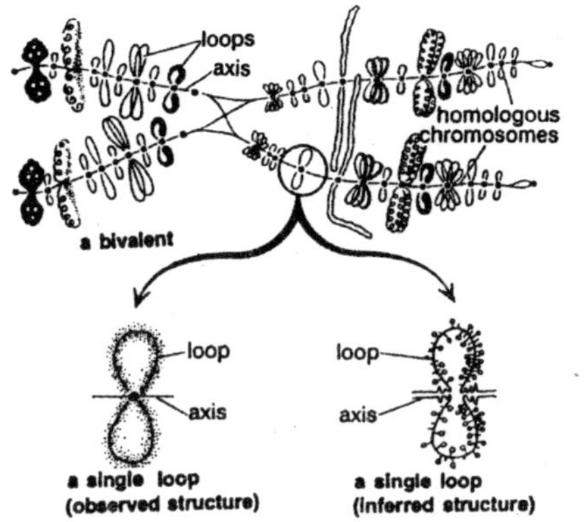

Lampbrush chromosomes showing details of structures (redrawn from Lewis and John: Chromosome Marker, 1963).

Salivary Gland Chromosomes: In salivary gland cells of dipleran species, giant chromosomes were observed by *E.G.* Balbiani for the first time in 1881. The availability of these chromosomes greatly helped the study of cytogenetics in fruitfly *(Drosophila).* These chromosomes may reach a size up to 200 times (or more) the size of corresponding chromosomes at meiosis or in nuclei of ordinary mitotic cells.

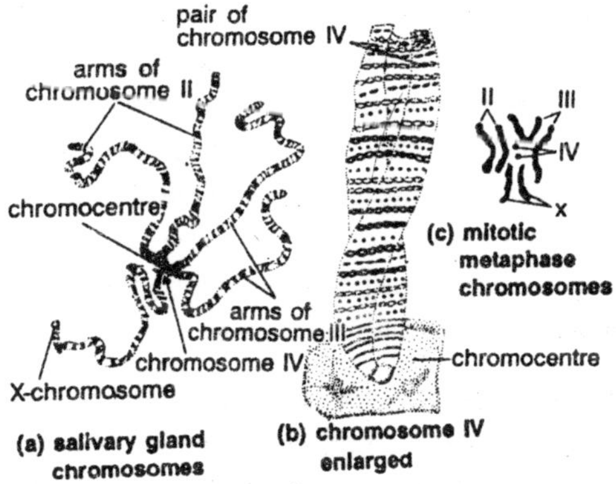

Salivary gland chromosome (a,b) and mitotic chromosomes (c) of Drosophila melanogaster (redrawn from Swanson: Cytology and Cytogenetics, 1957).

Another characteristic of these giant chromosomes is that they are somatically paired. Consequently the number of these giant chromosomes in the salivary gland cells always appear to be half that in the normal somatic cells. The giant chromosomes have a distinct pattern of transverse banding which consists of alternate chromatic and achromatic regions. These bands have greatly helped in the mapping of chromosomes in cytogenetic studies. The bands occasionally form reversible puffs, known as chromosome puffs or Balbiani rings, which are associated with differential gene activation.

The giant chromosomes represent each a bundle of fibrils which arise by repeated cycles of endo-reduplication of single chromatids. Endo-reduplication means that the chromatin replicates without cell division, as a result of which the number of chromonemata keeps on increasing. This is why these chromosomes are also popularly known as polytene chromosomes and the condition is described as polyteny. The number of chromonemata (fibrils) per chromosome may reach upto 2000 in extreme cases. Some workers placed this figure as high as 16,000.

In *D. melanogaster*, the giant chromosomes are found in the form of five long and one short strands radiating from a single more or less amorphous mass known as chromocentre (Fig.). One long strand corresponds to the X chromosome and the remaining four long strands are the arms of II and III chromosomes. The centromeres of all these chromosomes fuse to form the chromocentre. In the male flies the Y chromosome is also found fused within the chromocentre and is therefore not seen as a separate strand.

How an enormous increase in size of these chromosomes is brought about in salivary glands is not known and various hypotheses are available to explain this issue. The reader should consult Swanson's book, *Cytology and Cytogenetics*, to get a relatively detailed account of these hypotheses. It should,

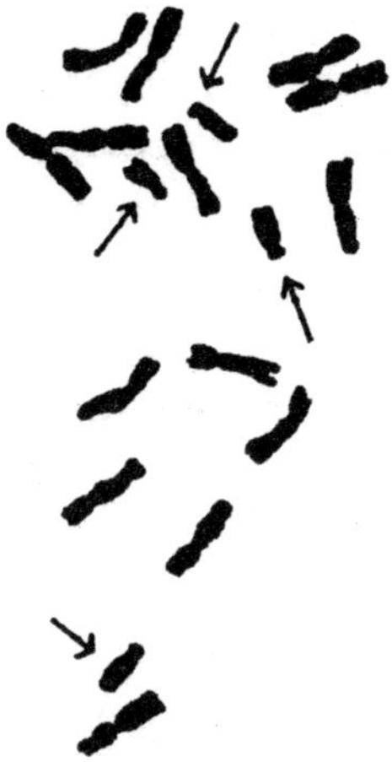

A mitotic metaphase plate showing the presence of 4 B chromosomes (arrowed).

however, be emphasised that these giant chromosomes though, commonly found in salivary glands, have also been found in malpighian tubules, fat bodies, ovarian nurse cells, gut epithelia and some other tissues.

B-chromosomes: B-chromosomes are a particular kind of supernumerary chromosomes, that may or may not be found in an organism as extra chromosomes over and above the standard diploid or polyploid chromosome complement (Fig.). The standard complement consists of chromosomes described as A-chromosomes, including sex chromosomes, if any.

The B-chromosomes are found in the natural populations of many plant and animal species and are recognised on the basis of their following characteristics: (i) they are dispensable (they are not found in all individuals of a species and may not be found in all cells of an individual organism); (ii) they are not homologous with any of the basic A chromosomes; (iii) their inheritance is non-Mendelian, sometimes due to non-disjunction during pollen mitosis (as in some plants); (iv) they are usually smaller than A-chromosomes and have their own unique pattern of heterochromatin distribution;

(v) in general, they are genetically inert, but may rarely organise nucleoli and carry functional genetic material; (vi) when present in high number, they suppress vigour and fertility; (vii) their origin and function are largely unknown.

B-chromosome in plants have been reported in more than 1000 species distributed over bryophytes (including mosses), ferns, gymnosperms and angiosperms (both monocotyledons and dicotyledons). Mostly, they are found in out-breeders (cross pollinated species). In the family Gramineae, they are found in 200 species including cereals, and forage grasses belonging to genera *Agrostis, Anthoxanthum, Avena, Bromus, Calamogrostis, Dactylis, Deschampsia, Festuca, Koeleria, Lolium, Pennisetum, Phleum, Secale, Sorghum* and *Zea*.

These B-chromosome are often absent in well adapted agronomic strains, and are perhaps eliminated due to selection. The B-chromosomes may sometimes be restricted only to aerial parts (absent in roots *e.g., Aegilops speltoidas, Ae. mutica)* and may also be eliminated during meiosis due to their division at anaphase I followed by elimination at anaphase II. B-chromosomes may also increase in number due to a drive involving non- disjunction during pollen mitosis, thus leading to the production of plants with an increased number of B-chromosomes in the progeny of a cross 0B♀ × 1B♂.

The most significant effect of B-chromosomes is on seed and pollen fertility. Flowering time is generally delayed by B-chromosomes and several characters (plant height, plant weight and tiller number) are adversely affected. A very important effect of B-chromosomes relates with their effect on pairing of A chromosomes in (i) plants carrying these B-chromosomes and in (ii) species hybrids involving a parent carrying B-chromosomes.

In rye, although 0-6 B-chromosomes did not influence the chiasmata frequencies, 8 B-chromosomes drastically influenced the range of chiasma frequencies among pollen mother cells

(PMCs) and among bivalents within individual PMCs. In maize, the use of various A/B interchange stocks demonstrated that the genetic elements affecting meiotic pairing of A-chromosomes appeared to be widely distributed throughout the length of B-chromosomes. The effect of B-chromosomes in suppressing or promoting meiotic pairing has been shown in a number of intergeneric or interspecific hybrids (wheat x *Aegilops* sp.; wheat × rye, *Lolium* × *Festuca;* interspecific hybrids within the genus *Lolium,* etc.). For more details, the readers should consult the book B-chromosomes written by R.N. Jones and H. Rees (1982).

Prokaryotic Nucleoids (Bacterial and Plasmid Genomes): As indicated earlier, the light microscope could not show any nucleus in the cells of prokaryotes *i.e.,* the bacteria and the blue green algae. These individuals are also designated as the akaryobionta as against the karyobionta having better differentiated nuclei. However, feulgen positive bodies are seen in bacteria and blue-green algae, a reaction meant for the nucleus or chromosomes. These bodies can be clearly observed with the help of electron microscope. It has also been demonstrated that these bodies consist of a network of fine threads (Fig.), making a single chromosome.

Bacterial Genome

Bacterial genome varies from 585kb in mycoplasma to 9,454kb in *Myxococcus* and therefore is much smaller to that in eukaryotes, where it can vary from 14 million kb in yeast to 102 million kb in lungfish. For many years it was believed that bacterial chromosome is circular. Only as late as 1990, a linear chromosome was described in *Borrelia burgdorferi* (a spirochaete).

However, more recently, using newer technique of pulse field gel electrophoresis (PEGE) and its variant transverse alternating field electrophoresis (TAFE), linear chromosomes were discovered in several other cases. Consequently, now we know that although generally a single circular DNA is found as a chromosome in a bacterial cell, there are following variations: (i) 2 or 3 circular chromosomes, (ii) one circular and one linear chromosome, (iii) one linear chromosome. The details of these exceptions to the paradigm of a single circular bacterial chromosome are listed in Table.

The exact three dimensional arrangement, by which 1100-1400 microns long DNA chain, forming 80% of the chromosome by mass (remaining 20% is protein + RNA), is packed in a one micron long nucleoid of a bacterial cell, has also been established for some time now. Atleast two proteins,

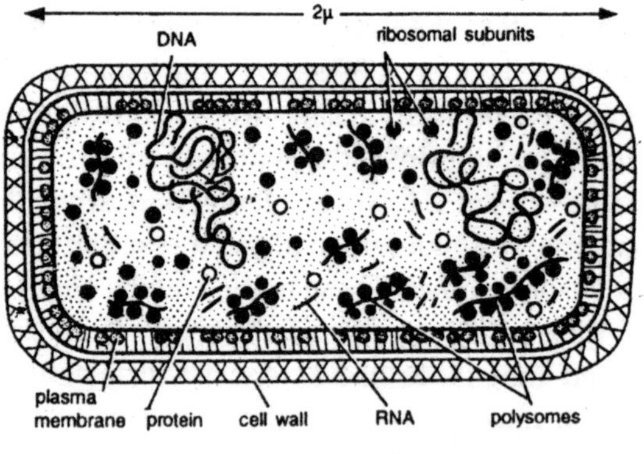

A bacterial cell showing details of internal structure (redrawn from De Robertis et. al., Cell Biology, 1975).

Exceptions to the Concept of Single Circular Bacterial Chromosome

Bacterium	*Number & conformation of chromosomes*	*Size of chromosome (kb)*
1. *Brucella melitensis*	2 (both circular)	2100,1150
2. *Leptospira* interrogans	2 (both circular)	4400-4600, 350

Contd...

Bacterium	*Number & conformation of chromosomes*	*Size of chromosome (kb)*
3. *Rhodobacter sphaeroides*	2 (both circular)	3046, 914
4. *Pseudomonas cepacia*	3 (all circular)	3400, 2500, 900
5. *Agrobacterium tumefaciens*	2 (one circular, one linear)	3000, 2100
6. *Streptomyces (six species)*	1 (linear)	8000

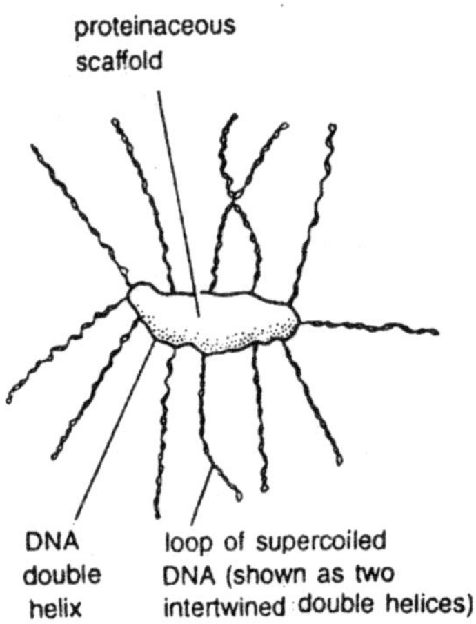

Diagrammatic representation of the organisation of DNA and proteins in bacterial chromosome.

which bind DNA, resemble histones of eukaryotes and organise the DNA into structures comparable to nucleosomes of eukaryotes. It has been shown that the chromosome of *E. coli* is organised in about 45 loops, which radiate out from a dense proteinaceous scaffold, which is assumed to anchor the DNA

(Fig.). In each of the 45 loops, DNA is supercoiled and complexed with protein. The functional significance of looped domains is not clear but they do not represent units of transcription as in case of lampbrush chromosomes.

Plasmid Genome: Plasmid genomes were also believed earlier to consist of only small supercoiled circular DNA molecules. Exceptions to this general paradigm have also been available recently due to the demonstration of the presence of linear DNA molecules in the plasmid genomes.

Although plasmid genome is usually a small molecule, very large circular molecules have also been shown to be present in the plasmids of *Rhizobium meliloti*. Some of these exceptions are listed in Table.

Centromere and Telomere Like Structures in Bacteria and Plasmids: The bacterial chromosome is characterised by the presence of a number of essential genes, rather than by its size, because sometimes, the bacterial chromosome is smaller in size than the plasmid DNA.

These essential genes include ribosomal genes, *oriC, dnaA* and several other genes which are found on bacterial chromosomes, but are missing in the plasmid genome which is considered to be accessary rather than essential.

In *E. coli,* after chromosome replication, structures called catenanes are formed, which are resolved into monomers with the help of two topoisomerases (DNA gyrase and topoisomerase IV) and xer CD recombinase. After this, partitioning of monomers into newly formed daughter cells takes place with the help of proteins MukB (a motor protein) and FtsZ.

In plasmids P1 and F, contromeres have been identified which are called *parS* (for P1) and *sopC* (for F). They are needed for proper segregation of plasmids into daughter cells.

Exceptions to the Concept of Small Circular DNA in Bacterial Plasmids

Plasmid origin	*No. & conformation of DNA molecules*	*Size of DNA molecule (kb)*
1. *Bacillus polymyxa*	1 (linear)	16
2. *Borrelia sp.*	3 (linear)	50,55,56
3. *Rhizobium meliloti*	2 (circular)	1340, 1700
4. *Rhodococcus sp.*	2 (linear)	270, 280
5. *Streptomyces coelicolor*	1 (linear)	390-630, 550, 1700
6. *S. violaceoruber*	1 (linear)	70
7. *Thiobacillus versatus*	1 (linear)	3.7

Structures homologous to eukaryotic telomeric sequences are also found in prokaryotes and are perhaps responsible for stability, maintenance and segregation (particularly in their replicons). In the linear molecules, two types of ends are identified— (i) 'hairpins' (*e.g.*, in *Borrelia* linear plasmids) with AT-rich perfect palindrome with a conserved 19-bp inverted repeat at the end and (ii) 'invertons' (*e.g.*, in *Streptomyces)* with the inverted terminal repeats.

8

Plant Cells

Most plant cells possess a cell wall, and this feature distinguishes them from animal cells. The cell wall is a nonliving structure which is formed by the living protoplast. It has a supportive and protective function. Three layers can be distinguished in the cell wall. These are the *middle lamella* the *primary cell wall* and the *secondary cell wall* (Fig.). Occasionally a *tertiary cell wall* may be present.

Cell Cover

The middle lamella is formed between adjacent cell walls during cell division. It consists of a comparatively thin layer of intercellular material. It is a viscous and jelly-like substance and acts as a cementing material between the primary cell walls of adjacent cells. The middle lamella is composed of pectin, cellulose, calcium and polymers of various types. Pectin is a hydrophilic colloidal substance.

The primary cell wall is formed during the early stages of growth and development. It is found in all plant cells, and is 1 to 3 mm thick. It is composed chiefly of cellulose, hemicellulose and pectic compounds. The primary cell wall is elastic, and undergoes extension with the growth of the cell. In many roots, fleshy stems, fruits and leaves the cells contain only the primary cell wall and the middle lamella. The *cellulose* fibrils of the primary cell wall are loosely interwoven, with a degree of polymerisation of 8,000 to 12,000 glucose units. They are about 100A in diameter.

The secondary cell wall is laid down on the primary cell wall when the latter has finished its growth. It is found only in certain mature and highly specialised cells. It is about 5 to 10 μ m thick. After the formation of the secondary cell wall the protoplasm disappears in many cell types. The secondary cell wall commonly has three layers. These are known as the *outer layer* the *middle layer* and the *inner layer*. The secondary cell wall consists of many layers of closely packed *micro-fibrils.* The succeeding layers are laid down at different angles to one another. In green plants the microfibrils are most often of *cellulose,* although they may contain other polysaccharides as well. In some algae there are many fibrils of *xylan* and *mannan.*

In some tissues a *tertiary cell wall* is formed on the inner surface of the secondary cell wall. This layer is very thin and is found in the xylem tracheids of Gymnosperms. It is composed mainly of *xylan,* instead of cellulose.

Organisation of cellulose. The structure of the cell wall is based on cellulose. The cell wall is composed of *macrofibrils,* 0.5 μ m in width, which are visible under the light microscope (Fig.). The macro-fibril consists of a bundle of *microfibrils,* each of which is about 250A in diameter. The microfibril is visible only under the electron microscope. The microfibril in turn consists of a bundle of *micelles* or *elementary fibrils,* each about 100A in diameter. The micelle contains about 100 *cellulose chains.* Cellulose is a polymer of *glucose* molecules. In the primary cell wall the macrofibrils are arranged at random. In the secondary cell wall they are closely packed and are arranged parallel to one another. They are oriented in different directions in the different layers of the cell wall.

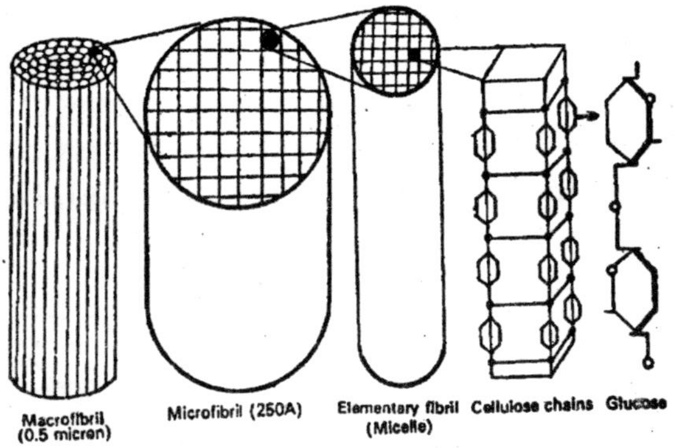

Structural elements of cellulose.

Matrix: The microfibrils of cellulose and other polysaccharides are embedded in a *matrix* which consists largely of polysaccharide material. The substances present in the matrix vary with the growth phase of the plant. In the earlier stages *pectic substances (polygalacturonic acid* derivatives) are predominant. In later stages *xylans* and several neutral polysaccharides *('hemicelluloses')* appear.

In dicots the primary cell wall contains complex polysaccharides linked to each other and to the cellulose microfibrils by covalent linkages. They include: (1) *xyloglucans* which contain a linear glucan chain with *xylose, galactose* and *fucose* units in its branches, (2) *arabinogalactans* and (3) *rhamnogalacturonans,* which consist of chains of *galacturonic* acid, with *rhamnose* rings inserted at intervals.

A *glycoprotein* called *extensin* is also present in plant cell walls along with the carbohydrates. Like collagen, extensin is rich in *4-hydroxy-proline*. It consists of a protein chain, to the hydroxyl groups of which are linked the sugars *arabinose* and *galactose* in the form of oligosaccharides of about 9 units each. During the later stages of growth large amounts of *lignin* are laid down in plant cells, and the walls harden into wood.

Primary Pit Fields and Primary Pits: Primary pit fields are found in cells which contain only the primary cell wall. In certain areas the primary cell wall is thin and contains a group of pores. These areas are called *primary pit fields.* In some plants the secondary cell wall has depressions or cavities called *pits.* Pits are usually found in nonliving cells like tracheids and fibres, whose function is conduction and support. Pits are of two types, *simple pits* and *bordered pits* (Fig.).

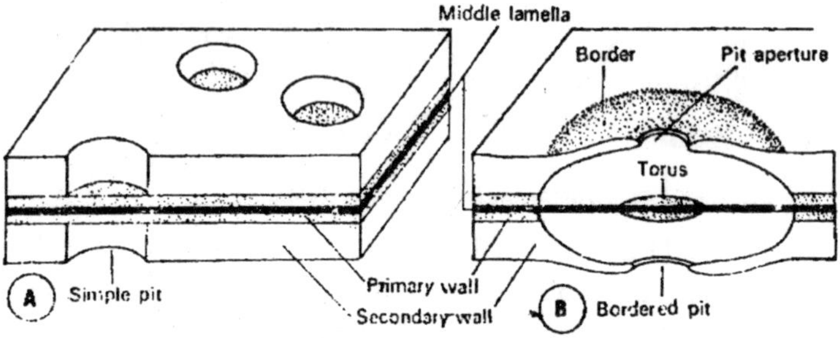

(A) Simple pits. (B) Bordered pit.

In a bordered pit the secondary cell wall projects over the cavity of the pit, enclosing a *pit chamber,* which opens outside through a *pit aperture.* In a simple pit there is no projecting margin. Adjacent pits are separated by the middle lamella and the primary cell wall, which together form the *pit membrane.* The pit membrane may have a thickening called the *torus* which is formed by circular deposition of microfibrils. The part of the membrane surrounding the torus is called the *margo.*

It is flexible and has radially arranged microfibrils which are anchored in the surrounding primary wall and hold the torus in position. The margo has small openings between the fibrils, through which aqueous substances flow from one cell to another. If the torus is pressed against the pit aperture due to pressure of aqeous substances in the cell, it stops the passage of substances. The pit and the pitted areas help in the passage of material from one cell to another.

Plasmodesmata: The primary cell wall contains many small openings or pores situated in the primary pit fields. The cytoplasm of adjacent cells communicates through the pores by means of cytoplasmic bridges called *plasmodesmata*. Tubules, which are in continuity with the endoplasmic reticulum, have been observed within the plasmodesmata. The plasmodesmata permit circulation of fluid and passage of solutes between cells.

Chemical Composition: The main components of the middle lamella are *pectic substances (pectin)*. Pectin is a hydrophilic colloidal substance. The primary cell wall is composed mainly of *cellulose, hemicellulose* and *pectic compounds*. The chief components of the secondary cell wall are *cellulose, hemicellulose* and *lignin*. Cellulose is thus the most important component of the cell wall in most plant groups. In fungi and lichens, however, the cell wall is composed of *chitin, glucans* and a *mannan-protein* complex.

Lignin is derived from carbohydrates and gives rigidity and strength to the cell wall. It is found in woody tissues. During the process of lignification, lignin is added to the matrix of the cell wall. Lignin is present in all the three layers of the cell wall. The process of lignification starts with the primary cell wall, and then extends to the middle lamella and the secondary cell wall.

Lipids like *suberin, cutin* and *waxes* are also found as structural components of the cell wall. A *suberin* lamella is found in the suberised cells of cork tissue. It is separated from the contents of the cell by a cellulose wall. A layer of *cutin* is found on the surface of epidermal cells. Cutin is also mixed with the cellulose layers beneath. The two layers together from the *cuticular membrane*. A thin pectic layer separates the cuticular membrane from the cutin-free inner part of the cell wall. The cuticular layer may be produced into *cuticular pegs* which extend between epidermal cells.

Formation of the Cell Wall: Immediately after nuclear division the *phragmoplast* or *cell plate* appears across the equator of the cell. At the end of mitosis granules arising from the Golgi complex arrange themselves on the equator of the cell. They then fuse to form the cell plate. The cell plate grows in thickness by addition of new material from the complex. Narrow openings, the plasmodesmata, are left in the cell plate, and cytoplasmic connection between the cells is retained through them.

During the development of the cell wall the *middle lamella* is formed first. It consists of gelatinous material which is probably mainly calcium pectinate. The *primary cell wall* is then secreted against the middle lamella. It consists of intertwined fibres of cellulose. The primary cell wall is plastic and extends with the growth of the cell. After the period of growth is over a *secondary cell wall* may be laid down between the primary cell wall and the cytoplasm of the cell. The secondary cell wall consists of up to three layers of parallel fibres. The direction of the fibres shifts through 120 degrees in each layer. The orientation of the fibres is, therefore, the same every fourth layer.

Golgi Intricate

Historical: In 1890 Camillo Golgi described the *apparato reticulare interno* (internal reticular apparatus) in the nerve cells of the barn owl as a special cytoplasmic area impregnated with silver nitrate. This structure had however, been discovered earlier by la Valette St. George (1865, 1867), Plattner (1885) and Hermann (1891).

Holmgren (1900) described a system of clear canals, which he called the *trophospongium*. Though this structure was earlier described as being homologous with the internal reticular apparatus (Cajal referred to the Golgi nets as the Golgi-Holmgren canals) this comparison was later dropped. The trophospongium may in fact be the *endoplasmic reticulum*.

Perroncito (1910) used the term *dictiyokinesis* to describe the division of the Golgi apparatus, and recorded that it divided into smaller units, which he called *dictyosomes.*

Raman y Cajal (1914) studied the Golgi apparatus in a wide variety of cell types. His work is important because he directed attention to the functional aspects of the apparatus by introducing experimental methods.

Gatenby (1917) showed the similarity between the Golgi apparatus and the dictyosomes of invertebrates.

Parat and Painleve (1924) attempted to equate the Golgi apparatus with the *vacuome* of French cytologists. According to the vacuome theory the two fundamental units of the cell were the *vacuome* and the *chondriome.* Later Parat (1928) divided the chondriome (mitochondria) into two classes, active and inactive. He assumed that the inactive mitochondria were a part of the Golgi apparatus.

Nassonov (1923, 1924) and Bowen (1929) finally established the relation of the Golgi apparatus to the process of secretion.

Palade and Claude (1949) thought that the Golgi apparatus was an artifact, but later discarded this interpretation. Baker and his colleagues (1944-1963) denied the existence of the reticulum and concluded that there was no evidence for a Golgi substance. Baker later modified his views and stated that many cellular organelles might react to the Golgi method. The introduction of electron microscopy in the early 1950s, however, clearly established the existence of the Golgi apparatus. In 1963 Baker also accepted its existence.

Important Terms

Baker (1951, 1953) referred to the Golgi apparatus as *lipochondria* because of the presumed lipid content. Structures similar to the Golgi complex have been found in plants. Botanists refer to them as *dictyosomes.*

Dalton (1952) observed parallel membranes and vacuoles under the electron microscope, and identified them as elements of the Golgi apparatus. Baker (1959) had preferred the use of the term *Dalton complex* for the structures described as Golgi bodies by the light microscopists. He did not accept the term Golgi apparatus earlier, but did so in 1963. Sjostrand (1956) earlier proposed the term y *cytomembranes for the* Golgi system, but later preferred the term Golgi membranes. A number of joined Golgi systems is known as a polysystem.

Number: The Golgi complex is generally a single large structure. A *Paramoeba* species has two large Golgi complexes, while in the amoeba *Stereomyxa* there are many Golgi complexes. Nerve cells, liver cells and most plant cells also have multiple Golgi complexes, there being about 50 in liver cells. Cells with dispersed Golgi complexes may have hundreds scattered throughout the cytoplasm of the cell.

Shape and Position: The shape of the Golgi apparatus is quite variable in different somatic cell types of animals. Even in the same cell there are variations in different functional stages. The shape is however, constant with each cell type. It varies in form from a compact mass to a disperse filamentous network.

The position of the Golgi complex is also variable. In cells of ectodermic origin the Golgi complex is polarised between the nucleus and the periphery. In secretory (exocrine) cells it lies between the nucleus and the secretory pole.

In endocrine secretory cells the position is variable. In ganglion cells of the mouse the position is peri-nuclear.

Size: The Golgi complex is large in nerve and gland cells, but small in muscle cells. The size is linked to the functional state. The Golgi complex hypertrophies during hyper function and becomes reduced during hypo function.

STRUCTURE OF ELECTRON MICROSCOPE

The first electron micrographs clearly reveal the structure of the Golgi complex were by Dalton and Felix (1954). These workers described the Golgi complex in the epididymis of the rat as consisting of three components; flattened sacs or *cisternae, large vacuoles* and *small granules.* The following description of the Golgi complex is a composite one based on the work of several authors.

Electron microscope observations of thin sections reveal the presence of three membranous components: (1) flattened sacs or *cisternae,* (2) *small tubules* and *vesicles* and (3) *large vacuoles* filled with an amorphous or granular substance. These membranous structures are characterised by the absence of ribosomes, *i.e.* they are smooth membranes.

The *cisternae* or *lamellae* are the most constant elements of the Golgi complex. They consist of flattened, parallel sacs piled one upon the other to form *stacks.*

The number of cisternae in a stack varies from species to species, and sometimes from one developmental stage to another. In most animal 'and plant cells there are 3-8 cisternae in a stack. Other cell types may have as many as 25 to 30 cisternae.

Mollenhauer and Whaley (1963) suggested that in certain plant cells the Golgi complex is polarised and has a *"forming face"* and a *"maturing face"*. The forming or proximal face is on the outer side while the maturing or distal face is on the opposite side. It is believed that the smooth membranes of the ER bud off vesicles, which then become arranged on the forming face of the stack. It is also possible that a lamella of the ER may be converted into a Golgi lamella by loss of ribosomes. On the other side is the maturing or secreting face where the lamella bud off *secretory vesicles.* Thus new lamella are formed on the forming face and mature lamellae are lost on the maturing face. Chemical analysis shows the composition of the Golgi complex membranes is intermediate between those of the ER and the plasmalemma. The membranes at the forming face of the Golgi complex are similar to the ER membranes and those of the maturing face to the plasmalemma. The membranes of the Golgi complex are in dynamic equilibrium. They are continually receiving lamellae through budding of vesicles from the smooth ER, and losing membranes through formation of secretory vesicles.

In a section the cisternae unit appears as a pair of parallel membranes continuous at the ends. The two membranes enclose a thin cavity about 150A across. The cavities of the cisternae on the maturing face are generally wider. The cisternal units are usually placed 200-300A apart. There is usually a difference in the size of the cisternae at the forming and maturing faces. The cisternae may be flat, but are more usually slightly curved. This gives the whole stack convex and concave faces.

In a number of cases the cisternae show variation from the typical form. In goblet cells, at a certain stage of maturity, the cisternae are all transformed into *mucigen granules* which almost fill up the cell (Neutra and Leblond, 1966). In the multifid gland of the snail the stack breaks up into *small vesicles* during certain stages of development. The stack-like form is again reorganised from the vesicle in the secreting phase (Outracth, 1972).

Fenestration: The membranes of the cisternae may sometimes be *fenestrated, i.e.* may have small pores. The pores may be confined to the periphery or may occupy three-fourths or more of the cisterna. The cisternae are often *reticulate* structures and not simply flattened sacs. Reticulation of the cisternae may vary from one face of the stack to the other, or may also vary with different developmental stages. The extent of reticulation may also depend upon experimental techniques. Reticulation, however, does exist *in vivo,* as is evidenced from freeze-etch material. In some cases reticulation is so extensive that the cisternae appears like a network of interconnected tubules.

Intercisternal Elements: In a few cases dense material has been found between the cisternae of the Golgi complex, and has been called the *intercisternal material*. In the Golgi complex of *Nitella*. the intercisternal elements are elongated, 60-80-A in diameter, oriented in the same direction, and located towards the distal face (Turner and Whaley, 1965). In the Golgi complex (parabasal body) of *Trichomonas* the intercisternal material appears to be uniformly granular.

It is confined to the central region of the Golgi complex, there being no material between the proximal and the distal 5 to 6 cisternae (Amos and Grimstone, 1968). In *Distigma* the intercisternal material forms a dense conical core which does not involve a few proximal and a few distal cisternae (Mignot, 1965). The composition and function of the intercisternal material is not known. It has been suggested that it acts as a cementing substance, holding the cisternae together.

In rabbit epididymis cells the Golgi stacks are closely associated to form a continuous tube. Some stacks are also found within the tube. The *small vesicles*, are 400-800A in diameter. They are intimately associated with the cisternae and may show continuity with them. The small vesicles arise from the cisternae by budding or pinching off.

Large Vacuoles: The large vacuoles are clear, and generally lie at the edge of the Golgi complex. They represent modified and expanded cisternae in which the two membranes have become widely separated, and the vacuolar space enlarged. They contain clear material which reduces metallic salts.

The isolated Golgi complex (dictyosome) of plant cells has been studied by gluteraldehyde fixation, followed by negative staining with phosphotungstic acid. It is composed of stacks of flattened, fenestrated cisternae. Many anastomosing tubules,

300-500A in diameter, are given off from the cisternae. Associated with the tubules are two types of vesicles, rough surfaced and smooth surfaced vesicles. The rough surfaced vesicles are spherical and about 600A in diameter. The smooth-surfaced vesicles vary in size. Between the cisternae are parallel *rods* or *fibers,* 70-80 A in diameter.

Biochemical Division

Morphologically the Golgi complex lies between the endoplasmic reticulum and the plasma membrane, the three membranes being linked by transitional structures and by secretory granules. This has led to the suggestion that the Golgi complex membranes are in an intermediate state of differentiation between the endoplasmic reticulum membranes and the plasma membrane. There is a gradation of many biochemical properties of the three membranes, *e.g.* the lipid content, phospholipid (lecithin and sphingomyelin) content and the fatty acid composition of phospholipids. Electrophoretic band patterns show that the membrane proteins are transitional between those of the ER and the plasma membrane.

Enzymatic activities of the three membranes have been mostly reported from rat liver:

1. Thiamine pyrophosphatase (TPPase) activity is greater in the Golgi fraction than in the other fractions.
2. 5'-Nucleotidase activity of the Golgi complex is lower than that of the plasma membrane.
3. Glucose-6-phosphatase activity is absent from the Golgi membranes, or very low (contamination?).
4. Acyl transferase and choline phosphotransferase are absent in the Golgi membranes, as distinguished from the condition in the ER membranes. Thus the Golgi membranes cannot synthesise *triglycerides* and *phosphatidylcholine.*

5. The Golgi membranes have a single electron transport chain, that containing *cytochrome* b_5. They lack *NADPH-cytochrome c reductase* activity and *cytochrome P450* activity, showing the absence of one electron transport chain. In this respect they differ from the ER membranes.
6. The characteristic feature of the Golgi membranes is that they have high *glycosyltransferase* activity. These enzymes catalyse synthesis of *glycoproteins.*

Generation of Golgi Intricate

The Golgi complex is constantly being formed, changed, broken down and reformed. It has been variously described as being formed from the plasmalemma, nuclear envelope, annulate lamellae and the endoplasmic reticulum.

(1) *From the Plasmalemma*: In the amoeba *Pelomyxa illionoisensis* the Golgi cisternae are described as originating from the plasmalemma vesicles (Daniels, 1964). These vesicles are formed by pinocytosis and phagocytosis of the plasmalemma.

(2) *From the Nuclear Envelope:* In the brown algae there is a close association between the nuclear envelope and the Golgi complex. Bouch (1965) has described vesicles, similar to those on the formative face of the Golgi complex, arising from the nuclear envelope.

(3) *From the Annulate Lamellae:* In the study of oocyte maturation in the frog, Ward (1965) has described vesicles apparently derived from the annulate lamellae eventually fusing and giving rise to the Golgi membranes.

(4) *From the Endoplasmic Reticulum:* Essner and Novikoff (1962) have described the formation of Golgi cisternae from the endoplasmic reticulum in certain hepatomas. Beams and Kessel (1968) have suggested that the Golgi

lamellae may be derived from the ER by loss of ribosomes.

It is believed that the Golgi complex arises from the granular ER, which changes to smooth ER, and then becomes the Golgi cisternae. The cisternae on the forming face are constantly being formed by fusion of vesicles derived from the ER. The cisternae on the maturing face are believed to form secretory vesicles. The presence of the nucleus is necessary to maintain the Golgi complex. In the absence of the nucleus the Golgi complex decreases in size and disappears. In enucleated amoebae the Golgi complex is formed within 30 minutes to one hour after nuclear transplant, and grows during 6-24 hours.

ROLE OF THE GOLGI INTRICATE

Several functions have been attributed to the Golgi complex. Most of the functions are based either on indirect observations or deductions.

Role in Secretion; General: There are numerous works describing secretory products in the cisternae of the Golgi complex. In the earlier works it was not clear whether secretory products were actually synthesised in the Golgi complex or whether the complex played a secondary role in secretion. Many electron microscope studies show that during vitellogenesis in oocytes, yolk products first become visible in the cisternae of the Golgi complex. However, in these studies it is not clear whether yolk is actually synthesised the Golgi complex or only packaged there. In certain oocytes the Golgi complex appears to give rise to cortical granules (Anderson, 1966).

In some cell-formed products appear in the expanded ends of the Golgi lamellae. In others, the secretory product completely fills the cisternae. The secretory products within the Golgi lamellae are very similar to the contents of the secretory granules near the Golgi complex. In some cases the ends of the Golgi cisternae may be pinched off to form *small secretory granules.* These may then fuse to form *larger granules.* In other cases the individual cisternae on the "maturing face" may be completely filled with secretory products, and then become rounded to form secretory granules. New cisternae would then apparently be formed on the "forming face". It is possible that the lamellae of the ER may become Golgi lamellae by loss of ribosomes.

Role in Protein Secretion: In pancreatic exocrine cells the distribution of secretory proteins (digestive enzymes) has been investigated by Siekevitz, Palade et al, (1962). (1) Proteins are formed on the ribosomes attached to the ER. (2) These nascent proteins are then transferred into the ER. (3) From here they go to the Golgi complex. There is morphological evidence that the ER may bud off vesicles which travel towards the Golgi complex.

The vesicles may then fuse with the membranes of the Golgi cisternae and release their contents into the latter. (4) In the Golgi complex the proteins are concentrated (possibly by water withdrawal) and transformed into *zymogen granules.* The zymogen of the granules consists of enzyme precursors of the pancreatic juice.

The membrane of the Golgi vacuole becomes the limiting membrane of the zymogen granule. (5) The zymogen granules released from the Golgi complex migrate to the surface of the cell. Here the limiting membrane of the zymogen granule fuses with the plasmalemma, thus discharging its contents. This process is a form of ' reversed pinocytosis.

From the above account it is apparent that the Golgi complex acts as a condensation membrane for proteins formed on the ribosomes. The concentrated material is then packaged for secretion.

Synthesis and Secretion of Polysaccharides: Studies on goblet cells by autoradiography and electron microscopy have established the interrelationship between protein synthesis, carbohydrate addition and sulphation. The goblet cells of the colon produce *mucigen.* This secretory material contains a large proportion of carbohydrate. The Golgi complex is found just above the nucleus. Towards the free surface of the cell are gradually enlarging *mucigen granules.* The proximal cisternae of the Golgi complex do not show any swelling, but at some distance across the stack the distal cisternae are quite suddenly converted into mucigen granules. The distal cisternae continually convert into mucigen granules every 2-4 minutes. New proximal cisternae are formed in compensation.

Studies by autoradiographic *^{3}H-glucose* and *^{3}H-galactose* labelling have provided direct evidence of polysaccharide synthesis in the Golgi complex (Peterson and Leblond, 1964; Neutra and Leblond, 1966). Five minutes after injection of ^{3}H-glucose the label is found over the Golgi complex. After 40 minutes the label crosses over to mucigen granules adjacent to the Golgi cisternae. Four hours after injection the label is found over the more apical mucigen granules. Neutra and Leblond also confirmed that sulphation takes place in the Golgi apparatus.

On the basis of these observations the following scheme was proposed by Neutra and Leblond (1969). (1) Precursors enter the goblet cells from the capillaries of the vascular system. (2) The *amino acids* are synthesised into *proteins* on the ribosomes of the endoplasmic reticulum. (3) The proteins are then transferred to the cisternae of the Golgi complex. (4) The simple sugar molecules go directly from the blood stream to the Golgi complex cisternae, where they are complexed with protein to form *glycoprotein.* (5) The glycoprotein is then sulphated in the Golgi complex to form *mucigen.* (6) The distal cisternae become rounded off and are transformed into *mucigen granules.* (7) The mucigen granules are progressively displaced towards the apex of the cell. During this process the mucigen undergoes further modification. (8) The mucigen granules are secreted into the intestine by exocytosis during which the vesicle membrane fuses with the plasma membrane.

Glycosylation: In many cells the protein released from the endoplasmic reticulum is combined with carbohydrate to produce complex carbohydrates like glycoproteins, mucopolysaccharides, glycogen and glycolipids. Addition of the carbohydrate components to the proteins occurs in the Golgi complex as well as the rough endoplasmic reticulum. Both the Golgi complex and the rough endoplasmic reticulum contain enzymes called *glycosyl-transferases* (Fig.). The nonglycoproteins formed on the ribosomes move into the

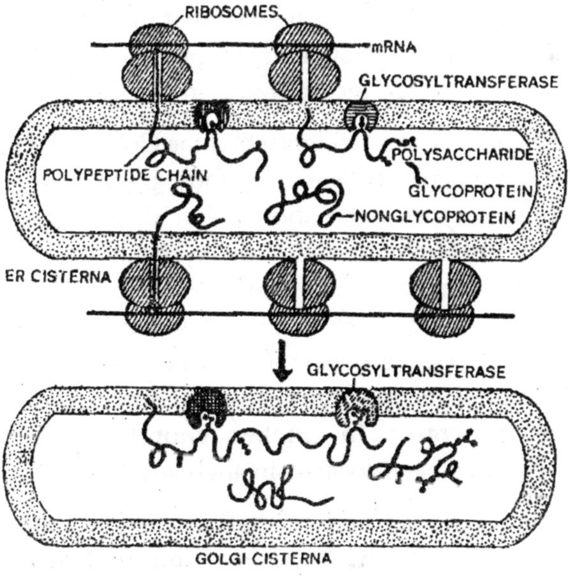

Diagram showing glycosylation of proteins. Above. Polypeptide chains synthesised on the ribosomes are glycosylated by glycosyltransferases in the ER. Non-glycoproteins move into the lumen of the ER. Below. Completion of glycosylation in the Golgi complex cisterna and release of glycoprotein into the lumen.

lumen of the ER cisternae immediately after polypeptide chain synthesis. Proteins destined for glycosylation remain attached to the ER membrane which contains glycosyltransferases. These enzymes catalyze glycosylation of proteins. The first sugars may by attached to the polypeptide chain in the ER cisternae even while the chain is attached to the ribosome.

The polypeptide chains are then transported to the Golgi complex. In the Golgi complex cisternae additional carbohydrate units (sugars) are added either to the polypeptide chain, or the sugar units already attached to the polypeptide chain. Glycosylation thus begins in the ER and is completed in the Golgi complex. After completion of glycosylation the glycoprotein is released into the lumen of the Golgi complex cisternae. Autoradiography studies of thyroglobulin synthesis by the thyroid follicle in the rat show that incorporation of the sugar *mannose* in the protein takes place in the ER, while *galactose* and *fucose* are incorporated in the Golgi complex.

Sulphation: There is evidence that the Golgi complex takes part in sulphate metabolism. Autoradiography experiments on several cell types have shown that there is radioactive sulphur (^{35}S) uptake in the Golgi region (Neutra and Leblond, 1966). Compounds containing active sulphur are formed in a two-step process. Sulphate is first activated by ATP in two stages, the process requiring two separate enzymes. The activated sulphate is then transferred to the acceptor molecule by *sulphotransferases.* In chicken chondrocytes sulpho-transferases have been located in the Golgi membranes.

(5) Plasma membrane formation. Secretory granules originating from the Golgi complex fuse with the plasma membrane during exocytosis (Fig.). The membrane of the granules becomes incorporated into the plasma membrane, and thus contributes to the renewal of the membrane constituents. The Golgi complex plays an important part in the synthesis of the carbohydrate components of the plasma membrane. Autoradio-graphic studies using radioactive tritiated

sugars have shown that the tracer which is first localised at the Golgi complex migrates to the cell surface" and appears in the cell coat (Rambourg *et al*, 1971). The glycoproteins formed on the Golgi membrane remain attached to the secretory vesicle membrane after it fuses with the plasma membrane. Secretory glycoproteins on the other hand are released into the extra cellular space after fusion of the secretory vesicle membrane with the plasma membrane.

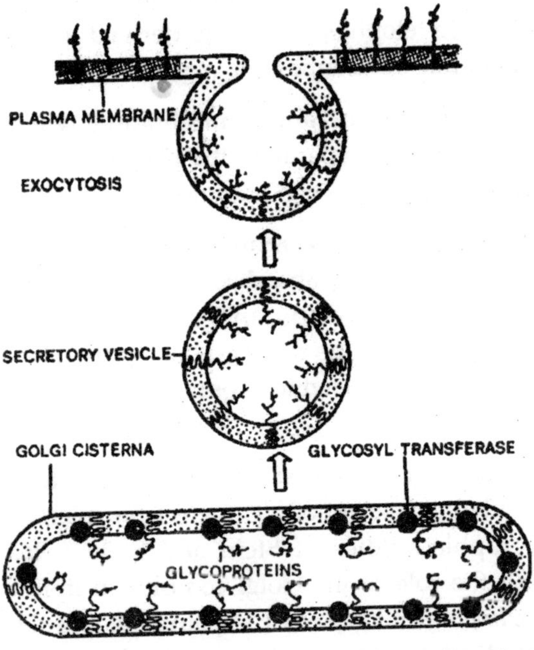

Diagram showing formation of a secretory vesicle from the Golgi complex cisterna and its subsequent fusion with the plasma membrane (exocytosis). The glycoproteins remains attached to the membranes.

It has been shown that in plant cells the plasma membranes of the cells resulting from cell division are contributed by the Golgi complex. The Golgi complex contributes to the biogenesis of the plasma membrane by supplying it with glycosylated molecules.

Plant Cell Wall Formation: The cell walls of plants are made up of fibrils which predominantly contain polysaccharides, along with some lipids and proteins. During cytokinesis a *cell plate* is formed between the two daughter nuclei, and has around it a membrane which later becomes the plasma membrane of the daughter cells. There is clear evidence that the polysaccharides are formed in the Golgi complex and transferred to the new cell wall which is laid down while the cells are still growing. In the root tip cells of *Spinacia* large and small vesicles are seen in the spindle region during anaphase-telophase. In the telophase the Golgi-derived vesicles fuse to form the new plasma membrane.

Substances like pectins and hemicelluloses, which form the matrix of the cell plate separating the plasma membranes, are also contributed by the Golgi complex.

Lipid Packaging and Secretion: Fats are broken down in the digestive tract and are absorbed into the epithelial cells of the intestine as fatty acids and monoglycerides. These substances are used in the synthesis of lipids. The epithelial cells secrete *chylomicrons* which contain lipids in the form of lipoproteins.

Earlier light microscopic studies had implicated the Golgi complex with lipid secretion. The electron microscopic and autoradiographic studies of Stein and Stein (1967) clearly brought out the role of the Golgi complex in lipid secretion. Labelled *palmitate* and *glycerol* (^{3}H-palmitate and ^{3}H-glycerol) were injected into fasted and ethanol treated rats. Two minutes after injection the labelled material, mostly triglycerides, was seen in the endoplasmic reticulum. Five minutes after injection it was seen in storage lipid droplets, and from 10 minutes onwards in the Golgi complex. This and other studies indicate that the endoplasmic reticulum is involved in triglyceride synthesis. The vesicles derived from the Golgi complex act as transport vesicles for lipids to the plasma membrane and the intercellular space. The Golgi complex may also be involved in adding the carbohydrate components of chylomicrons (Jones *et al*, 1967). Other studies, *e.g.* those on milk secretion in lactating mice, do not show labelled materials in the Golgi complex. Here the lipids may be released from the cell through a different pathway.

The overall role of the Golgi complex in lipid metabolism appears to be the concentration and modification of secretory material. These changes convert the lipid droplets into chylomicrons. The Golgi complex also provides a membrane for the envelopment of lipid so that it can be released from the cell.

On the basis of radio autography experiments Cohn and Benson (1965) have suggested that the Golgi region of phagocytes may be involved in the formation or storage of membranes containing phospholipids. Morre and Van Der Woude (1966) have also suggested that dictyosomes of plants are sites of active phospholipid metabolism.

Acrosome Formation: The acrosome vesicle lies in front of the nucleus in the sperm. The close association between the Golgi complex and acrosome formation was known since the early light microscopy studies on the subject. Bowen had pointed out the analogy between Golgi-produced vesicles in secretory cells and acrosomal content. The electron microscope studies of Fawcett and his co-workers (1955-1966) have established this relationship. Later electron-microscopy studies showed the derivation of the acrosomal membrane from the membranes of Golgi-derived vesicles (Susi *et al*, 1971).

In the early stages of the developing mammalian spermatid the Golgi complex appears as a spherical body with parallel flattened cisternae and many vacuoles. Later the complex becomes irregular and the cisternae dilate to form sacs. *Proacrosomic granules* appear in the centre of the Golgi complex and ultimately fuse to form the *acrosome.*

The acrosome has a high glycoprotein content, and some of the glycoproteins have lytic properties. Penetration of the sperm into the egg requires lytic substances to dissolve the egg coats. The lytic enzymes of the acrosome are believed to be of the nature of lysosomal enzymes. On this basis the acrosome has been considered to be a giant lysosome.

Recognition and binding between the egg and the sperm is due to the presence of substances with antigenic properties on the sperm membrane surface. Data suggest that the plasma membrane overlying the acrosome may be organised by the Golgi complex.

Lysosome Formation: Novik off and his co-workers (1961-1964) have proposed that *primary lysosomes* are formed by the Golgi complex in a manner similar to that of protein granules. Other workers have confirmed different phases of this activity. The entire process may be summarised as follows. The ribosomes synthesise lysosomal *hydrolases* (hydrolytic enzymes), which then enter the ER.

The ER forms small vesicles of these hydrolases by *blebbing* (budding), and the vesicles are transferred to the Golgi complex. The cisternae of the Golgi complex in turn form vesicles (the *primary lysosomes)* by blebbing.

The primary lysosomes fuse with pinocytic vesicles, or with autophagic vesicles, and form *secondary lysosomes.* It has also been suggested that the Golgi vesicles transfer acid hydrolases to *injection vacuoles (food vacuoles)*, converting them into *digestive vacuoles* (De Duve, 1963).

Because of the close functional relationships between the Golgi complex, endoplasmic reticulum and lysosomes, Novik off has denoted the system as the GERL (Golgi Endoplasmic Reticulum Lysosomes) system. Lysosomes can also arise directly from the ER without the Golgi complex taking any part, as in liver cells and in neurons.

Neurosecretion: A study of neurosecretory cells of many invertebrates and vertebrates has revealed that neurosecretory granules lie close to the Golgi complex. Precursors of neurosecretory products have been found between the lamellae of the Golgi complex in studies on the supra-oesophageal ganglion of the earthworm (Scharrer and Brown, 1961) and the hypothalamus of the mouse (Murakami, 1962). In many works it has been described that the neurosecretory material is synthesised in the Golgi complex. However, in later works *(e.g.* the review by Bargmann, 1966) it has been suggested that the material is synthesised in the ribosomes of the endoplasmic reticulum. It is then transferred to the Golgi complex, where it undergoes packaging to form neurosecretory granules.

Pigment Formation: In many mammalian tumour and cancer cells the Golgi complex has been described as the site of origin of pigment granules *(melanin).* The Golgi complex has also been associated with pigment formation in retinal pigment epithelium of chick embryos, in the test cells of the ovaries of certain tunicates and in the oocytes of the salamander (Beams and Kessel, 1968).

Regulation of Fluid Balance: A homology has been suggested between the Golgi complex and the contractile vacuole of lower Metazoa and Protozoa. In 1924 Nassonov observed that dictyosome-like bodies are situated near the contractile vacuole. Electron microscope studies have shown that the structure of these bodies is similar to the Golgi complex structure of Metazoa (Gatenby et al, 1955; Dalton and Felix, 1955). The contractile vacuole expels surplus water from the cell. In certain Protozoa the Golgi complex is also concerned with regulation of fluid balance.

9

Tissue Alterations

Variations in the structure and number of chromosomes have been observed in natural populations and could also be produced artificially in a variety of organisms. These variations have been extensively studied and can be due to either structural changes or numerical changes.

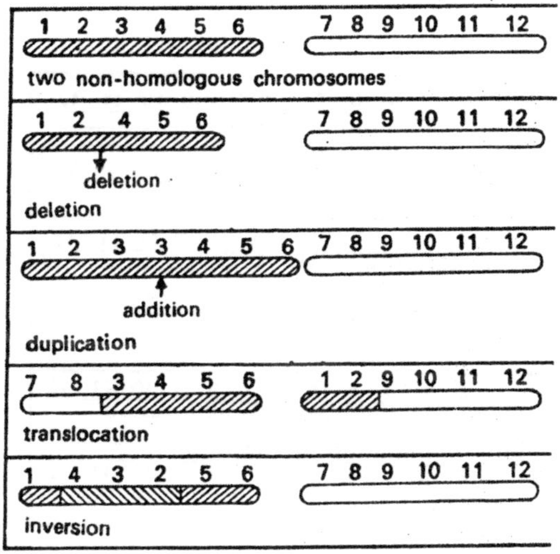

Different kinds of changes in chromosome structure.

Structural changes can be of following types: (i) deficiency which involves loss of a part of chromosome, (ii) duplication, which involves addition of a part of chromosome, (iii) translocation, which involves exchange of segments between non-homologous chromosomes, and (iv) inversion, which involves a reverse order of the genes in a part of chromosome.

These structural changes are diagrammatically represented in Figure, where two non-homologous chromosomes from the complete set are shown. Structural abnormalities may be found in both the homologous chromosomes of a pair, or in only one of them. When both homologous chromosomes are involved, these are called structural homozygotes *e.g.*, deficiency homozygote, duplication homozygote, etc. If only one chromosome is involved, this will be called a structural heterozygote. The constitutions of a translocation heterozygote and that of a translocation homozygote are shown in Figure. In this chapter, a brief and elementary account of different structural changes is presented. For a more detailed account of this subject, readers are encouraged to consult author's advanced book 'Cytogenetics'.

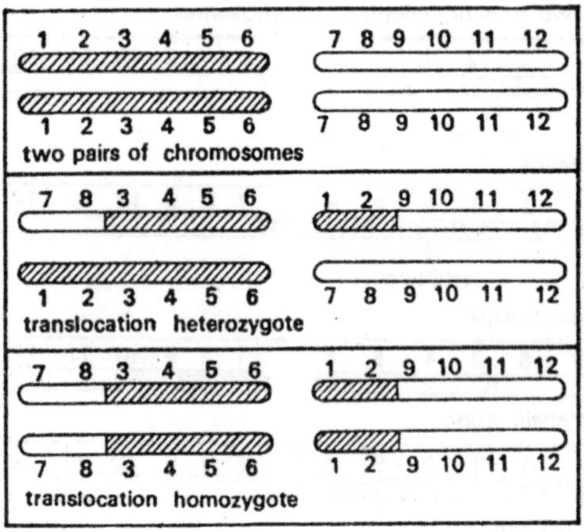

Chromosome constitution of a translocation heterozygote and a translocation homozygote.

THE DEFECTS

Deficiency is due to loss of a part of a chromosome. Smaller deficiencies, present in heterozygous condition (only on one of the two homologous chromosomes), can be tolerated by an organism. Such individuals at meiosis will form a loop in a bivalent that can be observed at pachytene stage (Fig.). Loops can also be observed in salivary gland chromosomes of *Drosophila* which are found in a permanent state of pairing, so that even small deficiencies could be detected in these chromosomes (Fig.).

Deficiencies have an effect on inheritance also. In presence of a deficiency, a recessive allele will behave like a dominant allele (pseudodominance). This principle of pseudodominance exhibited by deficiency heterozygotes has been utilised for location of genes on specific chromosomes in *Drosophila*, maize and other organisms. L.J. Stadler, who was a pioneer in radiation work in plants devised a method where a homozygous recessive stock was pollinated by irradiated pollen from dominant stock, so that if irradiation induced a deletion, recessive allele will express due to pseudodominance.

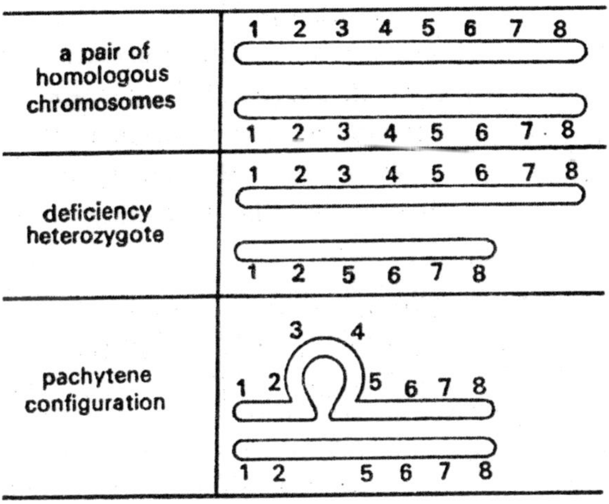

Chromosome pairing in a deficiency heterozygote.

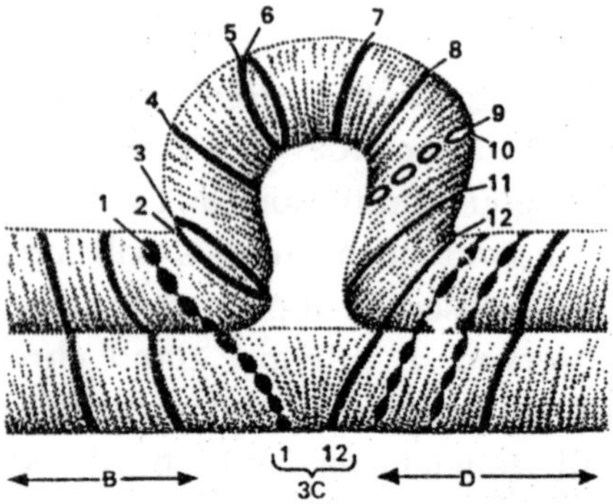

Diagrammatic representation of pairing of salivary gland X-chromosomes in a deficiency heterozygote in a♀ Drosophila, showing a loop. Note that the bands 3C2 to 3C11 are missing in one chromosome.

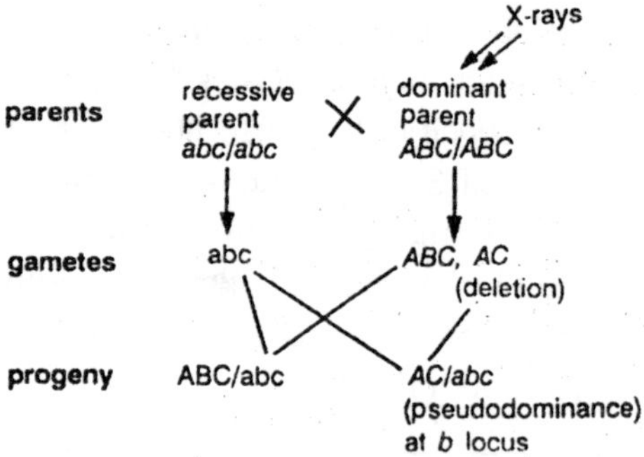

Detection of deletion due to pseudodominance.

As shown in Figure, if homozygote *abc* is pollinated by *ABC*, heterozygous F1 *(ABC/abc)* will be produced expressing only dominant characters. If pollen with dominant alleles *ABC* is irradiated, a deletion may be induced leading to expression of pseudodominance by one or more recessive alleles. If meiosis at pachytene is examined in such a deficiency heterozygote, presence of loop will indicate location of gene. Several genes were located on different chromosomes of maize and tomato, utilising deficiencies. In *Drosophila* also deficiencies were recorded particularly on X-chromosomes in regions of genes *w (white eye), fa (facet eye)* and v *(vermilion coloured eye)*. Deficiencies have also been recorded in waltzing mice in region of gene v inducing nervous abnormality. In human beings, a deficiency was discovered, which was associated with cat like-cry so that the child carrying this deficiency had a cat like cry and also had microcephaly (small head and low mental faculty). This deficiency was found in a segment of chromosome 5.

Copy or Transcript

Duplications are obtained due to addition of a part of a chromosome. If duplication is present only on one of the two homologous chromosomes, at meiosis (pachytene), cytological observations characteristic of deficiency will be obtained in duplication also. Duplication of a chromosome segment, may be brought about by addition in any of the following positions: (i) in adjacent region, (ii) at a displaced position of the same arm, (iii) on the different arm of the same chromosome or (iv) on a different chromosome. Sometimes the duplication may be found as a reverse repeat.

One of the classical examples of duplication in *Drosophila* is Bar eye. Bar eye is a character, where eyes are narrower as compared to normal eye shape. This phenotypic character is due to duplication for a part of a chromosome. By the study of giant salivary gland chromosomes, it could be demonstrated

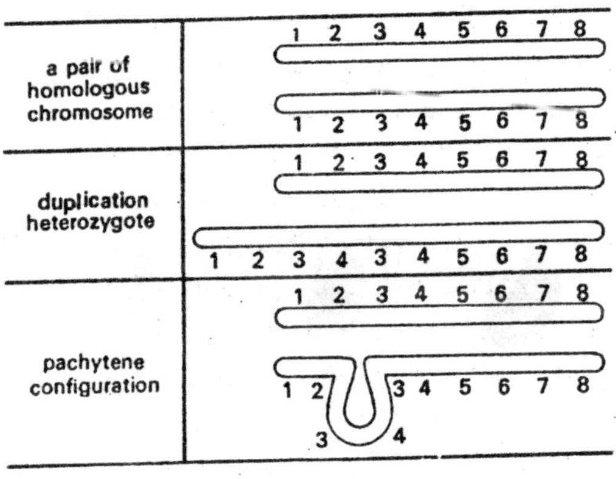

Chromosome pairing in a duplication heterozygote.

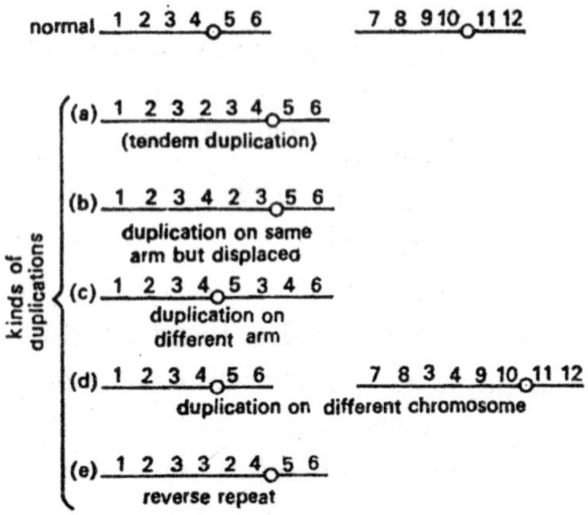

Different kinds of duplication in chromosome.

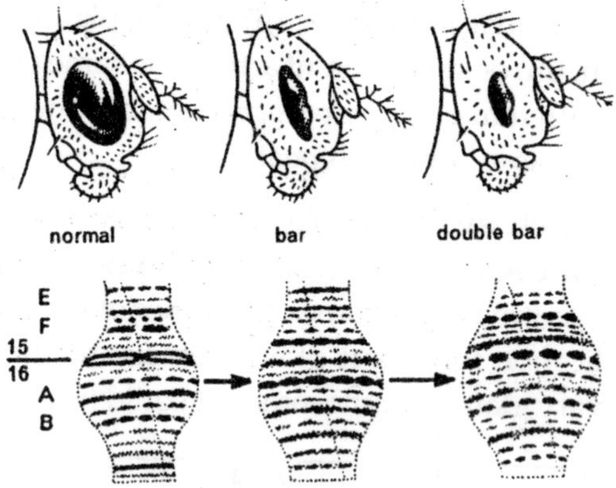

A normal eye, bar eye and a double bar eye with corresponding chromosome segments (salivary gland chromosomes) showing duplications.

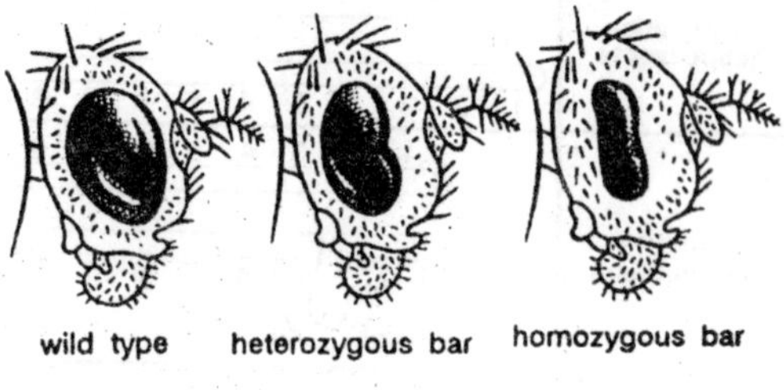

Shapes of eye in normal, heterozygous bar and homozygous bar Drosophila files.

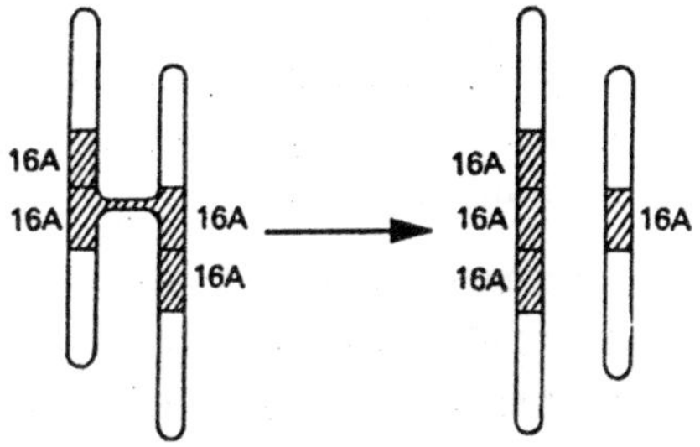

An ultrabar condition resulting from, 'Bar' due to unequal crossing over.

that 'Bar' character was due to a duplication in region 16A of X-chromosome. Barred eyes will have slightly different phenotype in heterozygous and homozygous individuals (Fig.). Barred individuals *(16A 16A)* gave rise to ultrabar *(16A 16A 16A)* and normal wild type *(16A)* due to unequal crossing over (Fig.).

Some other duplications known in *Drosophila* lead to following phenotypic effects: (i) a reverse repeat in chromosome 4 causes *eyeless* dominant *(Ey)*; (ii) a tandem duplication in chromosome 3 causes *confluens (CO)* resulting in thickened veins, and (iii) another duplication causes *hairy wing (Hw)*.

THE SUBSTITUTIONS

Translocation is a broad term including all types of unilateral or bilateral transfer of chromosome segments from one chromosome to another. An important class of translocations having evolutionary significance is known as reciprocal translocations or segmental interchanges, which involve mutual exchange of chromosome segments between two pairs of non-homologous chromosomes.

Cytology of a Translocation Heterozygote: If a translocation is present in one of the two sets of chromosomes, this will be a translocation heterozygote. In such a cell, normal pairing into bivalents will not be possible among chromosomes involved in translocation. Due to pairing between homologous segments of chromosomes, a cross-shaped (+) figure involving four chromosomes will be observed at pachytene (Fig.). This ring of four chromosomes at metaphase I can have one of the following three orientations:

Alternate: In alternate orientation, alternate chromosomes will be oriented towards the same pole. In other words, adjacent chromosomes will orient towards opposite poles. This will be possible by formation of a figure of eight.

Adjacent I: In adjacent I orientation, adjacent chromosomes having non- homologous centromeres will orient towards the same pole. In other words, chromosomes having homologous centromeres will orient towards opposite poles. A ring of four chromosomes will be observed.

Adjacent II: In adjacent II orientation, adjacent chromosomes having homologous centromeres will orient towards the same pole. A ring of four chromosomes will be observed.

As shown in Figure, alternate disjunctions will give functional gametes. Adjacent I and adjacent II disjunctions will form gametes, which would carry duplications or deficiencies and as a result would be non-functional or sterile. Therefore, in a plant having a translocation in heterozygous condition, there will be considerable pollen sterility. A ring of four chromosomes as described above is found under conditions when a single interchange is found.

If two interchanges are involving three non-homologous chromosomes, a ring of six chromosomes is found, and the size of ring can increase with additional interchanges. More than one ring can also be found if two or more interchanges are independently found, each involving two different non-homologous chromosomes.

The first case of translocation was found in *Oenothera,* which was originally described as a mutation by de Vries while working for his Mutation Theory. *Oenothera, Tradescantia* and *Rhoeo* are such cases, where translocations in heterozygous condition are frequently found in nature. In many other crop plants they have been artificially induced.

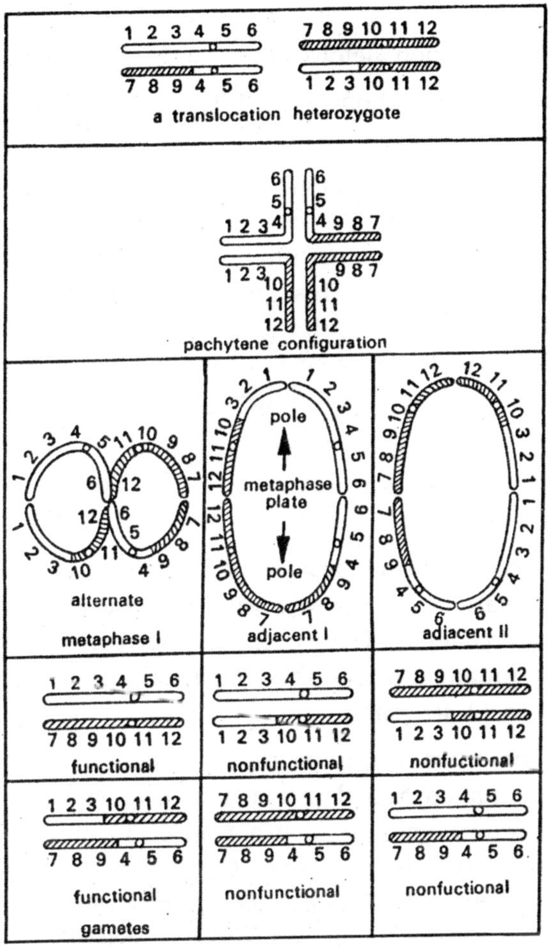

Chromosome pairing and different kinds of gametes formed in a translocation heterozygote.

Breeding Behaviour of a Translocation Heterozygote: Presence of translocation heterozygosity can be detected by presence of semi-sterility and low seed set. This can then be confirmed at meiosis by quadrivalent formation. As shown above only two types of functional gametes are formed which result from alternate disjunction. The functional gametes will give rise to three kinds of progeny (Fig.) namely:

(i) normal,

(ii) translocation heterozygote, and

(iii) translocation homozygote. These three types would be obtained in 1: 2: 1 ratio.

Interchange Heterozygosity in Oenothera: Subgenus *Euoenothera* of genus *Oenothera* has been studied during 1920-1930 and cytogenetic structure, leading to evolution in this group was examined. This group has $2n = 14$ and all 7 chromosomes of a haploid complement have median centromeres. Different species in the subgenus *Euoenothera,* can be classified in three groups:

(i) First group is represented by species showing bivalents or small rings at meiosis (*e.g. O. hookeri, O. grandiflora, O. argillicola).*

(ii) Second group is represented by species forming rings of various sizes at meiosis indicating the presence of interchanges. These rings are not permanent but are maintained due to their superiority in adaptive value (*e.g. O. irrigua).*

(iii) The third group is represented by those having permanent translocation heterozygosity involving all chromosomes, so that a ring of 14 chromosomes is regularly formed (*e.g. O. biennis, O. strigosa, O. parviflora).* In *O. lamarckiana,* a ring of only 12 instead of a ring of 14 chromosomes is observed (Fig.).

These three groups also differ in phenotypes like flower size, etc. and can be identified. The members of third category behave like pure lines and are actually permanent heterozygotes.

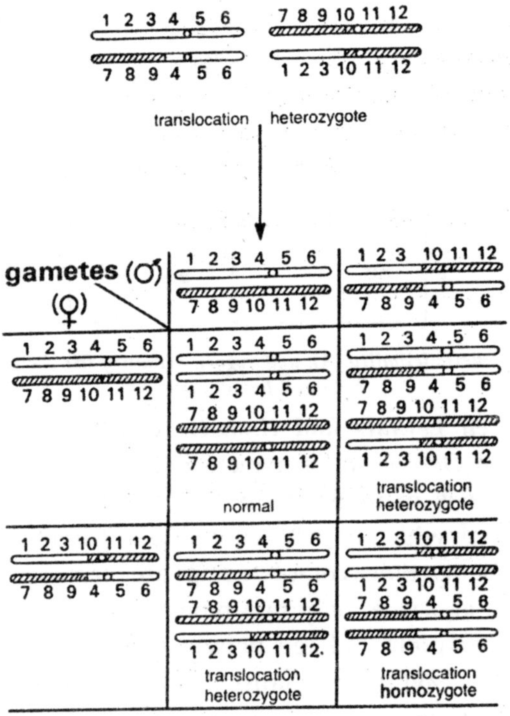

Different kinds of progenies obtained due to self fertilization in translocation heterozygote.

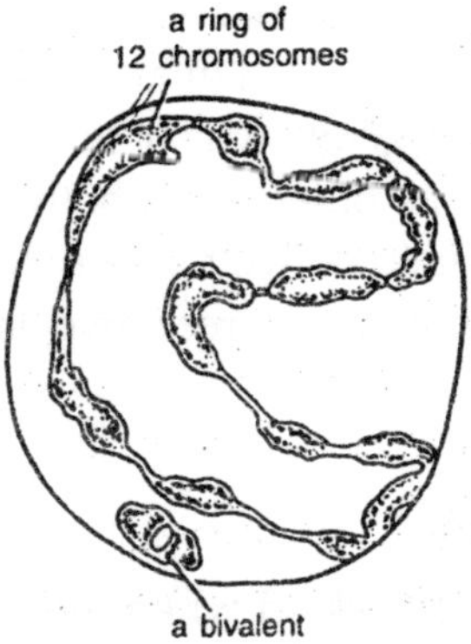

Chromosome complex in Oneothera Lamarckiana (2n = 14) showing formation of a ring of 12 chromosomes and a bivalent, as an evidence of multiple interchanges.

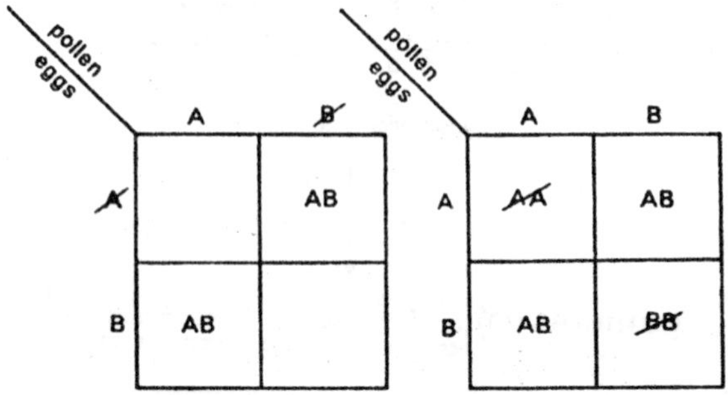

Gametic lethality (A), and zygotic lethality (B) showing balanced lethal systems.

Balanced Lethals and Gametic Complexes: Permanent hybridity in *Oenothera*. Permanent hybridity in some species of *Oenothera* is maintained due to operation of a balanced lethal system, which may function due to gametic lethality or zygotic lethality. Since complete rings are formed and alternate disjunction is a rule, only two types of gametes are formed showing complete linkage between 7 chromosomes. The gametic and zygotic lethality leads to survival of only heterozygotes (Fig.).

It may be noticed that in gametic lethality, only one of the two types of gametes will function on the male side, the other type being functional on the female side, thus giving rise to only one type of progeny, which will be heterozygous. In zygotic lethality on the other hand, both the types of gametes will function on male as well as on female side, but the homozygote progeny due to recessive lethal genes will not survive.

Change of Order

An inversion is produced when there are two breaks in a chromosome and the intercalary segment reunites in reverse order *i.e.*the segment rotates at 180°. Let us imagine that a chromosome *1-2-3-4-5-6-7-8* gives rise to another chromosome having the order *1-2-7-6-5-4-3-8*. The segment *3-4-5-6-7* has rotated here at 180° giving an inverted order of genes *7-6-5-4-3*. *A* similar hypothetical example using a chromosome *ABCDEF* has been shown in Figure, where due to coiling, breaks occur between *B* and C as well as between *D* and *E*. Reunion at broken ends may lead to inversion of the segment *CD* into *DC*.

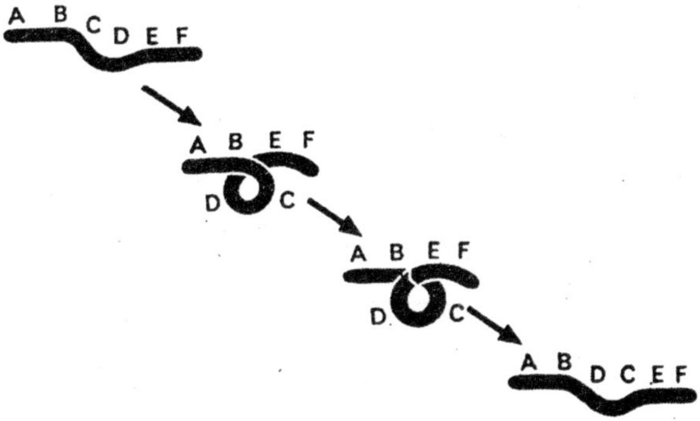

One of the possible mechanisms, which may give rise to chromosomal inversion.

The inversion can be of two types: (i) paracentric inversion, and (ii) pericentric inversion. Paracentric inversions are those inversions, where inverted segment does not include centromere. On the other hand, in a pericentric inversion, inverted segment includes centromere. In order to remember these terms and their meaning, one should bear in mind that pericentric means surrounding the centromere or on the periphery of centromere.

Cytology of Inversions: Due to an inverted segment in one of the two homologous chromosomes, the normal kind of pairing is not possible in an inversion heterozygote. In order to enable pairing of homologous segments, a shape of loop is formed by each of the two chromosomes as shown in Figures. This kind of configuration will be observed both in paracentric as well as in pericentric inversions. As will be observed, the products of crossing over and the subsequent stages of meiosis will differ in these two kinds of inversions.

Paracentric Inversion: A single crossing over or an odd number of crossovers in inverted region will result into formation of a dicentric chromosome (having two centromeres) and an acentric chromosome (with no centromere). Of the remaining two chromatids, one will be normal and the other will carry the inversion: The dicentric chromatid and acentric chromatid will be observed at anaphase I in the form of a bridge and a fragment. Double crossovers and crossovers within and outside inversion will give various kinds of deficiencies and duplications (Fig.).

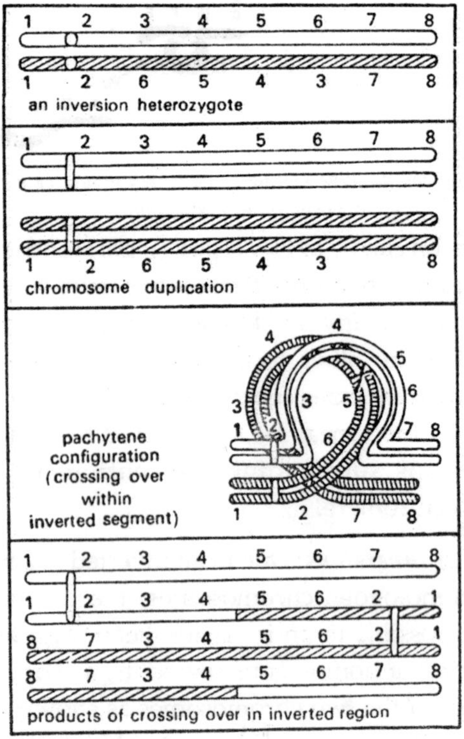

Chromosome pairing and products of crossing over in a paracentric inversion heterozygote.

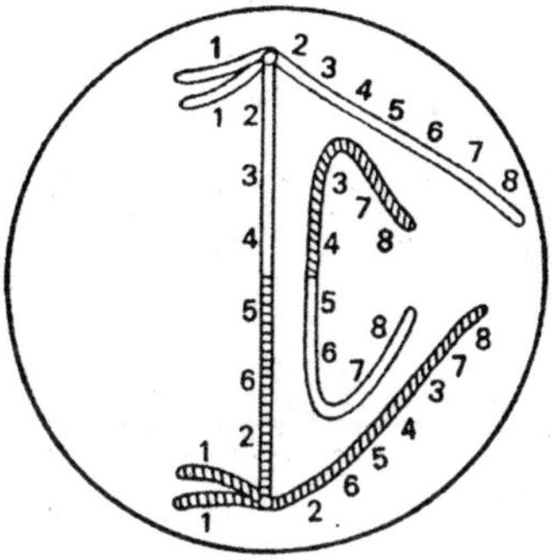

Dicentric bridge and an acentric fragment at anaphase I.

These will also give rise to a variety of characteristic configurations at anaphase I and anaphase II (Fig.; for details consult author's advanced text book *Cytogenetics).*

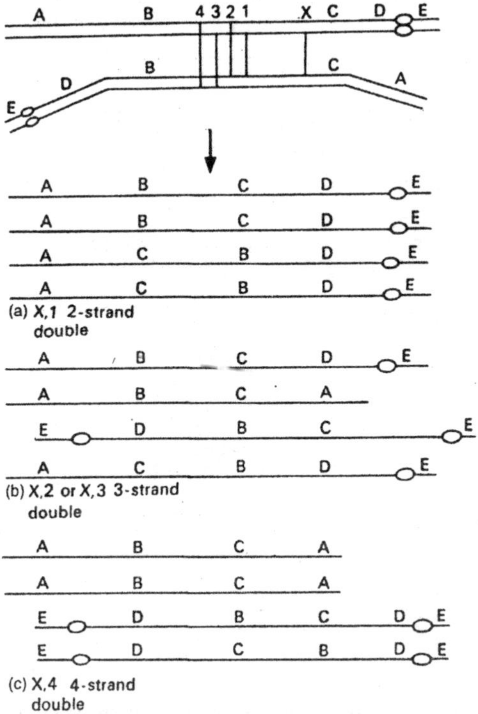

Consequences of 2-strands, 3-strands and 4-strands double crossovers within a paracentric inversion.

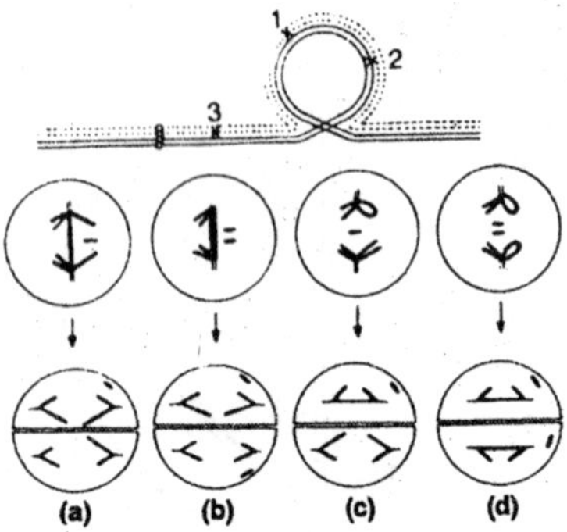

On the top is shown inversion loop in an inversion heterozygote. Below are shown anaphase I (AI) and anaphase II (AH) configurations (A-D) resulting from four different combinations of crossovers within and outside the inversion loop. A. single crossover at positions I or 2; B. 4-strand double crossovers at positions 1 and 2; C. 3-strand double crossovers, with one crossover at position I or 2 within inversion loop and the other crossover outside the loop at positions 3; D. 4-strand triple crossover at position 1, 2 and 3 (redrawn from McClintock, 1938).

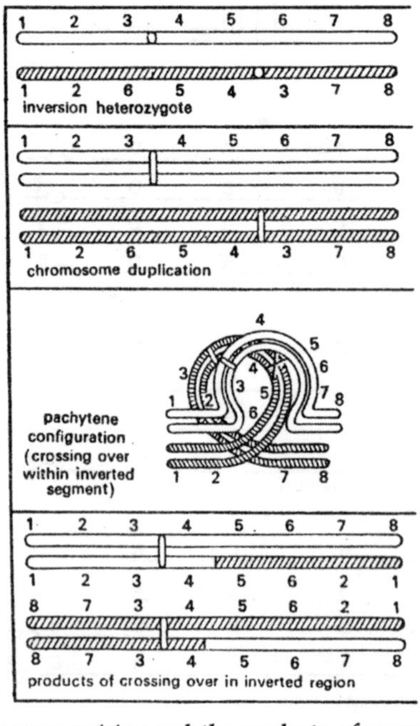

Chromosome pairing and the products of crossing over in a pericentric inversion heterozygote.

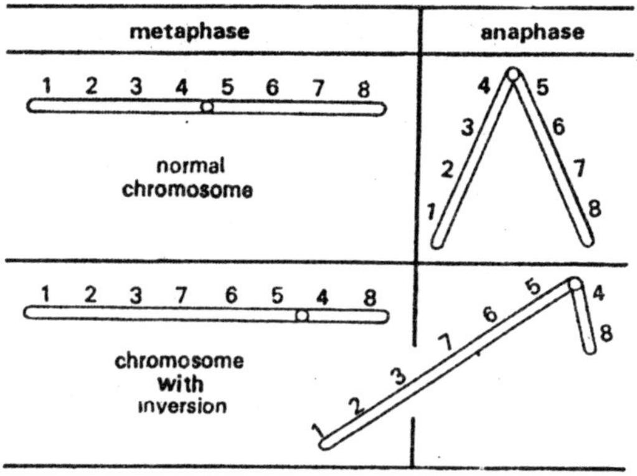

Change in chromosome shape due to pericentric inversion.

Pericentric Inversion: In a pericentric inversion (where centromere is present within the inverted segment), the pachytene configuration observed is similar to the one described above for paracentric inversion. However, the products of crossing over and configurations at subsequent stages of meiosis differ. In this case, two of the four chromatids resulting after meiosis will have deficiencies and duplications. However, unlike paracentric inversion, no dicentric bridge or acentric fragment will be observed (Fig.). Consequently, at anaphase I, no bridge or fragment will be seen.

However, in pericentric inversion, if two breaks are not situated equidistant from the centromere, this will result in a change in shape of the chromosome. For instance, a metacentric chromosome (with centromere in the centre) may become submetacentric and *vice-versa*.

Genetic Consequences of Inversion: Among four chromatids resulting after crossing over, the two chromatids resulting from crossing over would have deficiencies and duplications. The gametes having these chromosomes will not function. Therefore, there should be considerable gametic or zygotic lethality. In plants, there will be sufficient pollen sterility. (For details see author's book *Cytagenetics).* However, since the products of single crossover will not function and the only crossovers recovered will be double crossovers, the observed frequency of recombination between any two genes in question will be considerably reduced. Due to this reason, inversions, are often called crossover suppressors.

This reduction in crossing over is not the actual reduction in cytological crossing over, but is the result of lack of recovery of the products of single crossovers. This property of inversions has been utilised in the production of *CIB* stock, used by H.J. Muller for the detection of sex linked lethal mutations.

Overlapping Inversions: Sometimes a second inversion is induced in a chromosome which already has one inversion. This results in an overlapping inversion if the segments involved in first and second inversions contain a common region. The gene sequences and meiotic configurations found in an inversion heterozygote of this type are shown in Figure.

Inversions in Drosophila Populations: Inversions are known to have played a significant role in evolution of different species and races of *Drosophila*. This knowledge is particularly available in *Drosophila* due to the ease of identification of inversions in salivary gland chromosomes. They also occur in plants, but can not be so easily worked out in the absence of giant chromosomes.

In *Drosophila,* however, it is obvious that inversions occurred spontaneously in nature and became established in populations due to the adaptive benefit they conferred. Due to adaptive value, these inversions are restricted to definite localities and the different races actually derived their names after these localities. Th. Dobzhansky and A.H. Sturtevant even derived evolutionary relationships between races on the basis of overlapping inversions. These relationships are shown in the form of a tree in Figure.

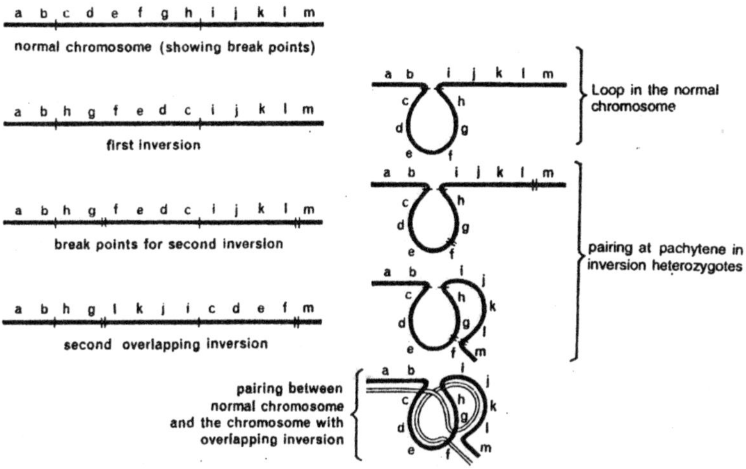

Steps leading to an overlapping inversion and corresponding pachytene configurations.

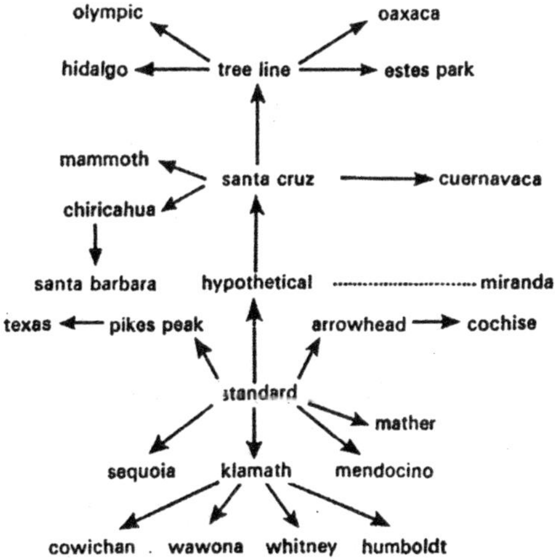

An evolutionary tree, showing derivation of a number of races due to simple and overlapping inversions in Drosophila.

Bibliography

Abbas, A.K, A.H. Lichtman and, J.S. Pober : *Cellular and Molecular Immunology,* Saunders, Philadelphia, 1999.

Ameisen, J. C. : *Tissue Culture,* Oxford, New York, 2000.

Anderson, S. : *Cell Biology,* Oxford University Press, London, 1981.

Atkins, J. F. : *Tissue Culture: an Introduction,* Oxford, New York, 1996.

Auerbach, C. : *Mutation Research: Problems, Results and Perspectives,* Chapman and Hall, London, 2002.

Baker, T.A. : *DNA Replication,* Freeman, New York, 2002.

Beale, G.H. : *Cellular Control Mechanisms and Cancer,* Oxford, New York, 2002.

Becker, W.M. and D.W. Deamer : *The World of the Cell,* Benjamin-Cummings, Redwood City, 2000.

Benjamin, Lewin : *Genes,* Oxford University Press, New York, 2000.

Bennett, R. H. : *Transcription, Processing and Editing in Plant Mitochondria,* Oxford, New York, 1992.

Bittar, E.E. : *Cell Biology in Medicine,* John Wiley, New York, 1999.

Branden, C. and Tooze, J. : *Introduction to Cell Biology,* Garland, New York, 1991.

Court, D. : *Regulatory Sequences Involved in the Promotion and Termination of RNA Transcription,* Cambridge, New York, 2003.

Darnell, J. E. : *Molecular Cell Biology,* Scientific American Books, New York, 1995.

Das, A. : *Control of Transcription Termination,* Routledge, New York, 1993.

Demidov, V. V. : *PNA and LNA throw Light on DNA, Trends,* Oxford, New York, 2003.

DeRobertis, E.D.P. : *Cell Biology,* Waverly Pvt. Ltd., New Delhi, 1988.

DuPraw, E. J. : *Cell and Molecular Biology,* Academic Press, New York, 1969.

Ebby, S. R. : *Non Coding RNA Genes and Modern RNA,* Oxford, New York, 2001

Edlin, G. : *Human Genetics : A Modern Synthesis,* Jones & Bartlett Pub., Boston, 1990.

Ellis, R. J. : *Chloroplast Protein Synthesis,* Oxford, New York, 1975.

Fincham, J.R.S. : *Genetic Complementation,* Benjamin, New York, 1999.

Fournier, M.J. : *The Small Nucleolar RNAs,* MacMillan, London, 1995.

Friedberg, E. C. : *Relationships Between DNA Repair and Transcription,* Oxford, New York, 1996.

Gilbert, W. and B. Muller : *Isolation of the Lac Repressor,* Oxford, New York, 1966.

Gilham, N. W. : *Genetic Analysis of the Chloroplast and Mitochondrial Genomes,* Oxford, New York, 1974.

Glick, B. and G. Schatz : *Import of Proteins into Mitochondria,* Oxford, New York, 1991.

Gray, M. W. : *The Evolutionary Origin of Organelles*, Oxford, New York, 1989.

Grunstein, M. : *Histones as Regulators of Genes*, Oxford, New York, 1992.

Gupta, P. K. : *Cell Biology*, Rastogi Publications, Meerut, 2000.

Hadjiolov, A. A. : *The Nucleolus and Ribosome Biogenesis*, Oxford, New York, 1985.

Henikoff, S. : *Cell Biology : A Reference Manual*, MIT Press, Cambridge, 2002.

Hoagland, M. G. : *The Present Status of the Adaptor Hypothesis*, MacMillan, London, 1959.

Holley, R. W. : *Structure of a Ribonucleic Acid*, McGraw Hill, London, 2002.

Hunt, T. : *The Cell Cycle*, Oxford University Press, Oxford, 2002.

Ingram, V. : *The Biosynthesis of Macromolecules*, Benjamin, New York, 2001.

Jacobson, M. : *Developmental Neurobiology*, Plenum Press, New York, 2002.

Jukes, T. H. : *Mitochondrial Codes and Evolution*, Oxford, New York, 2000.

Kaguni, L. S. : *Eukaryotic DNA Polymerase-primase : Structure, Mechanism and Function*, MacMillan, London, 1999.

Kaziro, Y: *Structure and Function of Signal Transducing GTP Binding Proteins*, Blackwell, London, 2001.

Kendrew, J. C. : *The Three-dimensional Structure of a Protein Molecule*, Sinauer, New York, 1991

Kramer, A. :*The Structure and Function of Proteins Involved in Mammalian Pre-mRNA Splicing*, Grandada, New York, 2001.

Kurland, C. G. : *Structure and Function of the Bacterial Ribosomes*, Oxford, New York, 2000.

Lehninger, A. L. : *Cell Biology,* Academic Press, New York, 2001

McKnight, S. L. : *Molecular Zippers in Gene Regulation,* Princeton, New York, 2002.

Merrick, W. C. : *Overview : Mechanism of Translation Initiation in Eukaryotes,* Longman, London, 2001.

Moore, P. B. : *Molecular Mimicry in Protein Synthesis,* Cambridge, London, 2002.

Noller, H. F. : *Ribosomol RNA and Translation,* Oxford, New York, 1999.

Olson, R. E. : *Enzymatic Synthesis of DNA,* John Wiley, New York, 2001.

Owen, L. : *DNA Synthesis,* Freeeman, San Francisco, 2001.

Pardee, A. B. : *Molecular Basis of Biological Regulation: Origins of Feedback Inhibition and Allostery,* Arnold, London, 2003.

Paszkowski, J. : *DNA and Histone Methylation in Plants,* MacMillan, London, 2002.

Razin, A. and A. D. Riggs : *DNA Methylation and Gene Function,* Longman, New York, 2002.

Reinbcrg, D. : *Common Themes in Assembly and Function of Eukaryotic Transcription Complexes,* MacMillan, London, 2002.

Rich, A. and S. H. Kim : *The Three Dimensional Structure of Transfer RNA,* Oxford, New York, 1999.

Robertson, M. : *RNA Processing : the Post-RNA World,* Oxford, New York, 1999.

Sauer, R. T. : *Transcription Factors : Structural Families and Principles of DNA Recognition,* Printice Hall, London, 1993.

Schmid, M. B. : *Structure and Function of the Bacterial Chromosome,* Granada, London, 1990.

Stryer, L. : *Cell Biology,* W.H. Freeman & Co., New York, 2002.

Temin, H. M. : *RNA Directed DNA Synthesis,* MacGraw-Hill, New York, 2002.

Threadgold, L.T. : *The Infrastructure of Animal Cell,* Pergamon Press, London, 1999.

Turner, B. M. : *Histone Acetylation and Control of Gene Expression,* MacMillan, London, 2002.

Ulrich, B. : *Mechanism and Regulation of Eukaryotic Protein Synthesis,* Oxford, New York, 2002.

Uptain, S. M. : *Basic Mechanisms of Transcript Elongation and its Regulation,* MacMillan, London, 1997.

Voinnet, O. : *RNA Silencing : Small RNAs as Ubiquitous Regulators of Gene Expression,* MacMillan, London, 2002.

Walbot, V. : *Structure of Plant Mitochondrial Genomes,* John Wiley, London, 1992.

Wallace, D. C. : *Diseases of the Mitochondrial DNA,* Blackwell, New York, 2002.

Wang, T. S. F. : *Eukaryotic DNA Polymerases,* MacMillan, London, 2002.

Wilkins, M. H. F. : *Physical Studies of the Molecular Structure of Deoxyribose Nucleic Acid and Nucleoprotein,* MacMillan, London, 2002.

Woese, C. R. : *The Genetic Code : The Molecular Basis for Genetic Expression,* Harper & Row, New York, 2003.

Wuthrich, K. : *A Hand Book of Cell Biology,* Oxford, New York, 2001.

Yanofsky, C. : *Introduction Tissue Culture,* Oxford, New York, 2001.

Yarus, M. : *Translational Efficiency of Transfer RNAs,* Oxford, New York, 2002.

Zetka, M. : *History of Tissue Culture,* Oxford, New York, 2002.

Index

N

O

P

❑❑❑